AF616419

Cone Beam Computed Tomography in Endodontics

Shanon Patel · Simon Harvey · Hagay Shemesh · Conor Durack

Shanon Patel · Simon Harvey · Hagay Shemesh · Conor Durack

Cone Beam Computed Tomography in Endodontics

Contributors

Francesca Abella Sans DDS, PhD
Program Co-ordinator of Restorative Dentistry and Endodontics, Universitat Internacional de Catalunya, Barcelona, Spain

Bhavin Bhuva BDS, MFDS RCS, MClinDent, MRD RCS (Edin)
Consultant in Endodontics, Endodontic Postgraduate Unit, Guy's and St Thomas' NHS Foundation Trust, London, UK and Specialist practice, London, UK

Conor Durack BDS, MFD RCSI, MClinDent, MEndo RCS (Edin)
Specialist in Endodontics, Limerick, Ireland

Simon C Harvey BDS, MA (MedLaw), MFDS RCS (Edin)
Specialist Registrar in Dental and Maxillofacial Radiology, Guy's and St Thomas' NHS Foundation Trust, London, UK

Shalini Kanagasingam BDS, MClinDent, MFDS RCS (Eng), MRD RCS (Edin)
Head of Operative Dentistry, National University of Malaysia, Kaula Lumpur, Malaysia

Shanon Patel BDS, MSc, MClinDent, FDS RCS (Edin), MRD RCS (Edin), PhD
Consultant/Honorary Senior Lecturer in Endodontics, King's College London Dental Institute, London, UK and Specialist practice, London, UK

Navid Saberi BDS, MFDS RCS (Edin), MSc
Private practice (limited to Endodontics), Brighton, UK

Hagay Shemesh DMD, PhD
Associate Professor and Chair, Division of Endodontology, Academic Centre for Dentistry Amsterdam (ACTA), Amsterdam, The Netherlands

Mitsuhiro Tsukiboshi DDS, PhD
General Practitioner and Chairperson of Tsukiboshi Dental Clinic, Aichi, Japan and Clinical Professor, Tohoku University, Graduate School of Dentistry, Japan

Cindy Verdegaal DMD
Postgraduate in Endodontics, Division of Endodontology, Academic Centre for Dentistry Amsterdam (ACTA), Amsterdam, The Netherlands

Eric Whaites MSc, BDS, FDS RCS (Edin), FDS RCS (Eng), FRCR, DDR RCR
Senior Lecturer/Honorary Consultant in Dental and Maxillofacial Radiology, King's College London Dental Institute, London, UK

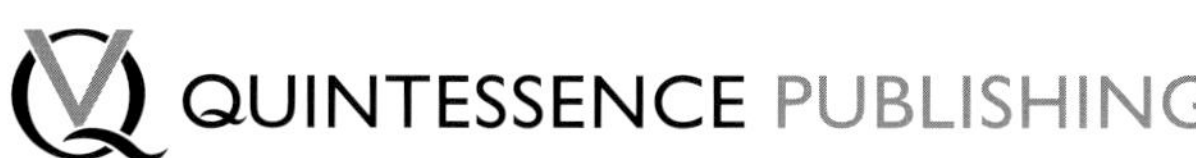

Berlin, Chicago, Tokyo, Barcelona, Bucharest, Istanbul, London, Milan, Moscow, New Delhi, Paris, Beijing, Prague, Riyadh, São Paulo, Seoul, Singapore, Warsaw and Zagreb

A CIP record for this book is available from the British Library.
ISBN: 978-1-85097-291-4

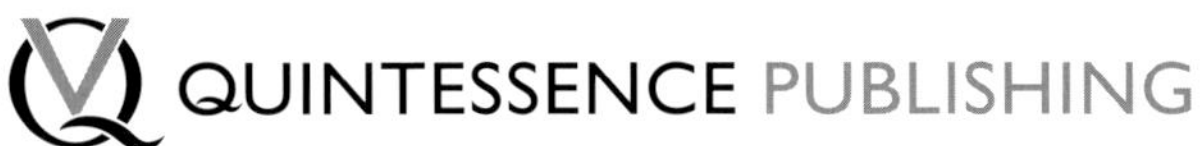

Quintessence Publishing Co. Ltd,
Grafton Road, New Malden, Surrey KT3 3AB,
United Kingdom
www.quintpub.co.uk

Editing: Quintessence Publishing Co. Ltd, London, UK
Layout and Production: Quintessenz Verlags-GmbH, Berlin, Germany
Index: Indexing Specialists (UK) Ltd
Printed and bound in Germany

Acknowledgements

To our families

The editors would like to thank the following:

Francesco Mannocci, *per i tuoi saggi consigli*;
Andrew Dawood for being ahead of the game, and introducing me to the 'third dimension' in 2006;
The endodontic staff and postgraduate team at King's College London Dental Institute.

Shanon Patel

Jackie Brown, Marta Varela, Eric Whaites and Georgina Harvey for their invaluable assistance.

Simon Harvey

JA Baart, Department of Maxillofacial Surgery, and JA Castelijns, Head and Neck Radiology, of the VU Medical Centre, Amsterdam, Netherlands.

Hagay Shemesh

Eilis Lynch at Ennis Periodontology and Implant Clinic, and my colleagues at Riverpoint Specialist Dental Clinic, Limerick.

Conor Durack

Foreword

The primary objectives of Restorative Dentistry are to relieve pain, prevent tooth loss and restore lost oral and dental tissues to meet the aesthetic, psychological and functional needs of patients. These key objectives often require the coordination of multi-professional teams, which in the context of this book include Endodontists.

The use of cone beam computed tomography (CBCT) in dentistry, and specifically endodontics, is controversial, and although several position statements and guidance documents have been published in recent years, there remains a lack of knowledge and a degree of misunderstanding about the benefits and risks associated with this diagnostic tool. Without doubt, there has been a need for a comprehensive and authoritative textbook that covers all the elements of this subject in relation to diseases of the pulp and periapical region. Thus, this new book on CBCT and endodontics is timely, and provides a rich resource for specialists in Endodontology and Maxillofacial Radiology. It is also an excellent reference book for general dentists, trainees on clinical training pathways, as well as students on specialist postgraduate programmes and undergraduates using CBCT.

The book is user-friendly and is divided into two sections. The initial chapters (1–4) cover the important and essential aspects of radiology in relation to CBCT, which is an area that is often underemphasised and misunderstood. The remaining chapters (5–11) are dedicated to the various applications of CBCT in endodontics. An essential focus running throughout the book is the understanding that, as CBCT is associated with a higher effective patient radiation dose, the ALARA principles are paramount.

Each chapter is written by subject specialists who have a wealth of research and clinical experience. The book is extensively illustrated with conventional radiographic and CBCT images, all with comprehensive legends.

CBCT is a relatively modern imaging method that provides a substantial amount of clinically relevant information. The book provides an excellent review of the subject, emphasises case selection and is supported by key references to provide an evidence-based approach and a framework for the use of CBCT in endodontics.

Professor Paul MH Dummer BDS, MScD, PhD, DDSc, FDS RCS (Edin), FHEA

Professor of Restorative Dentistry,
Dean of Education and Students, Cardiff University
Secretary of the European Society of Endodontology

Cardiff
October 2015

Preface

Endodontics relies on radiographic imaging for diagnosis, treatment planning and the assessment of healing. However, conventional radiographic imaging has several well-documented limitations, which can result in an impaired diagnostic yield, and potentially influence treatment planning.

In recent years, cone beam computed tomography (CBCT) has become much more widely available and utilised in all aspects of dentistry, including endodontics. CBCT overcomes many of the limitations of conventional radiography and has been shown to be essential for the diagnosis and management of complex endodontic problems.

The editors of *Cone Beam Computed Tomography in Endodontics* are all experienced users of CBCT. In their clinical practice and academic/teaching roles, they recognised the need for a guide to illustrate the applications of CBCT in endodontics using the latest evidence and principles.

The aim of the book is two-fold; firstly, to give the reader a thorough account of the radiological aspects of CBCT; and secondly, to comprehensively illustrate the applications of CBCT in endodontics. The book emphasises the fact that, inherent in the responsible use of CBCT is the understanding that, as CBCT is associated with a higher effective patient radiation dose than conventional radiographic imaging, the prescription of CBCT must be justified, and the associated radiation exposure be kept as low as reasonably achievable.

This book gives the reader a sound foundation on small field of view, high resolution CBCT and its applications in endodontics. However, one cannot overemphasise the fact that dental radiology is continuously evolving. As such, it is essential that CBCT users keep abreast of developments in dental radiology and maintain a contemporaneous core knowledge of both dental radiology and of CBCT, specifically.

Shanon Patel
Simon C Harvey
Hagay Shemesh
Conor Durack

Contents

Chapter 1

The Limitations of Conventional Radiography and Adjunct Imaging Techniques

Shanon Patel, Bhavin Bhuva, Eric Whaites

Introduction

Radiographic assessment is essential in every aspect of endodontics, from diagnosis to the management and assessment of treatment outcome (Forsberg, 1987a, b; Patel et al, 2015). Intraoral periapical radiography has historically been accepted as the most appropriate imaging system in endodontics. However, conventional periapical images yield limited information, which can potentially have an impact on diagnosis and treatment planning.

The purpose of this chapter is to describe the limitations of conventional periapical radiography, and to discuss the relative advantages and disadvantages of alternative imaging techniques.

Limitations of conventional radiographic imaging

Superimposition of three-dimensional anatomy

Conventional radiography results in three-dimensional (3D) structures being superimposed and displayed as a two-dimensional (2D) image (Nance et al, 2000; Cohenca et al, 2007). The resulting image allows complex dentoalveolar anatomy to be visualised only in the mesiodistal (clinical) plane, and provides limited information of the dental anatomy in the buccolingual (non-clinical) plane.

Radiographic 2D images prevent accurate assessment of the spatial relationship of the roots, and associated periapical lesions, to the surrounding anatomy (Cotti and Campisi, 2004). In addition, the location, nature, and shape of variations within the root under investigation (e.g. root resorption) may be difficult to assess (Patel et al, 2007; Whaites and Drage, 2013a). Diagnostic information in the missing 'third dimension' is of relevance when planning for endodontic surgery (Velvart et al, 2001; Bornstein et al, 2011). Useful information may include the position and angulation of the root/s in relation to the cortical plate, the thickness of the cortical plate itself, and the relationship of the root/s to adjacent anatomical structures, such as the inferior alveolar nerve, mental foramen or maxillary sinus (Lofthag-Hansen et al, 2007).

Additional parallax radiographic images, taken by changing the horizontal and/or vertical angulation of the X-ray beam in relation to the area under examination (Figs 1-1 and 1-2), may be used to enhance assessment of the spatial relationships of the imaged anatomical structures (European Society of Endodontology, 2006; Davies et al, 2015). However, these additional images will still only provide limited information (Soğur et al, 2012; Kanagasingam et al, 2015).

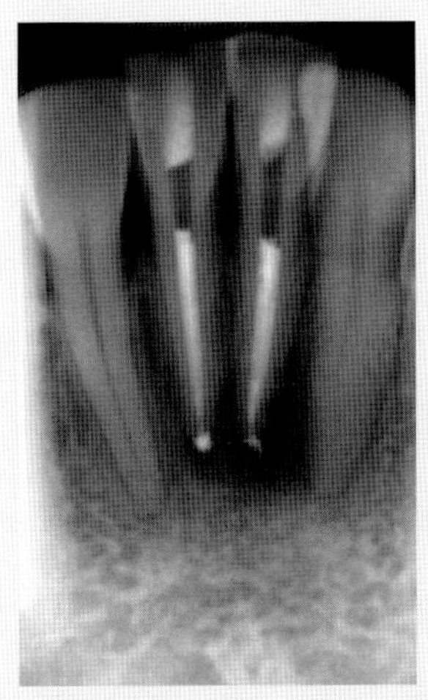

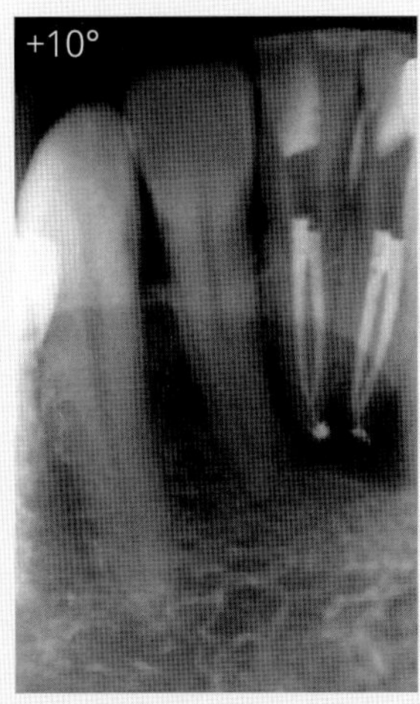

Fig 1-1 Horizontal parallax. The right radiograph has a 10-degree shift to aid visualisation of the two separate canals, which allows the quality of the root canal fillings to be assessed more accurately in the mandibular central incisors.

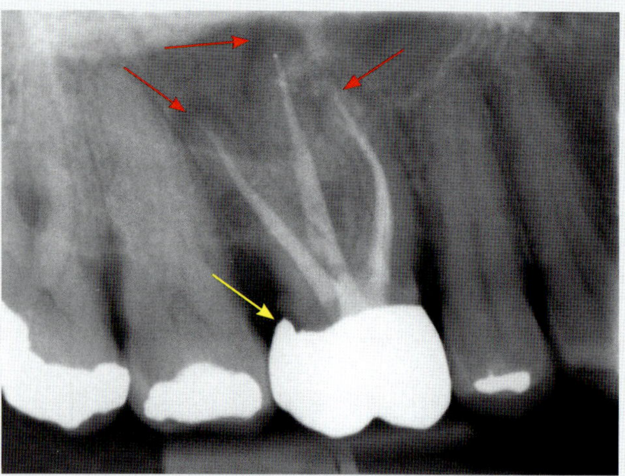

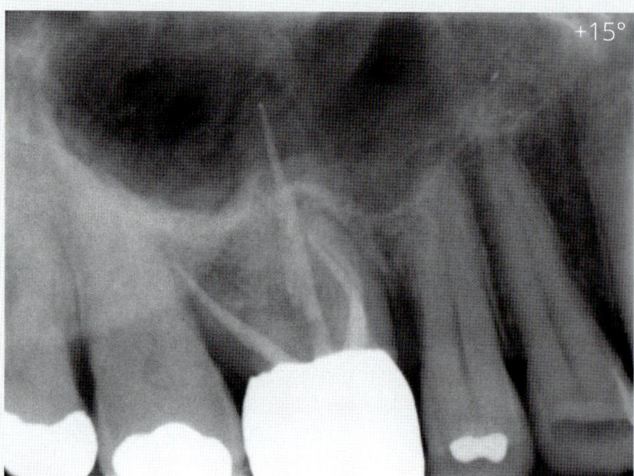

Fig 1-2 Vertical parallax. A vertical beam shift (change in inclination) has caused the periapical lesions (red arrows) associated with all three roots of this maxillary right first molar to disappear with the change of angulation in the right radiograph. Note that the defective distal margin on the left radiograph (yellow arrow) is also no longer visible on the right radiograph.

Geometric distortion

Intraoral periapical radiographic images should ideally be taken with a paralleling technique. The use of a biteblock to ensure the tooth and image receptor are parallel with one another, as well as the use of a beam aiming device to ensure the X-ray beam meets the tooth and image receptor at right angles, has been proven effective at creating a geometrically accurate image (Forsberg, 1987a, b, c).

An accurate image is obtained when the image receptor (X-ray film or digital sensor) is parallel to the long axis of the tooth, and the X-ray beam is perpendicular to both the image receptor and the tooth undergoing examination (Fig 1-3). This may be readily achievable in certain regions of the oral cavity, but may not be possible in some patients with e.g. small mouths or pronounced gag reflexes, and/or where the image receptor is poorly tolerated. Anatomical limitations, such as a shallow palatal vault, prevent the ideal positioning of the intraoral image receptor, causing incorrect long-axis orientation—which in turn results in geometric distortion (poor projection geometry) of the radiographic image (Figs 1-3 and 1-4). The ideal positioning of solid-state digital sensors may be even more challenging due to their size and rigidity, compared with conventional radiographic films and phosphor plate digital sensors (Patel et al, 2009a; Whaites and Drage, 2013a).

Ideal positioning of the image receptor may be possible when, firstly, the roots being imaged are relatively straight and, secondly, when there is sufficient space to position the image receptor correctly. If these objectives are not achieved (Fig 1-5), there will be a degree of geometric distortion and magnification. This may be particularly relevant in the posterior maxilla (Lofthag-Hansen et al, 2007). Over- or underangulated radiographs may reduce or increase the 'apparent' radiographic root length of the tooth under investigation (White and Pharaoh, 2014), and increase or decrease the size, or even result in the disappearance, of periapical lesions (Bender and Seltzer, 1961a, b; Huumonen and Ørstavik, 2002). A minimum 5% magnification of the imaged structures will occur, even when a 'textbook' paralleling technique has been employed (Vande Voorde and Bjorndahl, 1969).

Anatomical noise

Anatomical features within or superimposed over the roots being examined may obscure the area of interest, thereby preventing a thorough assessment of the imaged region (Gröndahl and Huumonen, 2004). These anatomical structures vary in radiodensity, and may be radiopaque or radiolucent. This phenomenon is sometimes referred to as 'anatomical noise' (Fig 1-6). The more complex the anatomical noise, the greater the reduction in contrast within the area of interest. The resulting radiographic image may be more difficult to interpret.

Fig 1-3 Geometric distortion. Although it may be possible to position the image sensor holder (and image sensor) parallel with the long axis of the crown and mid-third of the root, it is not possible to obtain a parallel relationship of the long axis of the entire tooth and root with the image sensor. The sagittal reconstructed CBCT image shows a parallel (and accurate) relationship of the mid-third root (green line) and the image sensor, and perpendicular X-ray beam (blue arrow). However, the apical third (red line) is not parallel to the image sensor or perpendicular to the X-ray beam, resulting in geometric distortion of the apical third of the root canal.

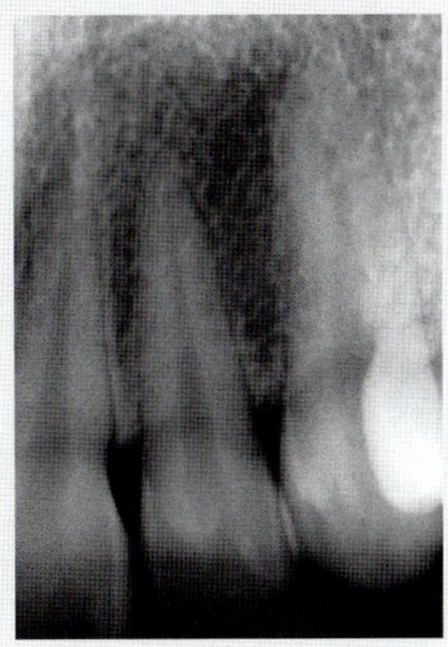

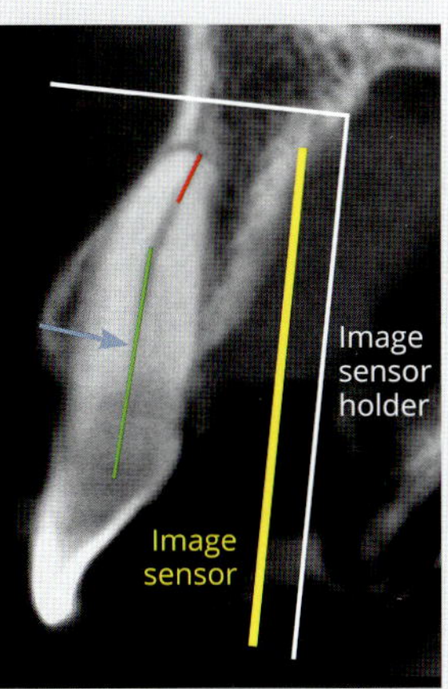

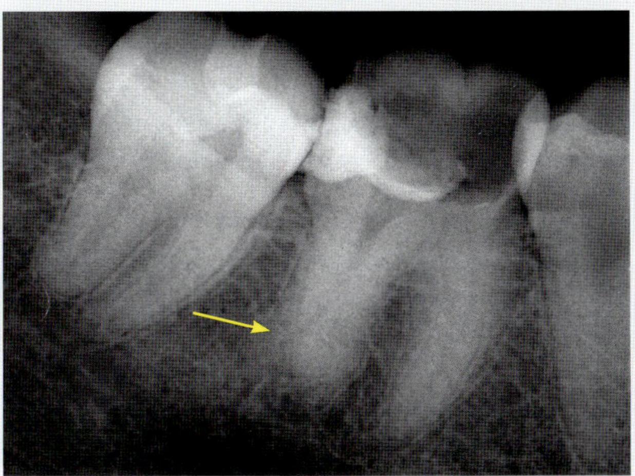

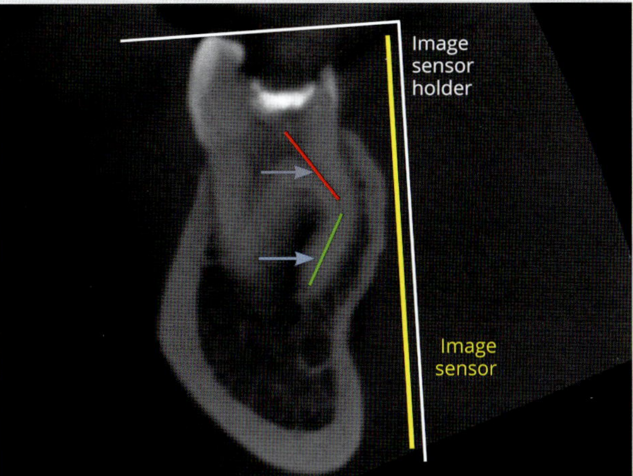

Fig 1-4 Geometric distortion. A distolingual canal (yellow arrow) can be seen on the intraoral radiograph (left). A coronal reconstructed CBCT image (right) clearly demonstrates how the distolingual root cannot be accurately assessed in the radiographic image. Neither the coronal (red line) nor apical (green line) halves of this root canal are parallel to the image sensor (yellow arrow), or perpendicular to the X-ray beam (blue arrow). This results in significant geometric distortion in this region of the image.

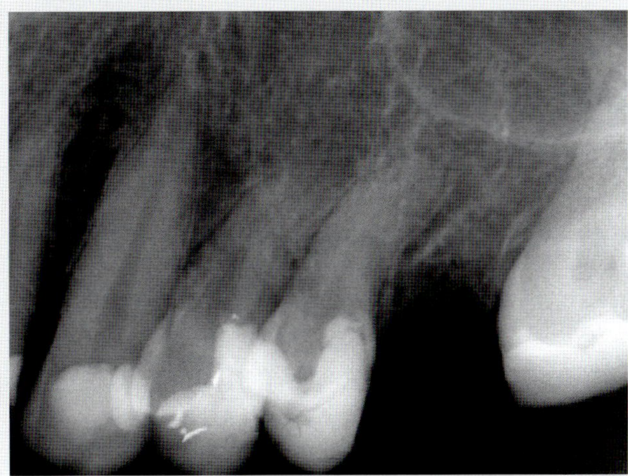

Fig 1-5 Geometric distortion. It may not be possible to position the image sensor in the ideal position, resulting in distortion of the resulting image. When imaging these maxillary left premolar teeth, the anatomical constraints of a shallow palate have prevented a paralleled image from being obtained.

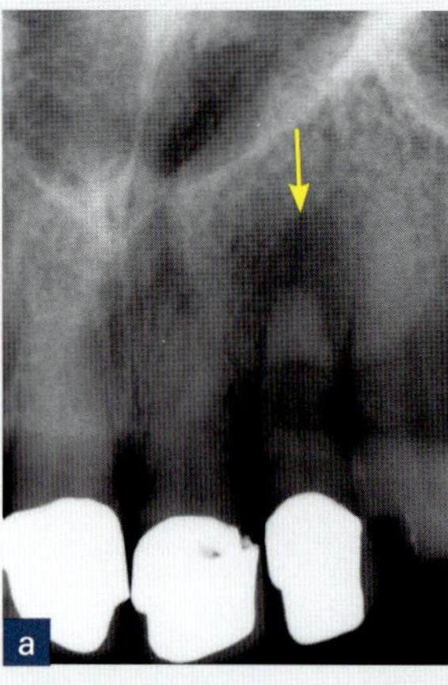

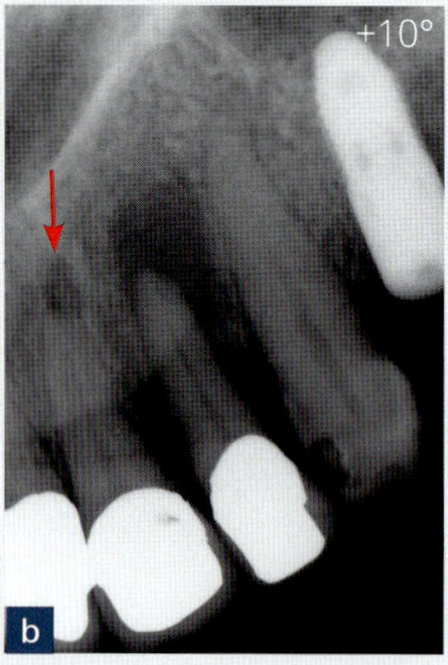

Fig 1-6 Anatomical noise. (a) A periapical radiolucency is clearly seen, and is associated with the maxillary left incisor (yellow arrow). (b) A second radiograph taken at a 10-degree horizontal shift reveals an additional periapical radiolucency (red arrow) associated with the maxillary left incisor. This 'new' radiolucency is the incisive foramen, which in this case creates radiolucent anatomical noise mimicking a periapical lesion.

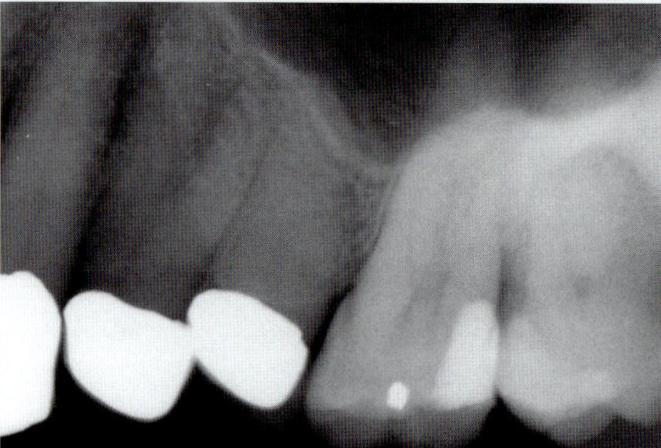

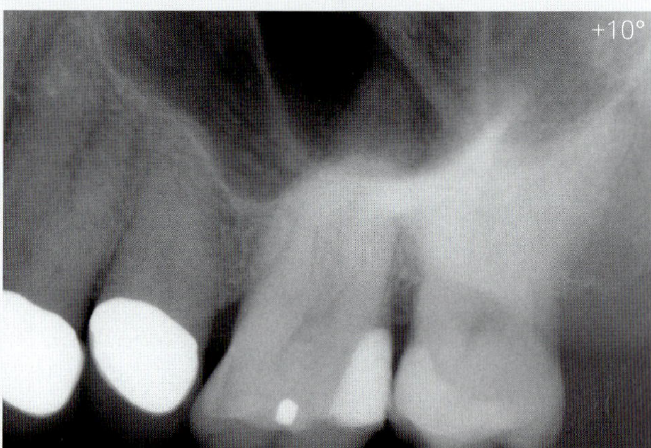

Fig 1-7 Anatomical noise. The superimposition of anatomical structures prevents complete and accurate assessment of the imaged teeth. As demonstrated in these parallax periapical radiographs, the maxillary sinus and zygomatic buttress may often create anatomical noise, which prevents visualisation of the periapical regions of the maxillary premolar and molar teeth.

Brynolf (1967, 1970a, b) demonstrated that superimposition of the incisive canal over the apices of the maxillary central incisors may complicate radiographic interpretation, i.e. the incisive foramen (anatomical noise) mimicked periapical lesions in healthy teeth.

Several studies have shown that periapical lesions confined to the cancellous bone may not be detected with conventional radiographic imaging (Bender and Seltzer, 1961a, b). It has been suggested that periapical lesions may be successfully detected when confined to cancellous bone, provided the cortical bone is thin and the anatomical noise minimal. Such lesions may go undetected beneath a thicker cortex. Anatomical noise also accounts for some underestimation of periapical lesion size in radiographic images (Shoha et al, 1974; Marmary et al, 1999; Scarfe et al, 1999).

The maxillary molar region is a complex anatomical region with a number of closely related structures, which include the maxillary sinus and zygomatic buttress (Fig 1-7).

Anatomical noise is dependent on several factors that may include: overlying anatomy; the thickness of the cancellous bone and cortical plate; and the relationship of the root apices to the cortical plate. Brynolf (1967) compared the radiographic and histological appearance of 292 maxillary incisor teeth to assess whether there was a relationship between the radiographic and histological features of the periapical lesions. Overall, there was a high correlation between radiographic and histological findings; this conclusion may have been related to the lack of anatomical noise in the specific area being assessed. The root apices of maxillary incisors lie very close to the adjacent cortical plate, and therefore erosion of this cortex may often occur soon after periapical inflammation ensues. In other areas of the jaws with increased anatomical noise, e.g. the posterior mandible with its thicker cortical plate, the correlation between histological findings and radiographic appearance may be less interrelated (Patel et al, 2009b).

Follow-up radiographs

Sequential radiographic images, taken over a period of time, are required when determining endodontic treatment outcomes (European Society of Endodontology, 2006). An accurate comparison can only be made when these images have been standardised with respect to radiation geometry, density, and contrast. Poorly standardised radiographs may lead to misinterpretation of the disease status (Bender et al, 1961a, b).

The use of customised bite blocks may be helpful in obtaining standardised images, but even then, no two images will be identical.

Advanced radiographic techniques for endodontic diagnosis

In order to overcome the limitations of conventional intraoral radiographs, a number of alternative imaging techniques to complement periapical radiography have been suggested. These include:

- magnetic resonance imaging
- ultrasound
- tuned aperture computed tomography
- computed tomography
- cone beam computed tomography.

Magnetic resonance imaging

Magnetic resonance imaging (MRI) is a specialised technique that utilises hydrogen atoms (one proton and one electron) and a magnetic field to produce an a magnetic resonance (MR) image. This imaging technique does not use ionising radiation.

For image acquisition, the patient is positioned within an MRI scanner that creates a strong magnetic field around the area being imaged (Fig 1-8a). Tissues that are composed of water contain protons (hydrogen atoms). Energy from the oscillating magnetic field is temporarily applied to the patient at the appropriate resonant frequency. This aligns the protons contained along the long axis of the magnetic field and the patient's body. A pulsed beam of radio waves, with a similar frequency to the patient's spinning hydrogen atoms, is then transmitted perpendicular to the magnetic field. This misaligns the hydrogen protons, resulting in an alteration of their axis of rotation from a longitudinal to a transverse plane (Fig 1-8b). The atoms behave like several mini bar magnets, spinning synchronously with each other. This generates a radio signal (resonance) that is detected by the receiver within the scanner (Fig 1-8c). Similar radio signals are detected as the hydrogen protons relax and return to their original (longitudinal) direction. A computer processes the receiver information, and an image is thereby produced (White and Pharaoh, 2014; Whaites and Drage, 2013b).

MRI has been used for the investigation of soft tissue lesions in salivary glands, the investigation of the temporomandibular joint, for tumour staging (Goto et al, 2007), and for the treatment planning of dental implants (Imamura et al, 2004; Monsour and Dhudia, 2008).

The MRI technique has been used to assess a cohort of patients with periapical disease. With MRI, it was possible to differentiate the roots of multirooted teeth, and smaller branches of the neurovascular bundle could be clearly identified entering apical foramina. The presence and nature of periapical lesions could also be determined, as could the remodelling of the cortical bone. An important advantage of MRI is that, unlike computed tomography (CT) imaging, it is not affected by artefacts caused by metallic restorations (Eggars et al, 2005).

There are several limitations to MRI, including poor resolution when compared with conventional radiographic images. The scanning times involved with the MRI technique are lengthy, and the cost and maintenance of the imaging hardware results in the scanners seldom being found anywhere but in dedicated radiology units. The dental hard tissues (e.g. enamel and dentine) cannot be differentiated from one another, or from metallic objects, as they all appear radiolucent. This currently limits the endodontic applications of MRI. Finally, MRI scanners need highly trained radiographers to take the image, and radiologists to interpret the resulting scan.

To make the MRI technique more applicable to the oral cavity, researchers have developed a technique that utilises an intraoral loop coil placed in the occlusal position. This technique has been shown to detect

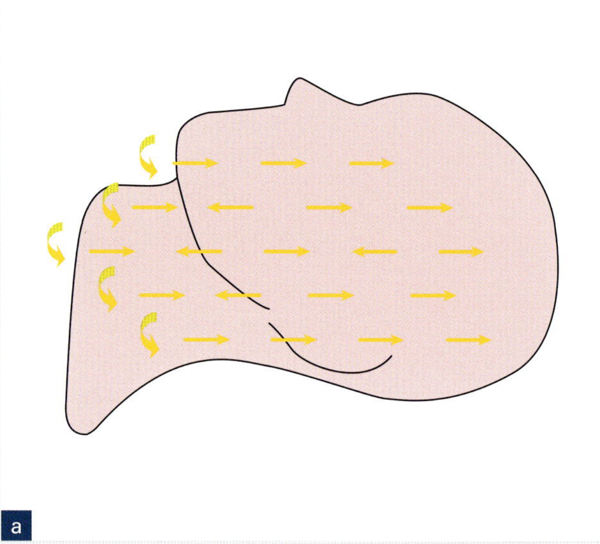

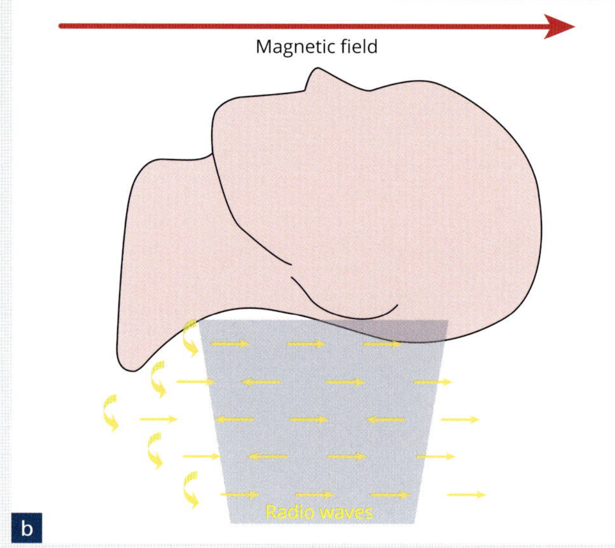

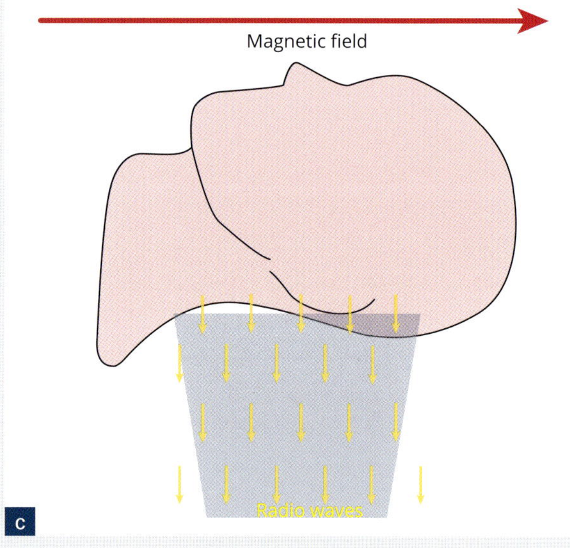

Fig 1-8 (a) The magnetic resonance imaging (MRI) technique involves the formation of a magnetic field around the area being imaged. The protons within the magnetic field and body then become aligned along the long axis. (b) A pulsed beam of radio waves is transmitted perpendicular to the long axis of the magnetic field, causing the protons to be disrupted, and altering their axis of rotation. (c) The disrupted protons spin synchronously with one another, producing a faint radio signal, which in turn is sent back to a receiver. A computer processes the resulting signal and the image is produced.

caries lesions *in vivo* (Tymofiyeva et al, 2009; Idiyatullin et al, 2011), and to differentiate between sound and carious dentine due to the porosity of the latter, which in turn has a higher water content (Tymofiyeva et al, 2009). Coil MRI has also been used to determine the distance from caries lesions to the pulp. While the potential applications of coil MRI show promise, problems are acknowledged due to patient movement and the effect of certain dental materials on image quality. However, it would seem that the MRI technique is less sensitive to dental materials than other techniques, such as CT imaging (Eggars et al, 2005).

One of the limitations of the conventional MRI technique is that the densely calcified dental tissues cause deterioration of the MRI signal before digitisation is achieved, which results in weakened or absent MRI signals. Thus, the majority of MRI studies in relation to dentistry have been on the dental soft tissues, including the pulp and periodontal ligament.

In addition to the limitations previously described, coil MRI lacks the ease of use of other imaging techniques. Furthermore, the costs involved with coil MRI are significant. As a result, access to suitable coil MRI scanning equipment is limited.

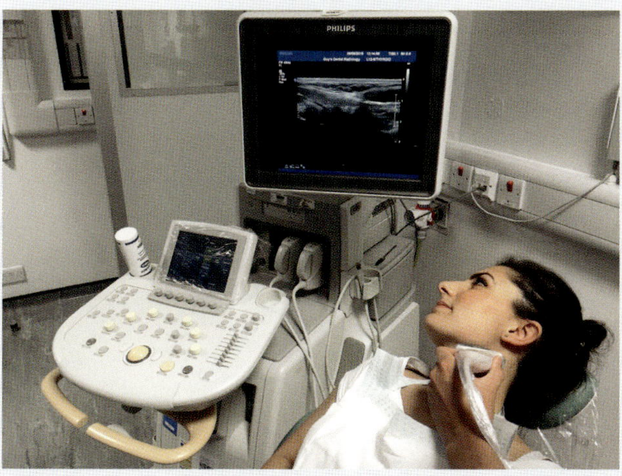

Fig 1-9 Ultrasound. An extraoral transducer probe emits and detects the ultrasound (US) signal. The US signal is created using the piezoelectric effect.

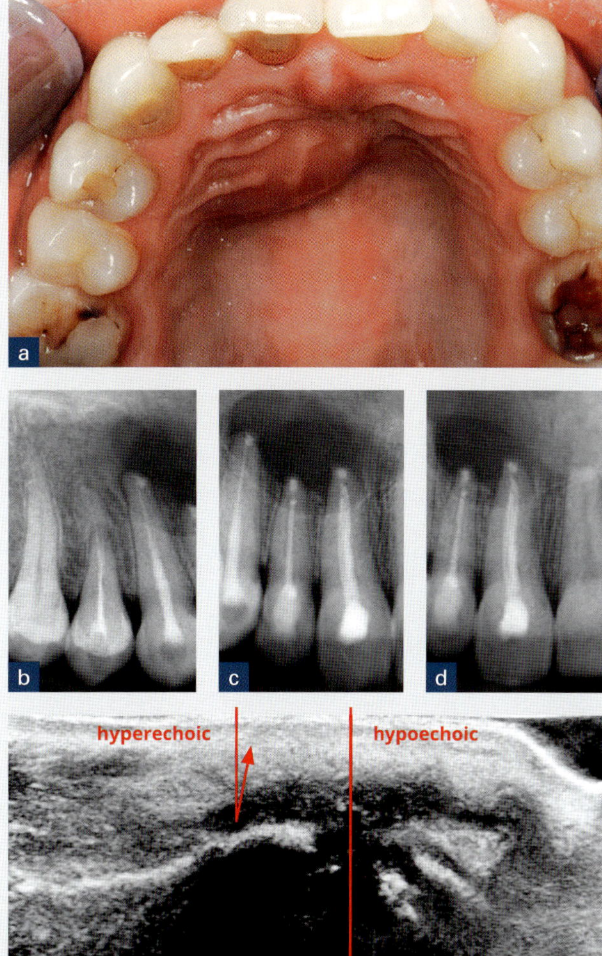

Fig 1-10 Ultrasound (US). (a) This patient presented with a large, fluctuant swelling palatal to the maxillary right anterior teeth. (b) Periapical radiographs demonstrated a large radiolucency encompassing the apices of the root-treated maxillary right central incisor, lateral incisor and canine teeth. Two-dimensional radiographs (b to d) fail to provide information on the depth of the lesion and the location of resorption of the respective buccal and palatal cortical plates. (e) A US scan of the area was conducted by placing a probe extraorally over the region of interest. The resultant scan images the relative hyperechoic and hypoechoic regions, demonstrating the buccolingual extent of the periapical lesion, as well as the locations where the cortical plates have been resorbed.

Ultrasound

The ultrasound (US) technique is based on the reflection (echoes) of US waves at the interface between tissues that have different acoustic properties (Gundappa et al, 2006). Ultrasonic waves are created using the piezoelectric effect via a transducer (probe). The beam of US energy is emitted and reflected back to the same probe (i.e. the probe acts as both emitter and detector). A transducer detects the echoes and converts them into an electrical signal (Fig 1-9). The resulting real-time image is composed of black, white, and shades of grey. As the probe is traversed across the area of interest, new images are generated in real time. The intensity or strength of the detected echoes is dependent on the difference between the acoustic impedance of two adjacent tissues. The greater the difference between the tissues, the greater the distinction in the reflected US energy, resulting in higher echo intensity. Tissue interfaces that generate high echo intensity are described as hyperechoic (e.g. bone and teeth). Anechoic tissues (e.g. fluid-filled cysts) are those that do not reflect US energy (Fig 1-10). Images consisting of varying degrees of hyperechoic and anechoic usually have a heterogeneous profile. The Doppler effect (the change of sound frequency reflected

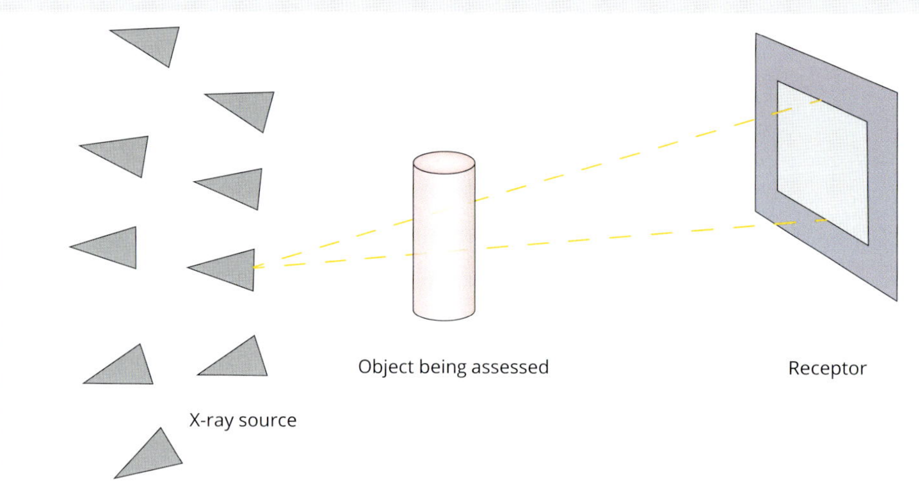

Fig 1-11 Tuned aperture computed tomography (TACT). With this technique, 8 to 10 digital radiographic images are taken at different defined projection geometries. The images are reconstructed to provide 3D data, which may be viewed slice by slice.

from a moving source) can be used to assess arterial and venous blood flow (Whaites and Drage, 2013b).

US has been used to diagnose the full nature of periapical lesions (Cotti et al, 2003). In this study, 11 periapical lesions of endodontic origin were assessed with US imaging. Provisional diagnoses were made according to the echo images (hyperechoic and hypoechoic). The evidence of vascularity within the lesions was determined using the colour laser Doppler effect. The provisional diagnoses (seven cysts, four granulomas) were successfully confirmed by histology in all 11 cases. A similar study also concluded that US was a reliable diagnostic technique for determining the pathological nature (granulomas versus cysts) of periapical lesions (Gundappa et al, 2006). However, in both of these studies the apical biopsies were not removed together with the root apices, therefore making it impossible to confirm whether the assessed lesions were true or pocket cysts. Furthermore, the lesions were not serially sectioned, making accurate histological diagnosis unreliable (Nair et al, 1996). Therefore, the ability of US to assess the true nature of periapical lesions is questionable.

Doppler flowmetry has also been used to assess the outcome of orthograde root canal treatment in maxillary anterior teeth (Maity et al, 2011). It was demonstrated that healing could be established earlier with the Doppler technique when compared with conventional radiographs. Evidence of healing was apparent in the majority of cases after just 6 weeks when assessed with Doppler flowmetry.

US energy is unable to penetrate bone effectively and is therefore only useful when assessing periapical lesions with little or no overlying cortical bone. While US may be used with relative ease in the anterior region of the mouth, the positioning of the probe is more difficult against the buccal mucosa of posterior teeth. In addition, the interpretation of US images is limited to radiologists who have received relevant training.

Tuned aperture computed tomography

Tuned aperture computed tomography (TACT) is based on the concept of tomosynthesis (Webber and Messura, 1999). A series of 8 to 10 radiographic images are exposed at different projection geometries using a programmable imaging unit with specialised software to reconstruct a 3D data set, which can then be viewed slice by slice (Fig 1-11).

The advantage of TACT over conventional radiographic imaging is that there is less superimposition of anatomical noise over the area of interest (Tyndall et al, 1997). The overall radiation dose of TACT is no greater than one to two times that of conventional periapical X-ray exposure, as the total dose is divided among the series of exposures (Nair et al, 1998; Nance et al, 2000). Additional advantages claimed for this technique include the absence of artefacts resulting from radiation interaction with metallic restorations (see later section on CT). The resolution is reported to be comparable to 2D radiographs (Nair and Nair, 2007).

TACT appears to have potential benefits that may make it useful in the future. For the time being, how-

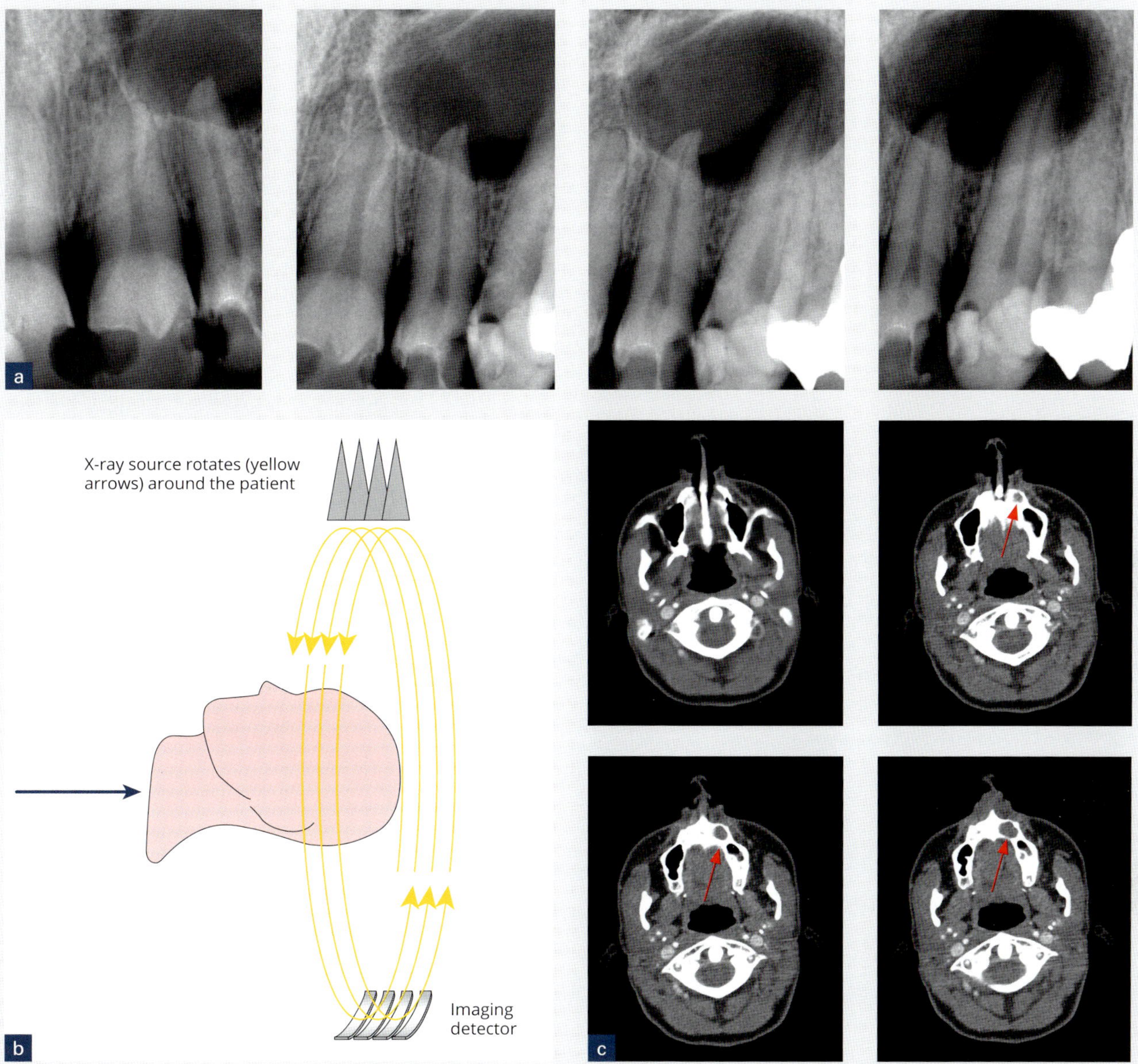

Fig 1-12 Computed tomography (CT). (a) A large periapical radiolucency associated with the maxillary left lateral incisor and canine teeth is revealed following periapical radiographic examination. (b) The gantry of the CT scanner contains the X-ray source and the imaging detectors. The patient is advanced through a circular aperture in the centre of the scanner. The patient is thereby scanned 'slice by slice' while being advanced through the scanner. (c) The reconstructed slices can then be observed individually in the imaged plane. In this case, the width and depth of the periapical radiolucency can be assessed at each of the axial sections (red arrows).

ever, the technique for the imaging of dentoalveolar anatomy should be considered as a research tool.

Computed tomography

Computed tomography (CT) is an imaging technique that produces 3D radiographic images using a series of 2D sectional X-ray images. Essentially, CT scanners consist of a gantry that contains the rotating X-ray tube head and reciprocal detectors. In the centre of the gantry is a circular aperture through which the patient is advanced. The tube head and reciprocal detectors within the gantry either rotate synchronously around the patient, or the detectors take the form of a continuous ring around the patient and only the X-ray source moves within the detector ring (Fig 1-12a and b). The data from the detectors produces an attenuation profile of the particular slice of the body being examined. The patient is then moved slightly further

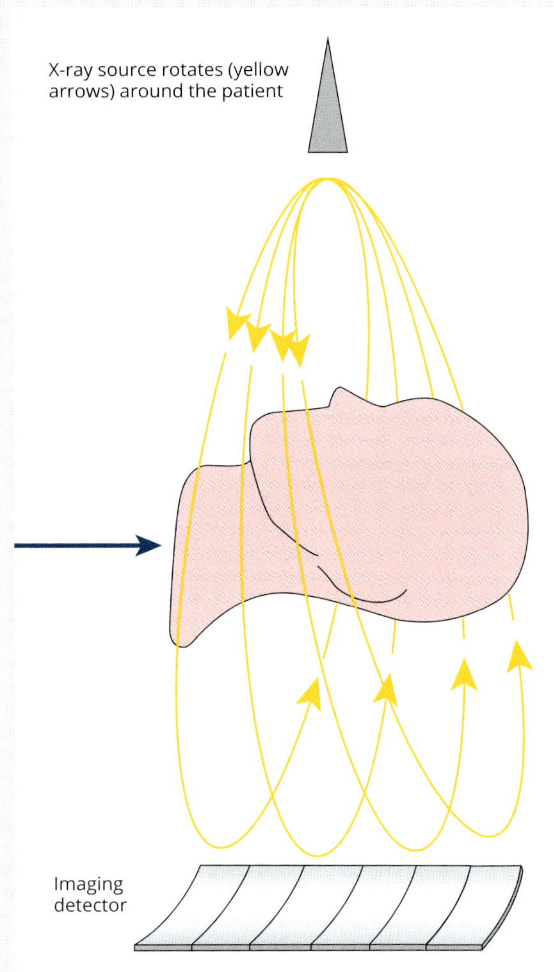

Fig 1-13 Multislice computed tomography (MSCT). To overcome the limitations of CT, the CT beam width is widened, and detectors are arranged in multiple rows, enabling the entire fan beam to be captured at any one time.

into the gantry for the next slice of data to be acquired. The process is repeated until the area of interest has been fully scanned.

Early generation CT scanners acquired 'data' in the axial plane by scanning the patient 'slice by slice', using a narrow collimated fan-shaped X-ray beam passing through the patient to a single array of reciprocal detectors. The detectors measured the intensity of X-rays emerging from the patient.

Over the past three decades, there have been considerable advances in CT technology (Yu et al, 2009; Runge et al, 2015). To overcome the problems of conventional (single slice) medical CT imaging, which results in relatively poor image quality, the technique of multislice computed tomography (MSCT) was developed. Here, the CT beam is widened in the z-direction (beam width), and instead of a single detector, multiple detectors are arranged in parallel rows, so that a number of slices can be obtained by capturing the entire fan beam at any one time (Fig 1-13). This reduces the number of rotations of the X-ray tube and therefore the radiation dose. The number of detectors on MSCT scanners has increased, facilitating a greater number of simultaneously acquired images.

A number of researchers have evaluated MSCT and compared it to cone beam computed tomography (CBCT). One autopsy study demonstrated that the quality of small-volume CBCT scans might be better or at least equal to MSCT in assessing delicate anatomical structures, such as the periodontal ligament and bone trabeculae.

In addition to providing multiplanar 3D images, CT has several other advantages over conventional radiography. These include the elimination of anatomical noise and high contrast resolution, allowing differentiation of tissues with less than 1% physical density difference, compared with the 10% variation in physical difference that is required with conventional radiography (White and Pharaoh, 2014).

A number of studies have used CT imaging to manage endodontic problems (Velvart et al, 2001; Huumonen et al, 2006). These were able to obtain additional information on the root canal anatomy when compared with plain film radiographs (Tachibana and Matsumoto, 1990). Valuable information on the relationship of the root apices with important anatomical structures, such as the maxillary sinus, was obtained using reconstructed axial slices and 3D reconstruction of the CT data. The information derived from CT scans has been compared with that obtained from periapical radiographs when planning periapical surgery (Velvart et al, 2001). Of the 50 mandibular molar teeth assessed, CT imaging detected the presence of a periapical lesion and the location of the inferior alveolar nerve in every case, compared with only 78% and 39%, respectively, with periapical radiographs. Furthermore, the buccolingual thickness of the cortical and cancellous bone, as well as the position and angulation of the root within the mandible, could only be assessed by CT. It was concluded that 'CT should be considered before the surgical treatment of mandibular premolars and molars when the mandibular canal

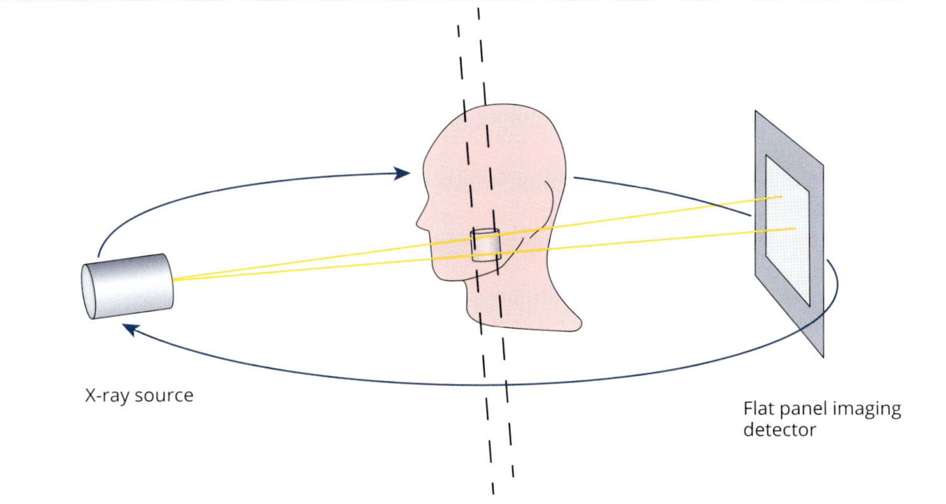

X-ray source

Flat panel imaging detector

Fig 1-14 Small volume CBCT imaging. The cone-shaped X-ray beam synchronously rotates around the patient, together with the imaging detector.

is not detectable or appears in close proximity to the periapical lesion or root with conventional radiographic techniques'.

The diagnostic value of CT and parallax periapical radiographs has been compared when assessing maxillary molar teeth for endodontic re-treatment (Huumonen et al, 2006). Periapical lesions were more reliably detected with CT when compared with periapical radiographs. In addition, the distance between the palatal and buccal cortical plates and the adjacent root apices could only be determined with CT. The authors of this study concluded that 'the information obtained from CT was essential for decision making in surgical re-treatment'. However, one should bear in mind that a high radiation dose is required to achieve an adequate resolution for assessing root canal anatomy.

The assessment of the 'third dimension' with CT imaging also allows the number of roots and root canals to be determined, as well as their anatomy in all three planes. The additional information may be extremely useful when diagnosing and managing persistent endodontic disease, which may remain undetected with conventional radiography. For example, CT has been used to detect the high incidence of unfilled second mesiobuccal canals in root-treated maxillary molars (Huumonen et al, 2006). Correspondingly, the majority of roots with unfilled canals had associated periapical lesions.

The uptake of CT in endodontics has been limited. This is primarily due to the high effective dose and relatively low resolution of the imaging technique. Other disadvantages of CT include the high costs of the scans, scatter due to metallic objects, poor resolution compared with conventional radiographs, and the limited availability of the scanners (e.g. hospital radiography units). Access for dentists in practice is therefore limited. CT technology has now been superseded by CBCT technology in the management of endodontic problems.

Cone beam computed tomography

Cone beam computed tomography (CBCT)—also known as digital volumetric imaging—is an extraoral imaging technique that was developed in the late 1990s to produce 3D scans of the maxillofacial skeleton at a considerably lower radiation dose than CT (Mozzo et al, 1998; Arai et al, 1999). CBCT differs from CT imaging in that the entire 3D volume of data is acquired in the course of a single sweep by the scanner, using a simple, direct relationship between sensor and source, which rotate synchronously around the patient's head (Fig 1-14).

The X-ray source and the detector rotate between 180 to 360 degrees around the patient. Unlike CT scans, most CBCT scans are taken with the patient sitting or standing up. The X-ray beam is cone-shaped (hence the name of the technique), capturing a cylindrical or spherical volume of data, described as the field of view (FOV). The FOV varies between different CBCT scanners (Pauwels et al, 2012). Each reconstructed image is comprised of a number of volumetric pixels, which are described as voxels. Voxel size typically ranges from between 0.08 to 0.125 mm^3.

Small FOV CBCT scanners usually have a lower effective dose than CT scanners. This is due, in part, to rapid scan times, a very low radiation dose for each X-ray image, and sophisticated image receptor sensors. The pulsed X-ray beam results in up to 950 'projection images' or basis exposures being taken, as the X-ray source and detector rotate around the patient. CBCT scanners are simple to use and take up about the same amount of space as panoramic radiographic machines, making them suitable for dental practices. Decreasing the size of the FOV, increasing the voxel size, and/or reducing the number of projection images taken as the X-ray source rotates around the patient may further reduce the radiation dose.

Sectional images or 'tomographic slices', as thin as 1 voxel thick, may be displayed in a number of ways. Typically, images are displayed in the three orthogonal planes—axial, sagittal and coronal—simultaneously. Coronal and axial views of the tooth are readily produced, allowing the clinician to gain a truly 3D view of the entire tooth and its surrounding anatomy. Surface rendering is also possible to produce 3D images.

The image quality of CBCT scans is superior to that of helical CT scans for assessing dental hard tissues. One study compared the image quality of an experimental CBCT scanner to a MSCT scanner and concluded that CBCT had a higher resolution for detecting small, high-contrast (i.e. hard tissue) structures such as 'nerve canals' carrying neurovascular bundles. Hirsch et al (2003) reached a similar conclusion when they compared limited CBCT to MSCT. However, the lower exposure settings of CBCT scans result in poor soft tissue contrast compared with conventional CT scans.

CBCT is undoubtedly a major breakthrough in dental imaging. For the first time, the clinician is able to use a patient-friendly imaging system to easily view areas of interest in any plane, rather than being restricted to the superimposed 2D images available with conventional radiography.

The radiographic aspects and specific applications of CBCT in endodontics will be described in the subsequent chapters.

Conclusions

- Images acquired using conventional intraoral radiographic techniques reveal information in two dimensions only (height and width). Valuable and relevant information in the third dimension (depth) is limited.
- Due to the inherent problems of positioning intraoral image receptors in the correct position in relation to the anatomical area of interest, it may not be possible to obtain an accurate, undistorted view of the area of interest.
- The detection and assessment of the true nature of endodontic lesions and other relevant features may be impaired by adjacent anatomical noise. The effect of this anatomical noise is unique for each patient and is dependent on the degree of bone demineralisation, size of the endodontic lesion, and physical nature of the anatomical noise (i.e. its thickness, shape, and the density of the overlying anatomy).
- Serial radiographs taken with the paralleling technique are not consistently reproducible. This may result in misinterpretation of the healing process or failure of the endodontic treatment.

Acknowledgement

This chapter has been adapted from: Patel S, Dawood A, Whaites E, Pitt Ford T. New dimensions in endodontic imaging: part 1. Conventional and alternative radiographic systems. Int Endod J 2009a;42:447–462.

References

Arai Y, Tammisalo E, Iwai K, Hashimoto K, Shinoda K. Development of a compact computed tomographic apparatus for dental use. Dentomaxillofac Radiol 1999;28:245–248.

Bender IB, Seltzer S. Roentgenographic and direct observation of experimental lesions in bone: I. J Am Dent Assoc 1961a;62:152–160.

Bender IB, Seltzer S. Roentgenographic and direct observation of experimental lesions in bone: II. J Am Dent Assoc 1961b;62:708–716.

Bornstein MM, Lauber R, Sendi P, von Arx T. Comparison of periapical and limited cone-beam computed tomography in mandibular molars for analysis of anatomical landmarks before apical surgery. J Endod 2011;37:151–157.

Brynolf I. A histological and roentenological study of the periapical region of human upper incisors. Odontologisk Revy 1967;18:(Suppl 11).

Brynolf I. Roentgenolgic periapical diagnosis. IV. When is one roentgenogram not sufficient? Sven Tandlak Tidskr 1970a;63:415–423.

Brynolf I. Roentgenolgic periapical diagnosis. III. The more roentgenograms—the better the information? Sven Tandlak Tidskr 1970b;63:409–413.

Cohenca N, Simon JH, Roges R, Morag Y, Malfaz JM. Clinical indications for digital imaging in dento-alveolar trauma. Part 1: traumatic injuries. Dent Traumatol 2007;23:95–104.

Cotti E, Campisi G, Ambu R, Dettori C. Ultrasound real-time imaging in the differential diagnosis of periapical lesions. Int Endod J 2003;36:556–563.

Cotti E, Campisi G. Advanced radiographic techniques for the detection of lesions in bone. Endod Topics 2004;7:52–72.

Davies A, Mannocci F, Mitchell P, Andiappan M, Patel S. The detection of periapical pathoses in root filled teeth using single and parallax periapical radiographs versus cone beam computed tomography - a clinical study. Int Endod J 2015;48:582–592.

Eggars G, Ricker M, Kress J, Fiebach J, Dickhaus H, Hassfeld S. Artefacts in magnetic resonance imaging caused by dental material. MAGMA 2005;18:103–111.

European Society of Endodontology. Quality guidelines for endodontic treatment: consensus report of the European Society of Endodontology. Int Endod J 2006;39:921–930.

Forsberg J. Radiographic reproduction of endodontic 'working length' comparing the paralleling and the bisecting-angle techniques. Oral Surg Oral Med Oral Pathol 1987a;64:353–360.

Forsberg J. A comparison of the paralleling and bisecting-angle radiographic techniques in endodontics. Int Endod J 1987b;20:177–182.

Forsberg J. Estimation of the root filling length with paralleling and bisecting-angle radiographic techniques performed by undergraduate students. Int Endod J 1987c;20:282–286.

Goto TK, Nishida S, Nakamura Y, et al. The accuracy of three-dimensional magnetic resonance 3D vibe images of the mandible: an in vitro comparison of magnetic resonance imaging and computed tomography. Oral Surg Oral Med Oral Pathol Oral Radiol Endod 2007;103:550–559.

Gröndahl HG, Huumonen S. Radiographic manifestations of periapical inflammatory lesions. Endod Topics 2004;8:55–67.

Gundappa M, Ng SY, Whaites EJ. Comparison of ultrasound, digital and conventional radiography in differentiating periapical lesions. Dentomaxillofac Radiol 2006;35:326–333.

Hirsch E, Graf HL, Hemprich A. Comparative investigation of image quality of three different X-ray procedures. Dentomaxillofac Radiol 2003;32:201–211.

Huumonen S, Ørstavik D Radiological aspects of apical periodontitis. Endod Topics 2002;1:3–25.

Huumonen S, Kvist T, Gröndahl K, Molander A. Diagnostic value of computed tomography in re-treatment of root fillings in maxillary teeth. Int Endod J 2006;39:827–833.

Idiyatullin D, Corum C, Moeller S, Prasad HS, Garwood M, Nixdorf DR. Dental magnetic resonance imaging: making the invisible visible. J Endod 2011;37:745–752.

Imamura H, Sato H, Matsuura T, Ishikawa M, Zezé R. A comparative study of computed tomography and magentic resonance imaging for the detection of mandibular canals and cross-sectional areas in diagnosis prior to dental implant treatment. Clin Implant Dent Relat Res 2004;6:75–81.

Kanagasingam S, Mannocci F, Lim CX, Yong CP, Patel S. Accuracy of single versus multiple images of conventional and digital periapical radiography in diagnosing periapical periodontitis using histopathological findings as a reference standard. Int Endod J 2015 (in press).

Lofthag-Hansen S, Huumonen S, Gröndahl K, Gröndahl HG. Limited cone-beam CT and intraoral radiography for the diagnosis of periapical pathology. Oral Surg Oral Med Oral Pathol Oral Radiol Endod 2007;103:114–119.

Maity I, Kumari A, Shukla AK, Usha H, Naveen D. Monitoring of healing by ultrasound with color power doppler after root canal treatment of maxillary teeth with periapical lesions. J Conserv Dent 2011;14:252–257.

Marmary Y, Koter T, Heling I. The effect of periapical rarefying ostetis on cortical and cancellous bone. A study comparing conventional radiographs with computed tomography. Dentomaxillofac Radiol 1999;28:267–271.

Monsour PA, Dhudia R. Implant radiography and radiology. Aust Dent J 2008;53(suppl 1):S11–S25.

Mozzo P, Procacci C, Tacconi A, Martini PT, Andreis IA. A new volumetric CT machine for dental imaging based on the cone-beam technique: preliminary results. Eur Radiol 1998;8:1558–1564.

Nair MK, Nair UP. Digital and advanced imaging in endodontics: a review. J Endod 2007;33:1–6.

Nair PNR, Pajarola G, Schroeder HE. Types and incidence of human periapical lesions obtained with extracted teeth. Oral Surg Oral Med Oral Pathol Oral Radiol Endod 1996;81:93–102.

Nair MK, Tyndall DA, Ludlow JB, May K, Ye F. The effects of restorative material and location on the detection of simulated recurrent caries. A comparison of dental film, direct digital radiography and tuned aperture computed tomography. Dentomaxillofac Radiol 1998;27:80–84.

Nance R, Tyndall D, Levin LG, Trope M. Identification of root canals in molars by tuned-aperture computed tomography. Int Endod J 2000;33:392–396.

Patel S, Dawood A, Ford TP, Whaites E. The potential applications of cone beam computed tomography in the management of endodontic problems. Int Endod J 2007;40:818–830.

Patel S, Dawood A, Whaites E, Pitt Ford T. New dimensions in endodontic imaging: part 1. Conventional and alternative radiographic systems. Int Endod J 2009a;42:447–462.

Patel S, Dawood A, Mannocci F, Wilson R, Pitt Ford T. Detection of periapical bone defects in human jaws using cone beam computed tomography and intraoral radiography. Int Endod J 2009b;42:507–515.

Patel S, Durack C, Abella F, Shemesh H, Roig M, Lemberg K. Cone beam computed tomography in endodontics—a review. Int Endod J 2015;48:3–15.

Pauwels R, Beinsbergera J, Collaert B, et al. Effective dose range for dental cone beam computed tomography scanners. Eur J Radiol 2012;81:267–271.

Runge VM, Marquez H, Andreisek G, Valavanis A, Alkadhi H. Recent technological advances in computed tomography and the clinical impact therein. Invest Radiol 2015;50:119–127.

Scarfe WC, Czerniejewski VJ, Farman AG, Avant SL, Molteni R. In vivo accuracy and reliability of color-coded image enhancements for the assessment of periradicular lesion dimensions. Oral Surg Oral Med Oral Pathol Oral Radiol Endod 1999;88:603–611.

Shoha RR, Dowson J, Richards AG. Radiographic interpretation of experimentally produced bony lesions. Oral Surg Oral Med Oral Pathol 1974;38:294–303.

Soğur E, Gröndahl HG, Baksi BG, Mert A. Does a combination of two radiographs increase accuracy in detecting acid-induced periapical lesions and does it approach the accuracy of cone beam computed tomography scanning? J Endod 2012;2:131–136.

Tachibana H, Matsumoto K. Applicability of X-ray computerized tomography in endodontics. Endod Dent Traumatol 1990;6:16–20.

Tymofiyeva O, Boldt J, Rottner K, Schmid F, Richter EJ, Jakob PM. High-resolution 3D magnetic resonance imaging and quantification of carious lesions and dental pulp in vivo. MAGMA 2009;22:365–374.

Tyndall DA, Clifton TL, Webber RL, Ludlow JB, Horton RA. TACT imaging of primary caries. Oral Surg Oral Med Oral Pathol Oral Radiol Endod 1997;84:214–225.

Vande Voorde HE, Bjorndahl AM. Estimated endodontic "working length" with paralleling radiographs. Oral Surg Oral Med Oral Pathol 1969;27:106–110.

Velvart P, Hecker H, Tillinger G. Detection of the apical lesion and the mandibular canal in conventional radiography and computed tomography. Oral Surg Oral Med Oral Pathol Oral Radiol Endod 2001;92:682–688.

Webber RL, Messura JK. An in vivo comparison of digital information obtained from tuned-aperture computed tomography and conventional dental radiographic imaging modalities. Oral Surg Oral Med Oral Pathol Oral Radiol Endod 1999;88:239–247.

Whaites E, Drage N. Periapical radiography. In: Essentials of Dental Radiology and Radiography, ed 5. London, UK: Churchill Livingston Elsevier, 2013a.

Whaites E, Drage N. Alternative and specialized imaging modalities. In: Essentials of Dental Radiology and Radiography, ed 5. London, UK: Churchill Livingston Elsevier, 2013b.

White S, Pharaoh M. Advanced imaging modalities. In: Oral Radiology: Principles and Interpretation, ed 7. St Louis, MO: Mosby, 2014.

Yu L, Liu X, Leng S, et al. Radiation dose reduction in computed tomography: techniques and future perspective. Imaging Med 2009;1:65–84.

Chapter 2

Radiation Physics

Simon C Harvey

Introduction

The aim of this chapter is, firstly, to explain what X-ray radiation is and, secondly, to describe the production and interaction of X-ray radiation.

The electromagnetic wave

The electromagnetic wave describes a wave of energy that has an electric field alternating (between positive and negative) along one axis. At right angles to this, a magnetic field alternates between north and south (Fig 2-1). The two are often drawn as one wave to make their depiction easier.

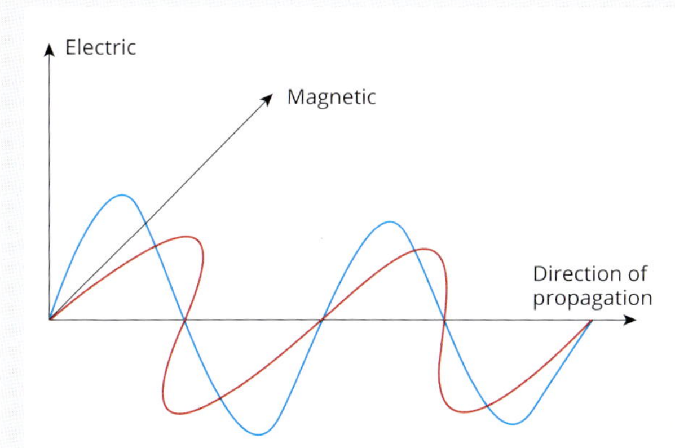

Fig 2-1 The electromagnetic wave.

All electromagnetic waves travel at the same speed in a vacuum, irrespective of their energy—the speed of light = 299 792 458 ms^{-1}. The speed of any wave is related to its wavelength and frequency by the following equation: speed = wavelength × frequency.

As the speed is known and constant (speed of light = c), the wavelength and frequency of different electromagnetic waves must change accordingly. At one end of the spectrum, the waves have a very long wavelength (and therefore low frequency) and are lower in energy. At the other end, the waves have a very short wavelength, high frequency, and are very high in energy (Fig 2-2).

The electromagnetic spectrum is continuous. Although we name different parts of the spectrum and provide cut-offs, these are arbitrary, and the different categories of waves differ only in the energy they possess.

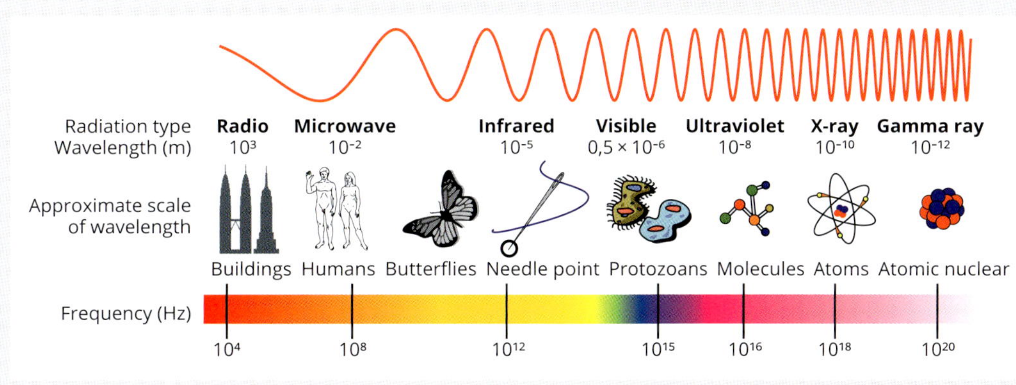

Fig 2-2 The electromagnetic spectrum (NASA).

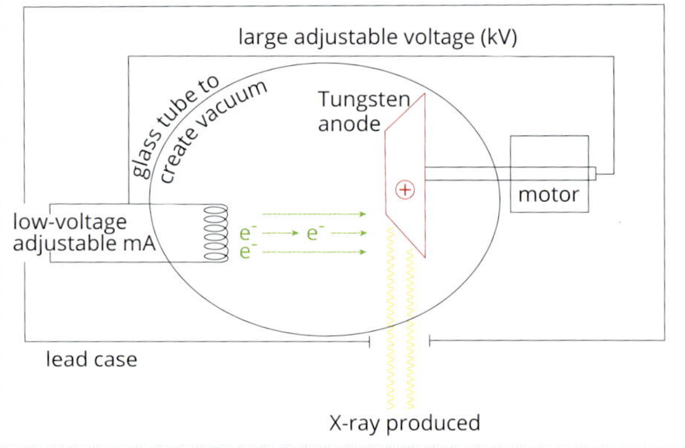

Fig 2-3 A rotating anode X-ray tube.

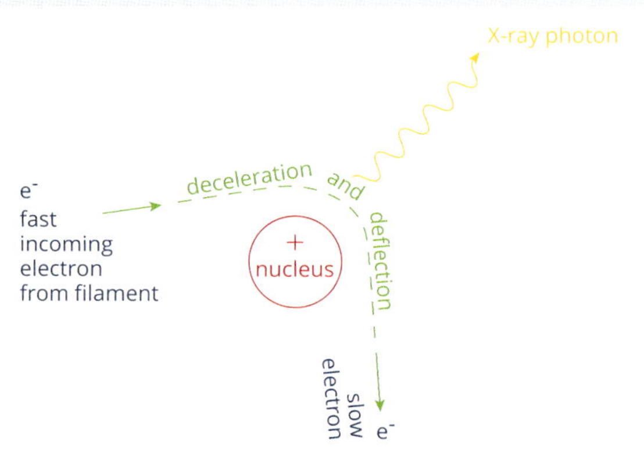

Fig 2-4 Bremsstrahlung radiation production.

It is noticeable that visible light only makes up a narrow band in the spectrum. Waves with frequencies below 4×10^{14} Hz are not visible to the human eye, and frequencies above 8×10^{14} Hz are equally invisible. Above a certain energy level, the waves can become ionising and cause damage to biological tissues. Higher-energy ultraviolet waves, X-rays, and gamma rays all have enough energy to damage human cells.

Individual photons or continuous waves?

We have seen that electromagnetic waves are a continuous wave: however, we often refer to 'photons', which have a particulate form and particulate properties. This is an alternative way of describing the interactions of electromagnetic waves more easily, and will appear throughout the book. It should be noted, however, that the photons have no mass, and even though they have particulate properties and can be described individually, they are in fact discrete packets of energy.

X-ray production

X-rays are high-energy electromagnetic waves or photons. They occur naturally and are emitted from some radioactive atoms; however, this is not amenable to everyday imaging, as the radioactive source would deplete, and be constantly irradiating, and the amount and energy of the radiation could not be easily controlled. Therefore, an artificial production method is needed.

An X-ray tube contains several essential components, as illustrated in Figure 2-3 and listed in Table 2-1, with a description of their purpose.

The X-rays are produced in two ways:

Bremsstrahlung

An incoming electron emitted from the Tungsten filament is accelerated through a vacuum towards the Tungsten anode. As it strikes and passes through the anode, it may be attracted to the positive nucleus of an individual Tungsten atom. This attraction will simultaneously deflect the trajectory of the fast-moving electron and cause it to slow down rapidly. This rapid deceleration and change of path results in energy loss, which is emitted as an X-ray photon. The greater the deflection and slowing of the electron, the greater the resultant X-ray photon energy. As each interaction between an individual electron and a nucleus of the Tungsten atom in the anode is different and the energy loss is dissimilar, the energy profile of the X-rays produced (the spectrum) is over a wide range.

The majority of X-rays—approximately 80%—from an X-ray tube are produced in this method. It should be noted that the interaction here is between an incoming electron released by the filament and the nucleus of the Tungsten atoms in the target (Fig 2-4).

Characteristic radiation

If the incoming electron passes close to the nucleus and has enough energy, it can knock out a tightly bound inner shell electron (K shell) from the Tungsten atom. This leaves a vacant inner shell, which is filled quickly by an outer shell (L or M shell) electron from the same atom. As the outer shell electron 'jumps down' energy shells, it loses energy in the form of X-ray radiation. In this case, the energy the outer electron needs to lose

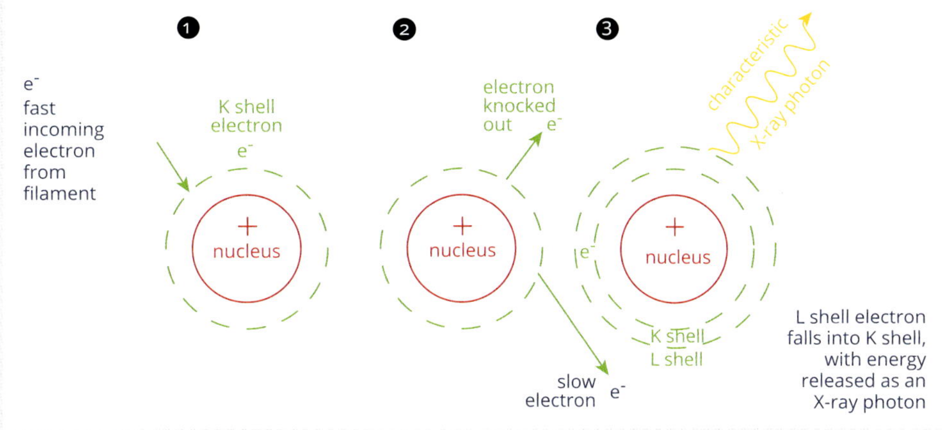

Fig 2-5 Characteristic radiation production.

when 'jumping' to the inner shell is a known amount for each different atom; so, the X-ray produced has exactly that amount of energy. The outer shell electron may come from an L or M shell, so the energy will differ slightly between the two. This is known as characteristic radiation—it is characteristic of that particular atom (Fig 2-5). For Tungsten, the values for characteristic radiation are 58 keV and 68 keV.

It should be noted that for characteristic radiation to be produced, the incoming electron must have enough energy to knock out the inner K shell Tungsten electron. The inner Tungsten electron needs 70 keV of energy to be knocked out; so only electrons with this amount of energy or more have the chance to produce characteristic radiation with a Tungsten target. This means that X-ray tubes operating below 70 kV will have no chance of producing characteristic radiation. Cone beam computed tomography (CBCT) sets generally use 80 to 120 kV, which is enough for characteristic radiation production with a Tungsten target.

Heat

The two interactions described above result in X-ray production; however, this is not the fate of every elec-

Table 2-1 X-ray tube components and their purpose.

Component	Purpose	Notes
Tungsten filament	Produces a supply of electrons by thermionic emission	Heats up via a low-voltage circuit to approx 2200°C
Tungsten anode/target for electrons	Large potential difference accelerates the electrons to a high speed, causing them to smash into the anode	Component
Vacuum	Ensures the electrons can be accelerated uninterrupted	This means excess heat created in the tube cannot be lost by convection as there is no convection medium (air)
Lead casing	Prevents X-rays leaving in other directions	
Oil in outer case	Helps with heat dispersal and insulates the unit electrically	An oil leak is very serious and the tube must not be used
Rotating motor	Rotates the anode, allowing a greater heat loading	Spins at up to 10 000 rpm
High-frequency generator	Provides a near constant high kV and therefore direct current	Older, smaller dental sets may use mains AC (alternative current), which is inefficient at X-ray production
Tube window	The only part of the lead casing that lets out X-rays	Often aluminium, and contributes towards filtration

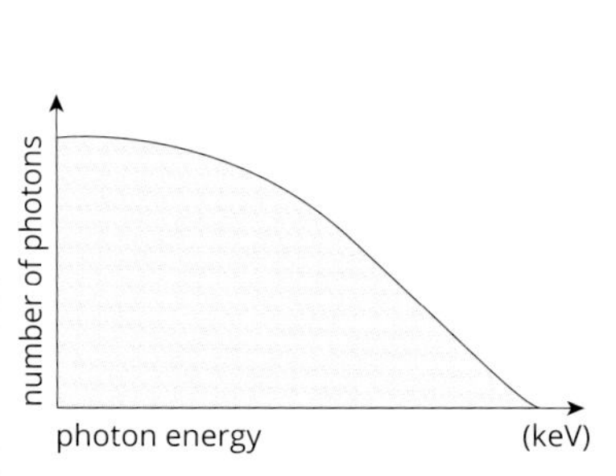

Fig 2-6 Bremsstrahlung spectrum profile.

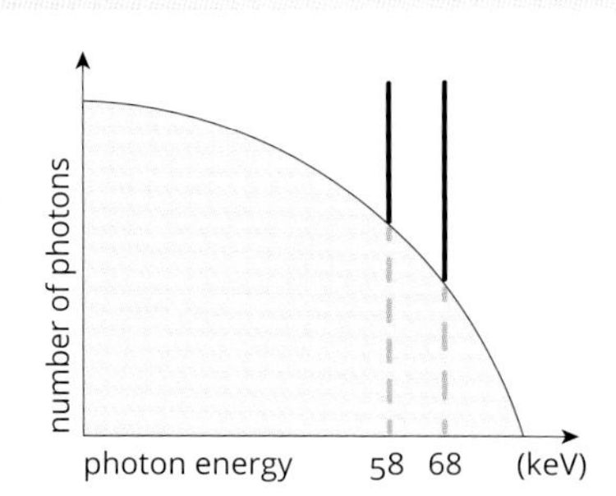

Fig 2-7 Bremsstrahlung plus characteristic radiation.

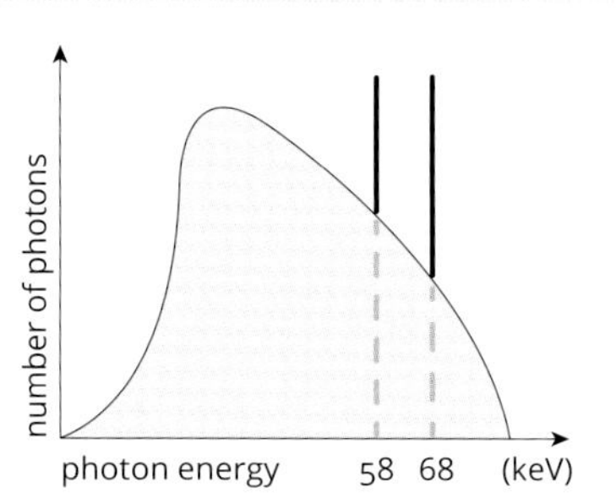

Fig 2-8 Filtered profile; note the lower-energy photons to the left have been removed.

tron released by the cathode that strikes the anode in the X-ray tube. About 99% of energy is converted to heat, so only 1% of energy results in X-ray production. Therefore, X-ray tubes are very inefficient at X-ray production. This large amount of heat energy is the reason for heat removing devices such as the rotating anode (see motor in Fig 2-3) and outer cooling oil.

Spectrum profile

Bremsstrahlung radiation is produced over a wide range of energies up to the maximum tube potential, as depicted in Figure 2-6.

If we use a tube operating at over 70 kV, then we also have characteristic X-rays, which are at specific values (see Fig 2-7).

Filtering

Only the higher-energy photons that have the potential to pass through the patient and record at the receptor are useful for imaging. The lower-energy photons are absorbed by the patient and only contribute to dose. This is discussed again later on. Filtering is the process whereby lower-energy photons are removed. The X-ray tube itself does some filtering by its inherent properties; the rest is added, usually in the form of aluminium. It is normal to have about 2.5 mm aluminium-equivalent filtration.

The spectrum of a tube operating at 120 kV with filtration then looks like Figure 2-8, with the lower-energy photons removed.

Altering the mA or kV

Changing the mA will result in more electrons being released from the cathode and accelerated into the anode; however, the maximum energy of these electrons is still the same. Therefore, an increase in mA causes an increase in the number of X-rays. The same effect is observed if the exposure time is increased (Fig 2-9).

Changing the kV has two effects; firstly, the maximum energy of the electrons increases, so higher-energy X-rays can be produced; secondly the anode pulls more electrons from the filament, so the number of X-rays increases (Fig 2-10).

Summary

- Double mA = double the number of X-rays
- Double time = double the number of X-rays
- Double kV = double the maximum X-ray energy and double the number of X-rays

For this reason, you may need to reduce the mA if you increase the kV.

Interaction with matter

When X-rays make contact with the patient, they can be absorbed, scattered or transmitted.

Absorbed X-rays

All the energy of the X-ray is deposited into the patient and the photon disappears completely. This is called photoelectric absorption. This process occurs when the photon hits a tightly bound inner electron of an atom in the patient. If the photon has more energy than the binding energy of the inner shell electron, the electron can be knocked free and shoots off. This then becomes a photoelectron (an electron with kinetic en-

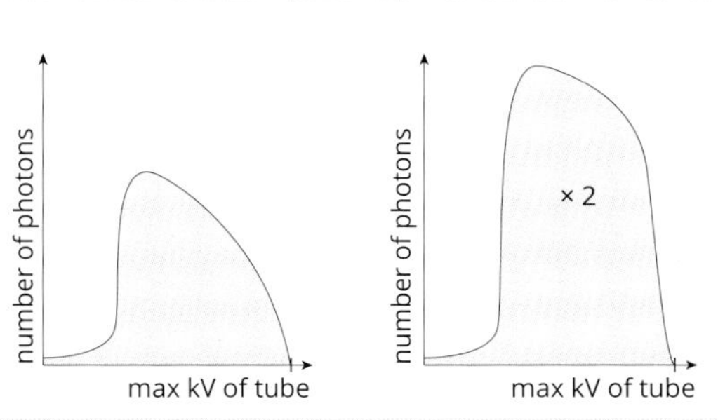

Fig 2-9 Double mA graph.

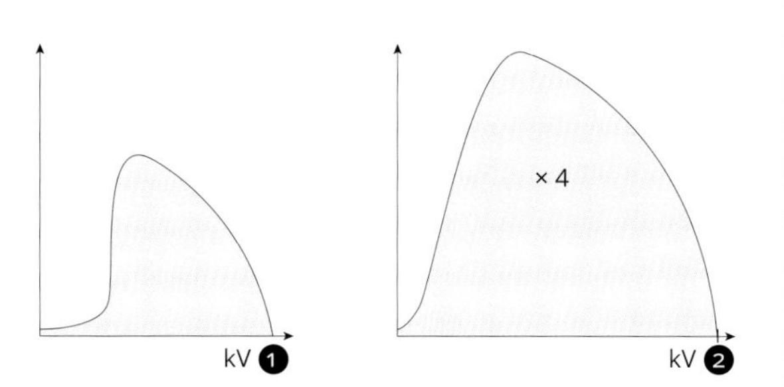

Fig 2-10 Double kV graph.

ergy from the photon), and the photon ceases to exist. An outer shell, electron from that atom will 'jump down' to fill the inner shell, releasing a very small amount of energy (as a low-energy photon), which is deposited in the tissue. The photoelectron will also deposit energy throughout the body tissues.

This interaction does not add to the image directly; however, in the areas where photons are absorbed the most (e.g. bone), there will be a lower signal, which will contribute to the image contrast (Fig 2-11a).

Scattered X-rays

There are two forms of scatter—Compton scattering and Rayleigh scattering. Rayleigh scattering has little or no effect during diagnostic radiography, so we will discuss Compton scattering only.

In this process, consider only the outermost electrons of the atoms in the patient; the ones that are so far from the nucleus that they are very weakly bound. The incoming photon hits one of these loosely bound electrons and gives up some energy to the electron. Thus, the electron heads off in a new direction with the extra energy. The initial X-ray photon is deflected in this collision, depending on the initial energy of the photon and how much energy it gives the electron.

Scatter adds X-ray dose to the patient, as the scattered electron has enough energy to ionise other cells and cause damage. The scattered X-ray photons also degrade the image as they have an altered course (Fig 2-11b).

Transmitted X-rays

The X-ray photons pass straight through the patient and hit the image receptor. These photons contribute directly towards the image (Fig 2-11c).

The chance of each process occurring depends on the energy of the incoming photon, the physical density of the tissue through which the X-ray passes, the atomic number of the tissue, and the electron density of the tissue.

Bone will attenuate X-rays more than soft tissue because it has a higher physical density, a higher average atomic number, and a higher electron density. This means that an incoming X-ray photon is more likely to be scattered in bone than in soft tissue, as there are more electrons to hit. It will also absorb more, as the atomic number of bone is higher, which means there is more likely to be photoelectric absorption (Table 2-2).

Table 2-2 X-ray and its various effects.

Factor	Effect	Notes
X-ray photon energy increases	Less likely to have photoelectric absorption = lower image contrast	Lowers dose, as the photons are more likely to be transmitted
Tissue is higher density	More likely to have Compton scatter	
Tissue has higher average atomic number	More likely to have photoelectric absorption = better contrast	

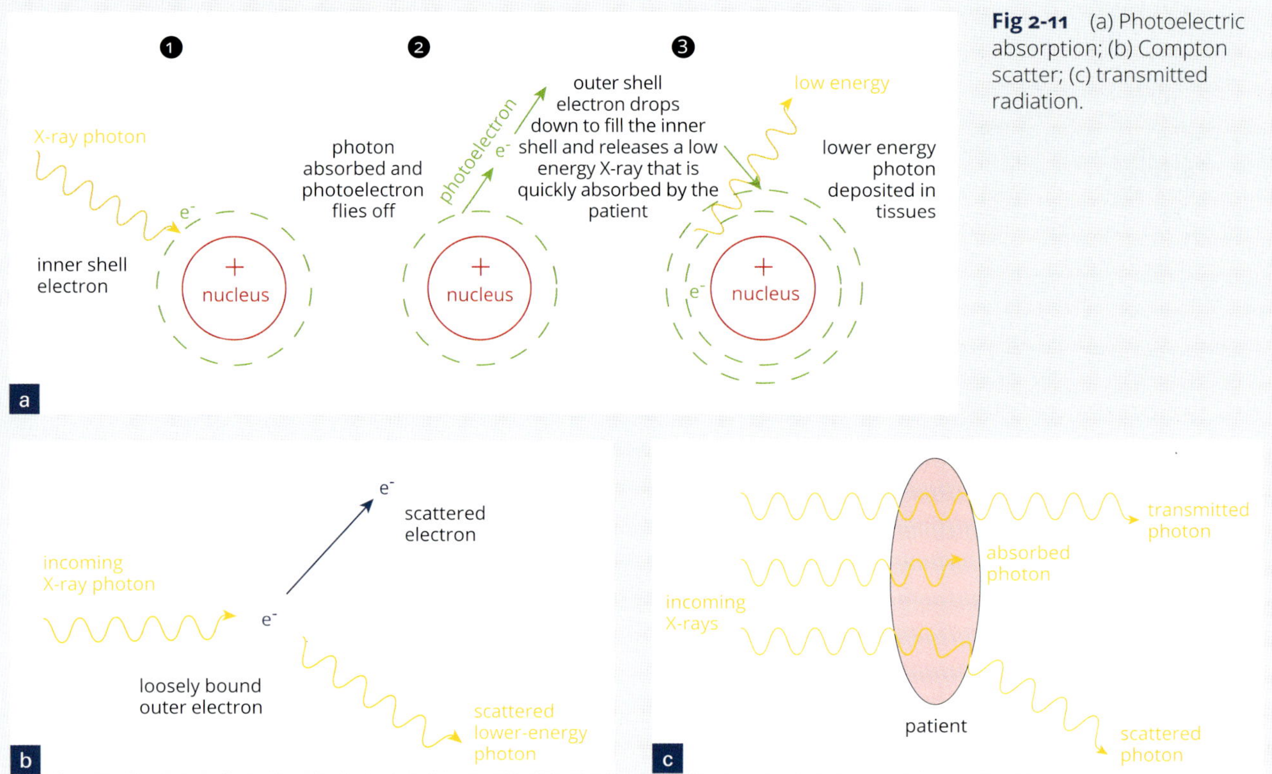

Fig 2-11 (a) Photoelectric absorption; (b) Compton scatter; (c) transmitted radiation.

Further reading

Ionising Radiation Regulations (1999): www.hse.gov.uk/radiation/ionising/legalbase.htm

Nemtoi A, Czink C, Haba D, Gahleitner A. Cone beam CT: a current overview of devices. Dentomaxillofac Radiol 2013;42:20120443.

Chapter 3

Cone Beam Computed Tomography

Simon C Harvey, Shanon Patel

The differences and similarities between multidetector computed tomography and cone beam computed tomography

Multidetector computed tomography

Modern multidetector computed tomography (MDCT) is a feature of the third generation of computed tomography (CT) machines. The description of the first, second, fourth and fifth generation CT machines is beyond the scope of this book, and they are already described in several available texts. The third generation CT machine came into existence around the late 1980s to early 1990s, and has been refined since then. In virtually all applications, the scanner consists of a gantry, which contains the rotating X-ray source and detector array. In the centre of the gantry is a circular aperture, through which the patient lying prone on a bed is advanced. Other than the slow-moving bed on which the patient lies, there are no visible moving parts. The basic layout is shown in Figure 3-1a.

CT in its most basic form uses a fan-shaped beam, takes individual axial slices of the patient, and stitches them together to form the 3D volume. The technique is also called helical scanning, due to the helical (spiral) nature of the rotation of the X-ray tube in relation to the movement of the patient bed (Fig 3-1b).

An advancement of this technique is used in the CT machines found in hospitals today, and is known as MDCT. The multidetector component describes several rows of detectors, which can gather several axial slices during one rotation. To do this, the beam needs a third dimension (Fig 3-2).

MDCT increases the speed of the exam compared to single slice CT; however, there are still groups of axial slices that are stitched together to make up the

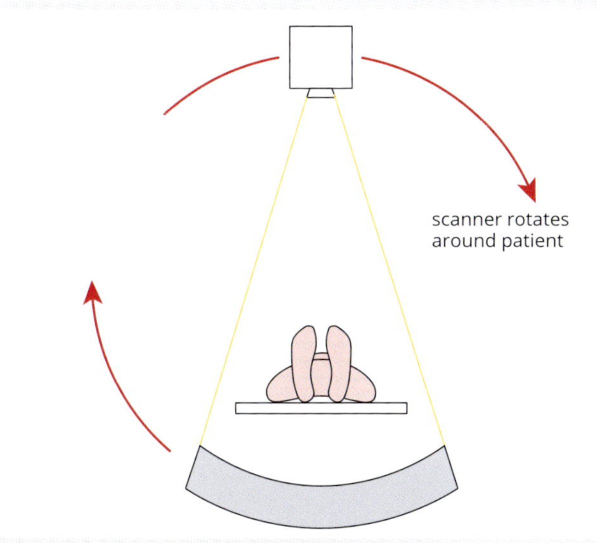

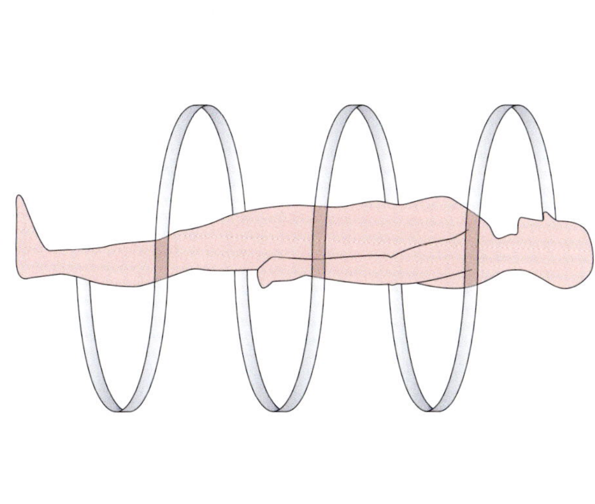

Fig 3-1 (a) CT scanner; note the fan-shaped X-ray beam and the rotating X-ray source. (b) Helical CT scanner.

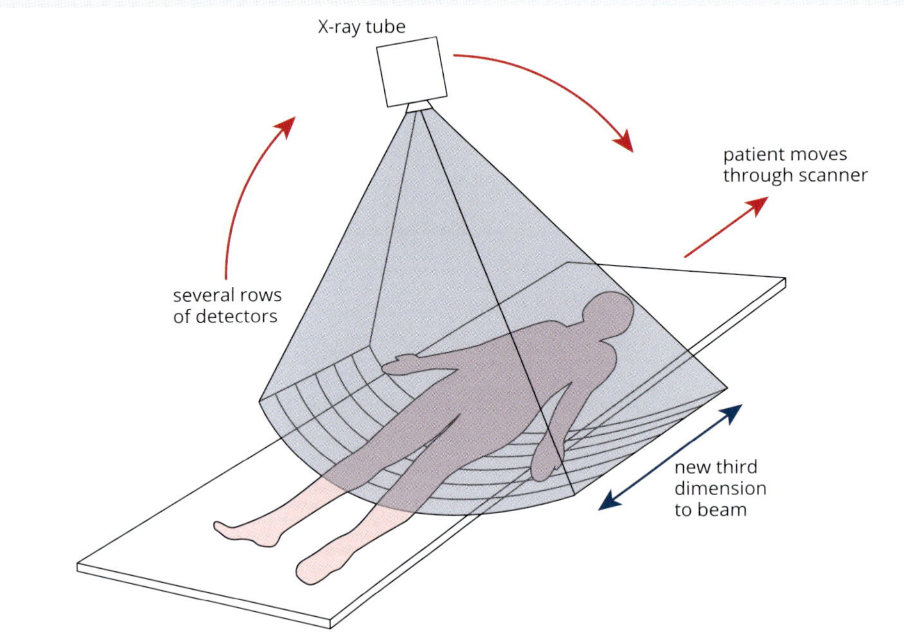

Fig 3-2 Third dimension to beam of MDCT.

3D volume. Thus, the detector and X-ray tube array must make several revolutions around the patient as s/he is advanced through the machine, to image the whole field of view. Modern machines spin at around 2 Hz, that is, two 360-degree revolutions per second. This is considerably faster than any CBCT machine on the market, which may take 20 seconds to complete a single revolution.

Most MDCT machines use reconstruction in much the same way as CBCT; that is, filtered back projection. More advanced systems might also use iterative reconstruction for final image processing, a reconstruction technique which currently is not used in CBCT.

CBCT

CBCT differs from MDCT in three main aspects. Firstly, it uses a cone- or pyramid-shaped beam as opposed to a fan-shaped beam. Secondly, it acquires all the data in a single rotation (or in some cases, even half a rotation—we will look at the 180-degree reduced dose later). Thirdly, a small volume of the patient can be imaged, rather than the entire axial slice of the patient.

This means there must be a detection area large enough to image the entire field of view required, as unlike MDCT the scanner needs to gather all the information in a single rotation. Fortunately, for endodontic use the CBCT scan volume is likely to be small, so machines with small detector plates are suitable. For maxillofacial applications, the detector plates may have to be significantly larger to capture the entire region of interest.

One may notice from the MDCT diagrams that the centre of rotation is in the middle of the patient and the X-ray fan-shaped beam and detectors are large enough to image the whole axial slice. For CBCT, the centre of rotation and volume can be adjusted to image only a small area of the patient—even a volume in the centre of the patient (Fig 3-3).

Most machines available on the market also scan with the patient standing or sitting, rather than lying down. The reason for this is for ease of use, and it allows CBCT machines to have a smaller footprint, similar to that of panoramic X-ray machines, making them relatively easy to accommodate in dental practices and imaging centres (Fig 3-4).

Detector types

There are presently three different types of detector plates in CBCT machines on the market: image intensifier; indirect digital flat panels; and direct digital flat panels.

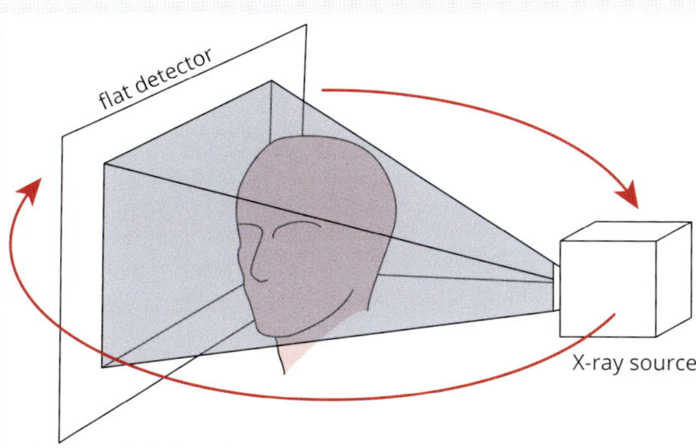

Fig 3-3 CBCT beam, showing cone-shaped X-ray beam against flat detector.

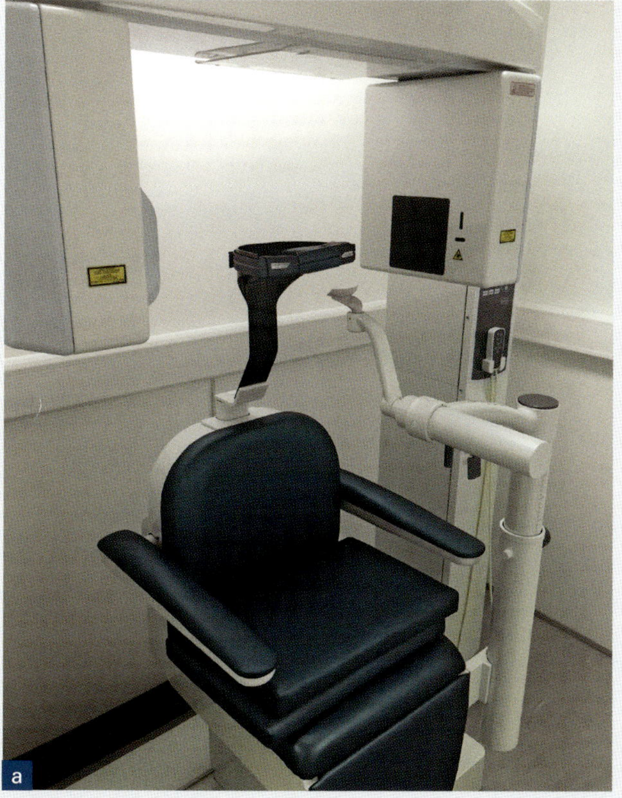

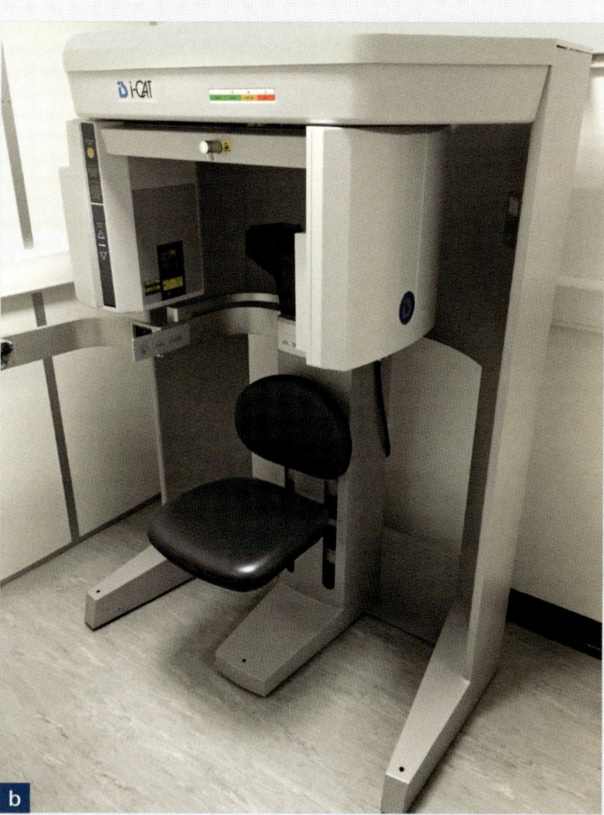

Fig 3-4 (a) Photograph of 3D Accuitomo 180 scanner (J Morita MFG, Osaka, Japan). (b) Photograph of i-CAT scanner (Imaging Sciences International, PA, USA).

Image intensifier

This is an older technology; however, it is still used daily in most general radiology departments in fluoroscopy suites. It works by increasing the size of the signal detected through acceleration of particles and minification of the image.

The first screen (scintillator) is made of caesium iodide and converts the X-rays into visible light via phosphorescence. This light is absorbed by the closely attached second layer (photocathode, which is made of antimony caesium) and is converted into electrons. The electrons are then accelerated along a vacuum tube and focused onto a small output screen, where the now high-energy electrons are converted back into visible light by the output phosphor (zinc cadmium sulphide). The picture can then be recorded by a camera system (most often a charge-coupled device [CCD]). Thus, the acceleration process and the minification

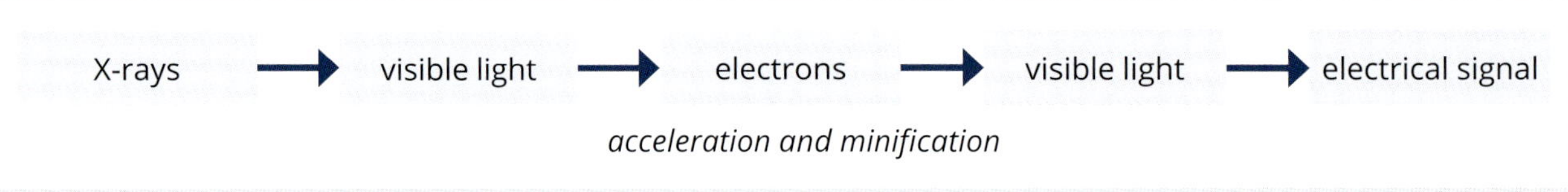

Fig 3-5 Image intensifier conversions.

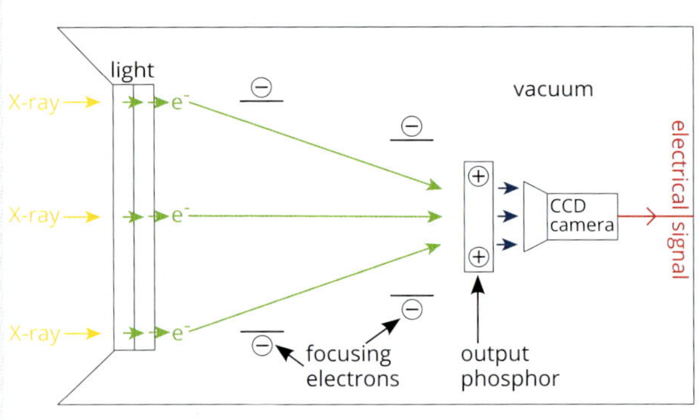

Fig 3-6 Diagram of an image intensifier.

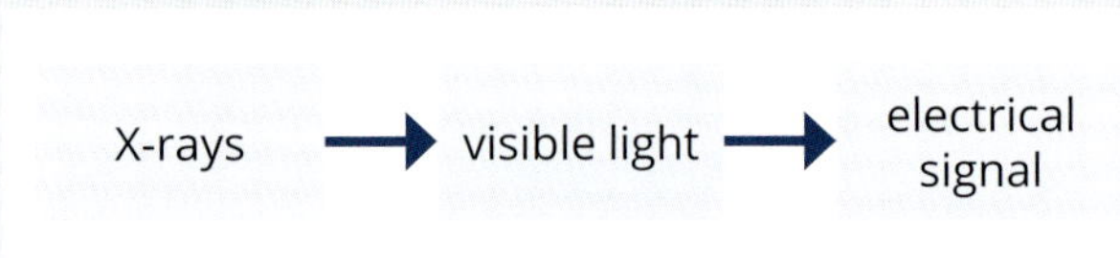

Fig 3-7 Indirect digital flat panel conversions.

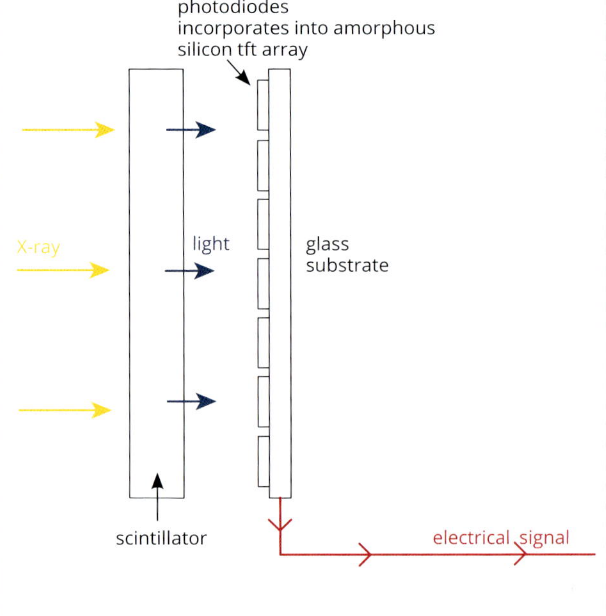

Fig 3-8 Indirect digital flat panel.

of the image means one incoming X-photon detected at the detector plate is converted to enough visible light to be detected by a CCD camera and viewed as an image.

The system involves a number of conversion processes, which are each inefficient—energy and therefore signal is lost at each stage. This means that fluoroscopy at low doses creates a noisy image. At higher dose rates, however, the pictures are very good quality. The nature of the image intensifier means pincushion and vignetting artefacts can occur; fortunately, for small-volume CBCT these artefacts are not a problem (Figs 3-5 and 3-6).

Indirect digital flat panels

While both digital systems involve the conversion of X-ray photons into an electrical signal, the method in which they do so is different. Indirect methods use a phosphor (often doped caesium iodide), which converts the X-rays into light, which is then detected by photodiodes in an amorphous silicon matrix (Figs 3-7 and 3-8).

Direct digital flat panels

Direct digital systems use amorphous selenium to convert the X-rays directly into an electrical signal (Figs 3-9 and 3-10).

Comparing the three detector types

The logical next question is—which detector is best for CBCT? There is no single right answer to this, as each detector in use has its own benefits and disadvantages, as depicted in Table 3-1.

An ideal image detector would:

- be cheap
- be stable
- show no degradation over time
- have a high detector efficiency

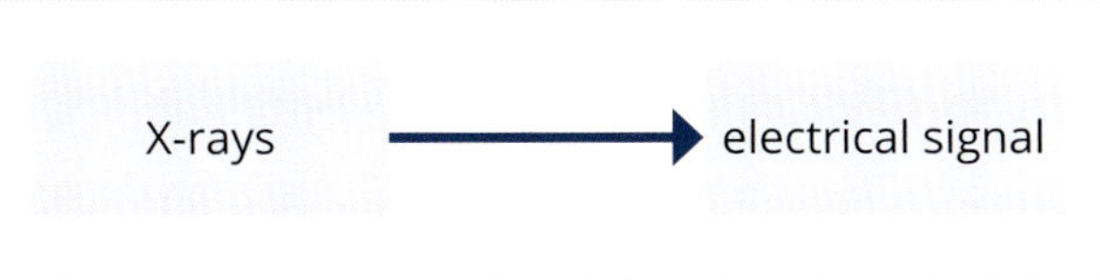

Fig 3-9 Direct flat panel conversions.

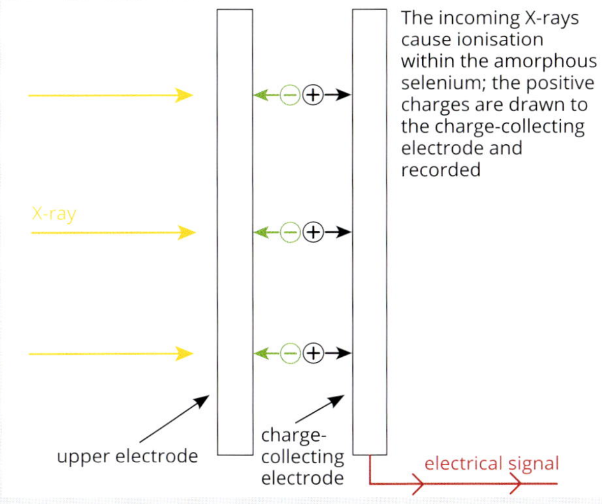

Fig 3-10 Direct flat panel.

Table 3-1 Pros and cons of certain scanner types.

Panel type	Pros	Cons
Image intensifier	Can work at very low doses Stable and hard wearing	Bulky Can produce noisy images at low doses
Indirect digital flat panel	Good value Can be built to cover large areas	The conversion of X-rays to light and then light to electric signal introduces noise
Direct digital flat panel	The highest detective quantum efficiency (DQE)	Expensive Difficult to build large detector areas

- have a large dynamic range
- have a quick recovery following the detection of an X-ray photon.

Detective quantum efficiency

The efficiency of the detector is called the detective quantum efficiency (DQE). This measures how effectively incoming X-ray photons are detected, and how little noise there is. Ideally, all photons would be detected and no noise added—this gives a DQE of 100%. The best direct digital systems have a DQE of around 65%.

Image reconstruction methods

In the related literature, it has been documented that the reconstruction process functions in several different ways. Essentially, the stages are:

1. Data capture at the image receptor.
2. Data filtering to remove very low or very high signals.
3. Image reconstruction—filtered back projection or iteration to produce 3D volume, sometimes called XYZ.
4. Multiplanar reconstruction (MPR) to alter the axis within the data.

Filtered back projection

Filtered back projection (FBP) is the most commonly used method for constructing 3D images from a series of 2D projections (Fig 3-11).

Let us consider the computer reconstructing a 3D volume from a series of 2D projections. The computer 'back projects' the data it received in that projection across the volume; that is, the signal at the image receptor is traced back along the path of the X-ray (Fig 3-11c).

The object's characteristics, however, can still not be recorded unless more projections are taken. Only

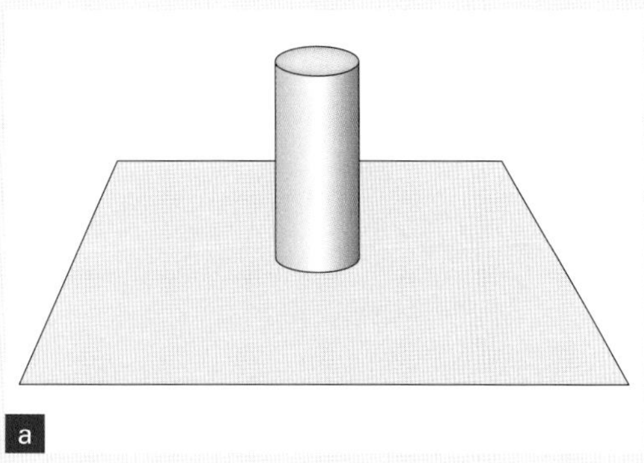

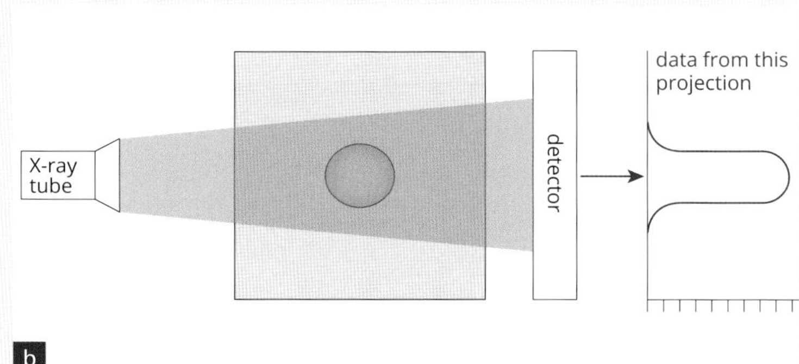

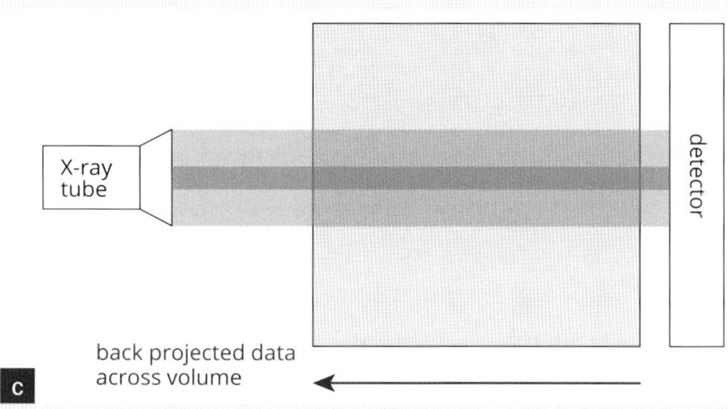

Fig 3-11 Object to be imaged and planned. (a) Object to be imaged. (b) First projection and data from that projection. (c) Single back projection.

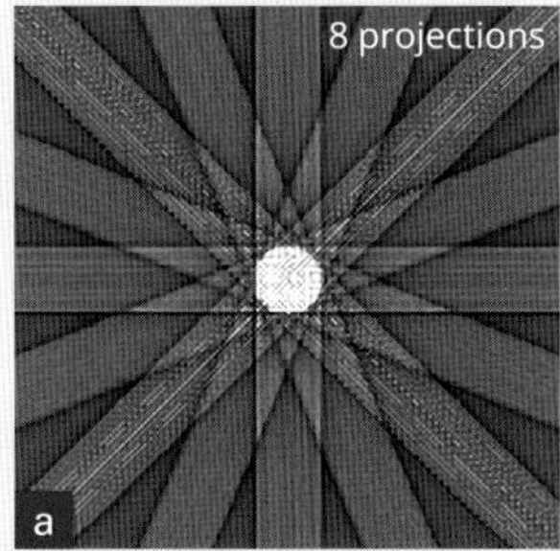

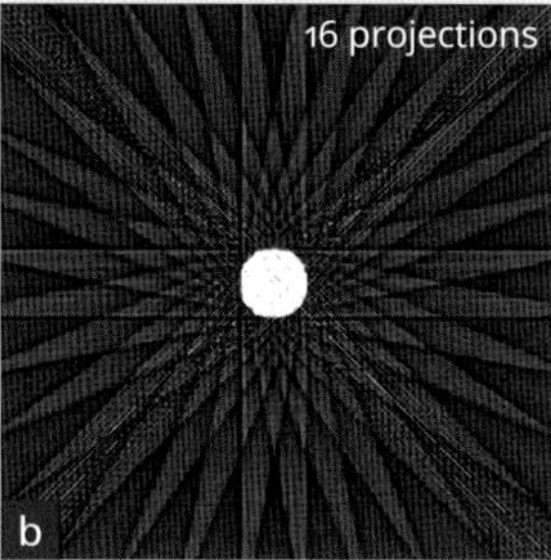

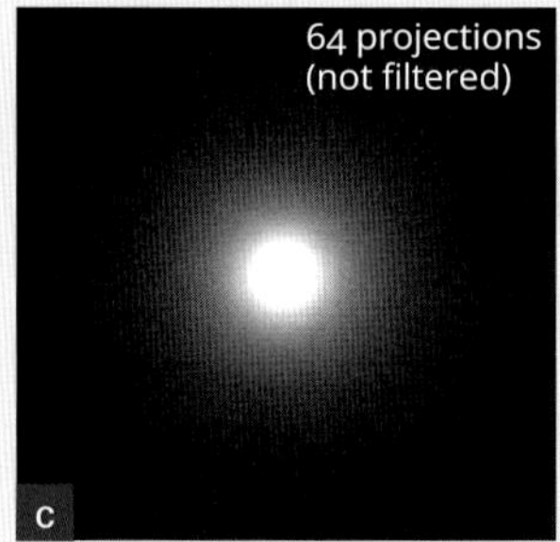

Fig 3-12 Back projections: (a) 8, (b) 16, and (c) 64 incidences.

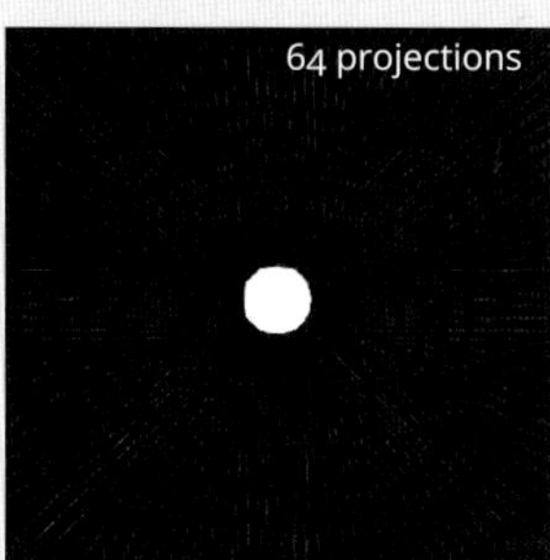

Fig 3-13 Back projections: 64 filtered incidences.

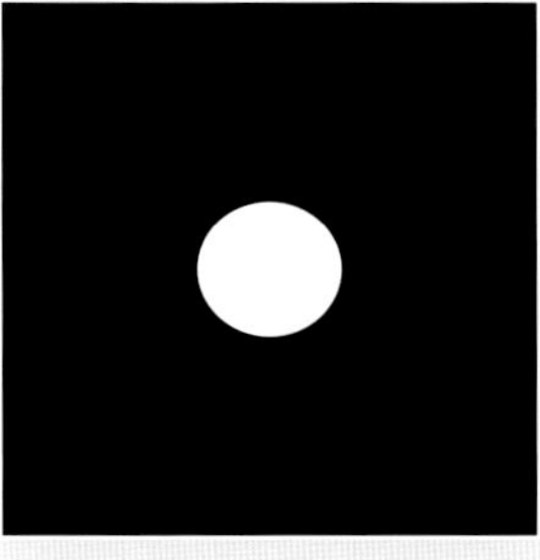

Fig 3-14 Iteration produced a perfect volume of data.

once all this data from different projection angles are back projected can one see roughly what shape the object is (Fig 3-12).

This method, however, is not good enough for medical use, as a star pattern/blurring appears around the object due to the back projected image, which was not there in the original. To remove this star pattern/blurring, filtered back projection is used (Fig 3-13). This creates a nearly completely accurate reconstruction of the original object.

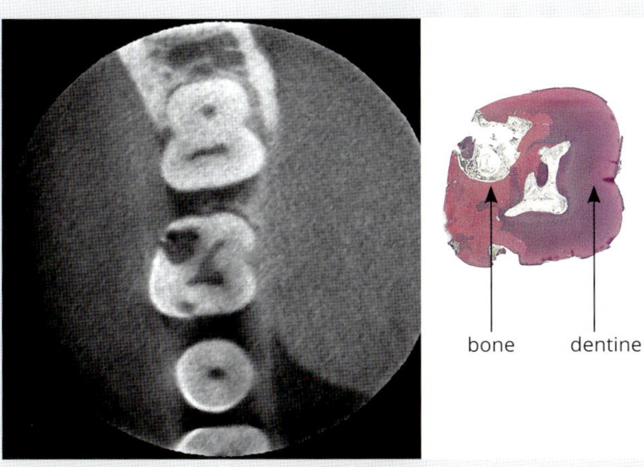

Fig 3-15 Contrast resolution. The replacement reposition in this tooth cannot be differentiated from dentine on the reconstructed CBCT slice due to the poor contrast resolution, but is clear on the histological slice (right).

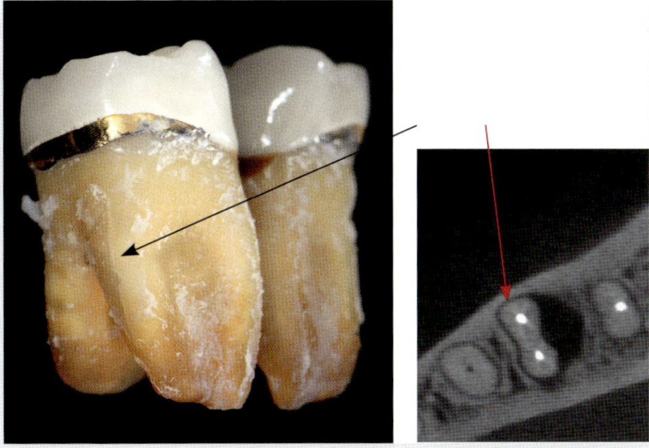

Fig 3-16 The root fracture on the spatial resolution. The mesial root (black arrow) cannot be detected on the same aspect of the reconstructed CBCT slice (red arrow) due to the poor spatial resolution.

Problems with filtered back projection and iteration

FBP is not a true representation of the original object because the filtering is a modification of the actual data received at the detector. The back projection is the reconstruction of the unmodified data, but as we have seen, this leaves a star pattern/blurring, which is not actually present. The filtering process could potentially remove useful data from the scan or add in data that is not actually present.

There is another, more accurate method for forming the 3D image, called iterative reconstruction.

Iteration is the act of repeating a process in order to achieve a certain result. Modern computers are particularly good at iteration as they are able to process thousands of functions every second. Iterative reconstruction works by first having a 'guess' at what the object may look like based on the data received. This guess could be based on FBP. The computer then compares its guess about the object with the actual data received. Any discrepancies can be changed in the new guess about the object, and then this new guess is compared to the original data. Then, any further discrepancies can be changed again and compared, and so forth. In this method one can see how the comparison to the actual data means this is a true image—if left long enough, the computer would eventually iterate enough times to produce a perfect representation of the original object (Fig 3-14).

Iterative reconstruction is more effective the more iterations there are, as the computer has more chance to make alterations in order to achieve the perfect image. This does take more time, however, as the computer completes more and more iteration cycles.

Upgrading the computer software to newer, better FBP algorithms or iterative methods will undoubtedly increase image quality and remove more artefacts.

Image quality

Contrast resolution

Contrast resolution is the ability to distinguish between two objects of different radiodensity. CBCT images are displayed as a greyscale from white through to black, with more radiodense areas appearing whiter and air appearing darker.

CBCT has poor contrast resolution, and therefore is unable to differentiate subtle changes in radiodensity (Fig 3-15).

Spatial resolution

Spatial resolution determines the ability to detect two structures close together as being separate. This is easiest to detect when the contrast is high, e.g. two small radiopaque pulp stones within the radiolucent pulp chamber. Visually, it can be harder to determine closely related structures (Fig 3-16) when the contrast is similar, e.g. incomplete vertical root fractures.

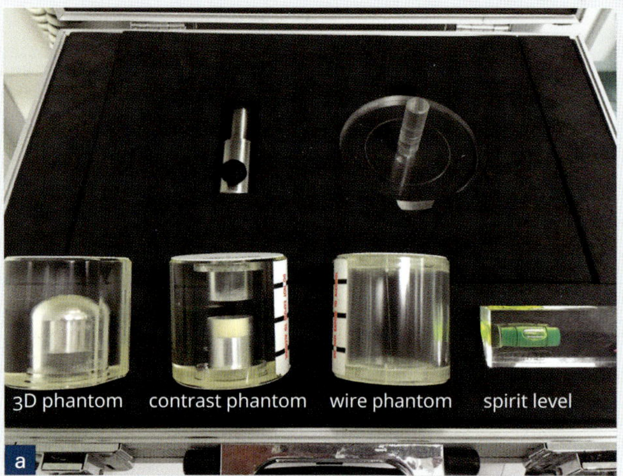

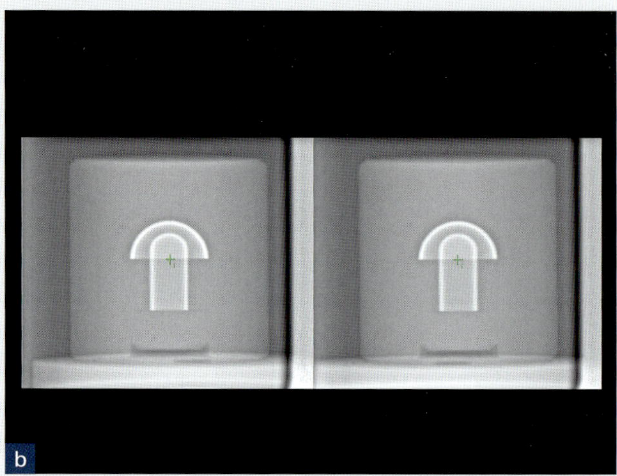

Fig 3-17 (a) Accuitomo test devices. (b) Scout scan the Accuitomo 3D phantom.

Testing contrast and spatial resolution

Contrast can be assessed with a step wedge. This has varying thicknesses of metal, which when scanned should appear distinct.

Spatial resolution can be assessed with a grid test device, which has lead or tungsten septa at known spacing. What is measured is the ability to distinguish separate septa as the gaps between get progressively smaller. This is measured in line pairs per millimetre—the pair being the metal septa and the gap. Manufacturers sometimes quote in terms of pixel size; however, the size of the pixel on the receptor plate is not necessarily the level of detail that can be seen.

The testing of a CBCT scanner (Fig 3-17) is part of the quality assurance (QA), which is a legal requirement under IRR99. Most manufacturers will provide the relevant test objects and instructions for use.

The performance of the viewing monitor is key, as a viewing monitor with fewer greyscale colours will suffer from contrast loss; likewise, a monitor with poorer spatial resolution than the scan will result in loss of fine detail.

A viewing monitor's performance can be assessed using the SMPTE test pattern, which incorporates both contrast resolution and spatial resolution. The authors would highly recommend setting up a radiology viewing area where the lights are dimmed and the monitor is placed at an ideal viewing height. Viewing images in brightly lit surgeries should be avoided (see page 51).

Noise

Noise degrades image quality and manifests as a scattering of grey pixels unrelated to the structure being imaged. Noise comes from three main sources:

Quantum noise

Sometimes also called quantum mottle, this is the random scattering of grey across an image. This is the most significant source of noise in imaging and is essentially due to the uncertainty inherent in the photon-detection process. If the number of photons detected increases, the mottle effect appears reduced.

Although quantum noise cannot be removed as it is inherent to imaging, its effects may be minimised by increasing the mA or kV. However, this increases the radiation dose, and also may have an impact on the diagnostic quality of the resulting image.

Structural noise

Variations in efficiency of the detector plate can cause structural noise, and as it is a physical difference, it will be in the same place in every image. This can be a problem with the less sophisticated (and usually less expensive) CBCT scanners. The more sophisticated (and usually more expensive) CBCT scanners are less likely to suffer from this type of noise due to higher quality control during manufacturing. Use of more complex reconstruction algorithms may also reduce the visibility of structural noise.

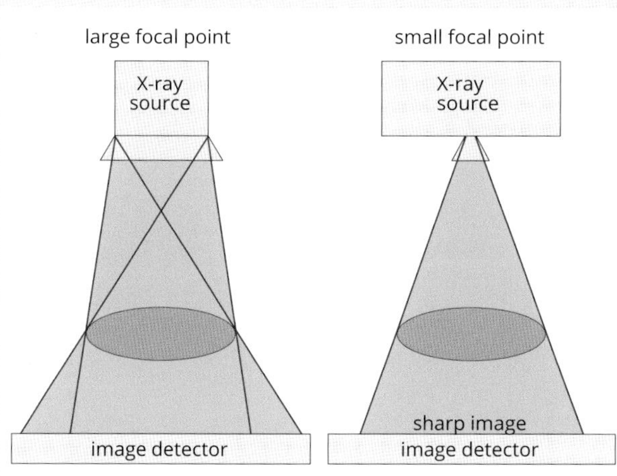

Fig 3-18 Penumbra effect diagram.

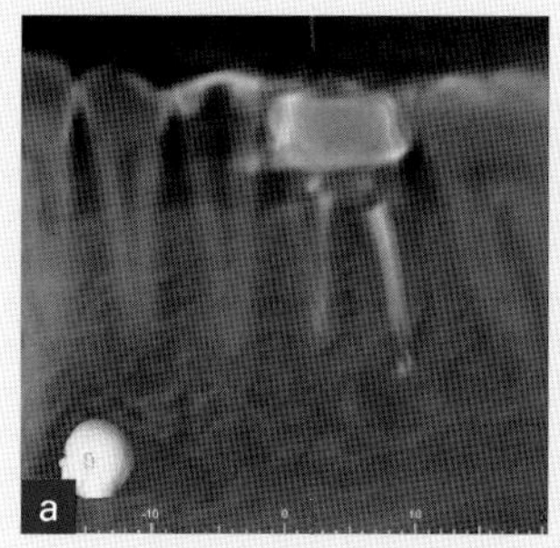
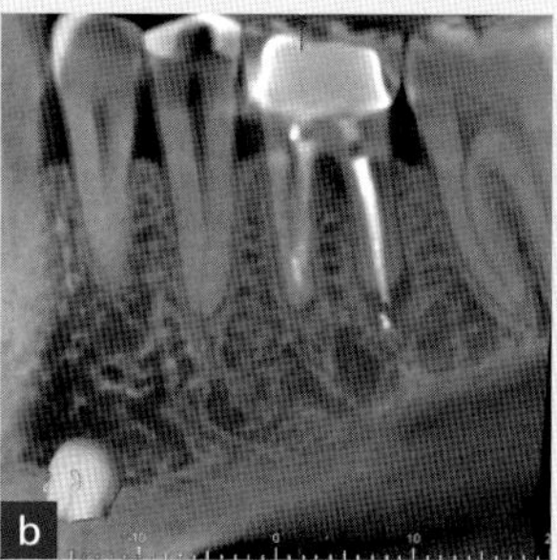

Fig 3-19 (a) Sagittal reconstructed CBCT image reveals movement unsharpness due to the 76-year-old patient moving during the scan. (b) The scan was retaken, resulting in a more diagnostically useful image.

Electronic noise

All computers suffer from electronic noise, which is the alteration of a signal as it passes through circuit boards. Fortunately, electronic noise is normally indistinguishable if a high-specification modern computer is used.

Signal-to-noise ratio

Signal-to-noise ratio (SNR) is a measure for the image quality and the effect of degradation by noise. Signal is useful and forms the image; however, noise is not useful and degrades the image—therefore, the higher the SNR, the better.

Unsharpness

Unsharpness is the loss of sharp edges between boundaries, which leads to a loss of spatial resolution. There are two main types of unsharpness seen in CBCT:

Geometrical unsharpness

This depends on the location of the imaging components—namely, the X-ray tube (specifically, the focus), the patient, and the receptor. Figure 3-18 demonstrates the effect of changing these parameters.

The geometrical unsharpness is reduced when the focal spot is small, the receptor is far from the source, and the receptor is close to the patient.

Movement unsharpness

This represents problems in CBCT, as the machine scan times are relatively long. Scan times vary from 5 to 40 seconds. Immobilisation devices should be used and clear instructions given to the patient. For paediatric patients or those who cannot stay still, the shortest possible scan time may be needed. Short scan times are usually associated with a higher mA.

If movement does occur early on in the scan, the operator may decide to terminate the exposure. If a movement artefact is only found after the scan is finished, then some software allow 180-degree reconstruction, which uses only the data from when the patient was still and discards the data from when the patient moved. This removes the problem of the movement artefact, but due to fewer X-rays being used to make the image, noise is more apparent.

It should be noted that scan time and acquisition time are not synonymous. The scan time is the total time it takes for the exposure to start and complete; the acquisition time is the total time taken when the machine is producing X-rays and receiving data at the receptor—many machines emit a pulsed X-ray beam as they pass around the patient as a dose-reduction feature (more on this later). Because of this, the acquisition time will be much shorter than the scan time. However, any movement during the scan time will cause movement unsharpness (Fig 3-19). Be sure to check with the manufacturer, as both these details are important—a shorter scan time reduces movement unsharpness, while a shorter acquisition time reduces dose.

Ideal machine characteristics

- Good value and easy to use
- Stable footprint
- Low dose
- Good software
- Adjustable field of view—reduces scatter and dose
- Adjustable exposure parameters—reduces scatter and dose
- Quick scanning—reduces movement artefact
- Good contrast and spatial resolution
- Small X-ray tube target—reduces penumbra/ geometric unsharpness
- Good detection efficiency (see Comparing the three detector types)
- Reliable
- Easily serviceable
- Easily upgradable
- Fully integrable into practice/hospital infrastructure
- DICOM compliant

Further reading

American Academy of Oral and Maxillofacial Radiology. Clinical recommendations regarding use of cone beam computed tomography in orthodontics. Oral Surg Oral Med Oral Pathol Oral Radiol 2013;116:238–257.

American Association of Physicists in Medicine (AAPM): Task Group 18. Assessment of display performance for medical imaging systems. [Updated 2006 Jan 10; cited 2006 Sept 29]. Available at: http://deckard.mc.duke.edu/~samei/tg18

Araki K, Fujikura M, Sano T. Effect of display monitor devices in intra-oral radiographic caries diagnosis; Clin Oral Investig 2015; DOI 10.1007/s00784-015-1401-z.

Brown J, Jacobs R, Levring Jäghagen E, et al. Basic training requirements for the use of dental CBCT by dentists: a position paper prepared by the European Academy of DentoMaxilloFacial Radiology. Dentomaxillofac Radiol 2014;43:20130291.

Guidelines on Patient Dose to Promote the Optimisation of Protection for Diagnostic Medical Exposures. NRPB, 1999.

Guidance on the Safe Use of Dental Cone Beam CT (CT) Equipment. Prepared by the HPA working party on Dental Cone Beam CT Equipment (HPA-CRCE-010), published 2010.

Hellén-Halme K, Petersson A, Warfvinge G, Nilsson M. Effect of ambient light and monitor brightness and contrast settings on the detection of approximal caries in digital radiographs: an in vitro study. Dentomaxillofac Radiol 2008;37:380–384.

IEC Annual Report, 2008. Available at: http://www.iec.ch/about/annual_report/pdf/perf2008.pdf

Ionising Radiation Regulations (1999). Available at: www.hse.gov.uk/radiation/ionising/legalbase.htm

Ionising Radiation (Medical Exposure) Regulations 2000 (IRMER). Available at: https://www.gov.uk/government/publications/the-ionising-radiation-medical-exposure-regulations-2000

Loubele M, Bogaerts R, Van Dijck E, et al. Comparison between effective radiation dose of CBCT and MSCT scanners for dentomaxillofacial applications. Eur J Radiol 2009;71:461–468.

Ludlow JB, Abreu M Jr. Performance of film, desktop monitor and laptop displays in caries detection. Dentomaxillofac Radiol 1999;28:26–30.

National Council on Radiation Protection and Measurements. Report No. 160. Ionising Radiation Exposure of the Population of the United States (2009).

Nemtoi A, Czink C, Haba D, Gahleitner A. Cone beam CT: a current overview of devices. Dentomaxillofac Radiol 2013;42:20120443.

NRPB guidance. Available at: https://www.gov.uk/government/uploads/system/uploads/attachment_data/file/337178/misc_pub_DentalGuidanceNotes.pdf

Patel S, Durack C, Abella F, et al. European Society of Endodontology position statement: the use of CBCT in endodontics. Int Endod J 2014;47:502–504.

SEDENTEXCT. Radiation Protection No 172. Cone beam CT for dental and maxillofacial radiology (Evidence based guidelines).

Shulze R, Heil U, Gross D, et al. Artefacts in CBCT: a review. Dentomaxillofac Radiol 201;40:265–273.

The 2007 Recommendations of the International Commission on Radiological Protection, IRCP Publication 103.

The Royal College of Radiologists, IT guidance documents. Picture archiving and communications systems (PACS) and guidelines on diagnostic display devices.

Chapter 4

Using CBCT: Dose, Risks and Artefacts

Simon C Harvey, Shanon Patel

Introduction

Cone beam computed tomography (CBCT) offers, among many advantages, a lower dose in comparison to other three-dimensional (3D) radiographic imaging techniques. Whatever the dose, however, it is still ionising radiation and, as such, should follow the principles of:

- justification
- optimisation
- limitation.

There is no doubt that the use of CBCT in dentistry is increasing, and therefore the population dose is growing. Any form of computed tomography (CT) is a higher-dose technique compared to plain film, so extra care must be taken to ensure that doses are as low as reasonably practicable (ALARP). This chapter covers the biological aspects of ionising radiation, dose reduction measures and artefacts.

Dose and risk

Ionising biological tissue

If the electromagnetic radiation has enough energy it can damage biological tissue. From Chapter 2, we know that X-rays have this potential because they are high energy. For damage to occur, however, the X-ray must be absorbed by the patient and therefore energy transferred to the biological tissue—if it is transmitted, then there is no energy deposited in the tissue.

Ionisation of the molecules inside the body eventually leads to cellular damage. The ionisation can occur in two ways—direct ionisation of a molecule or indirect ionisation through the creation of free radicals.

Indirect cell damage via ionisation of water

H2O + radiation → H2O+ + e-

H2O (decomposes) → H+ + OH

OH + DNA/enzyme → damaged DNA/enzyme

Direct cell damage

Molecules within cells + radiation → damaged molecules

It is the indirect damage that happens most frequently, because the human body is 70% water (Fig 4-1). The ionised water molecule quickly breaks down into free radicals (hydroxyl [OH] is particularly reactive), which can then damage important molecules—those most vulnerable are enzymes and DNA.

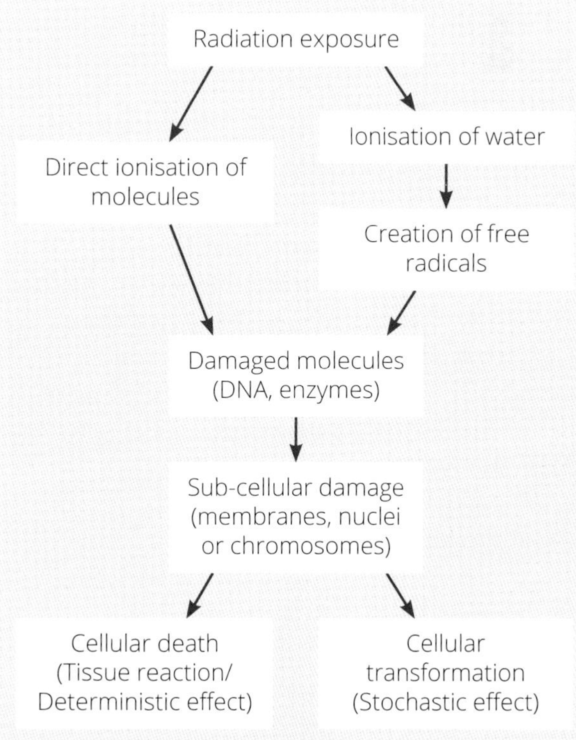

Fig 4-1 Biological radiation damage.

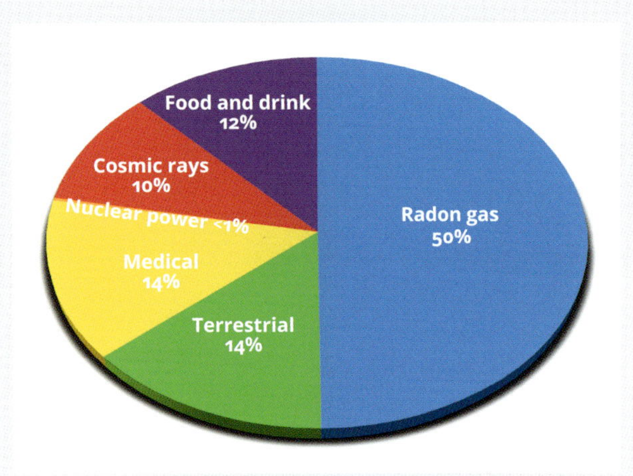

Fig 4-2 UK background radiation dose average per capita.

The damage can result in two possibilities—cellular death or transformation (potentially into malignancy). Fortunately, the cellular transformations can be repaired if the body has time.

Stochastic risk

This is the only important risk when discussing radiation in dental radiography. Stochastic comes from the Greek *stokhastikos* meaning 'to aim at' or 'guess'. Each X-ray photon has a chance of inducing a malignancy in the patient by the mechanisms we have explored earlier. Increasing the number of photons does not make a cancer induction certain—it may increase the chance, but there is no certainty. Conversely, because each individual photon has the chance of producing malignant change there is no safe dose, no matter how small. Thus, we describe the stochastic effects as occurring by chance; however, the more radiation the patient is exposed to, the greater the chance. There is neither a safe limit where one can guarantee no malignancies, nor an upper limit where one can guarantee malignancy.

Measuring dose

Dose is described in three ways, which will be discussed individually:

1. *Absorbed dose.* This is a measure of how much energy the radiation imparts into a given unit mass. It is measured in J/kg, also known as Gray (Gy). This is the most basic form of radiation dose measurement.
2. *Equivalent dose.* This takes into account the ionising power and linear energy transfer of different types of radiation and gives each a weighting factor. For diagnostic radiology and CBCT, the radiation is always X-rays, which have a weighting of 1. Equivalent dose is measured in Sieverts (Sv) and in diagnostic radiology (uses X-rays only): 1 Gy = 1 Sv.
3. *Effective dose.* This final step to measure dose takes into account the relative radiosensitivity of tissues in the body. An organ or tissue is given a weighting factor, which is multiplied by the equivalent dose. The effective dose should be thought of as a method to estimate stochastic (cancer) risk to the patient. It also uses the unit Sieverts (Sv). It should be noted that effective dose cannot be measured directly—it is a mathematical calculation from measurable absorbed dose and an estimation of which tissues are irradiated.

UK background dose

The average per capita background radiation dose in the UK is approximately 2.7 microsieverts (mSv) per year. Background dose can be divided into natural background dose and total background dose. Natural background radiation is estimated at 2.2 mSv and predominately comes from radioactive radon gas, although significant contributions come from foodstuffs, cosmic radiation, and terrestrial radiation. Medical and dental radiation dose is estimated at 0.5 mSv—however, as discussed, this figure will undoubtedly be rising.

The figure is also an average of everyone in the UK and of all medical exams conducted. There will therefore be a fairly large difference in annual total background radiation dose between a person who has had no radiographic exams living in the Norfolk Broads, and a person who has had several CT scans living in an area with a larger natural background dose, such as Cornwall (Fig 4-2).

Age and risk

Younger people are more at risk (i.e. more radiosensitive) to the effects of X-ray radiation than those who are older (Table 4-1). This is due to younger people having higher cellular turnover and a longer amount of time in which to develop a malignancy. This is a reason to particularly consider non-ionising radiation or low dose X-ray radiation techniques for young patients.

Table 4-1 Dose, risk and age.

Age	Risk multiplication
0–15	× 3
16–29	× 1.5
30–50	× 1
50+	× 0.3

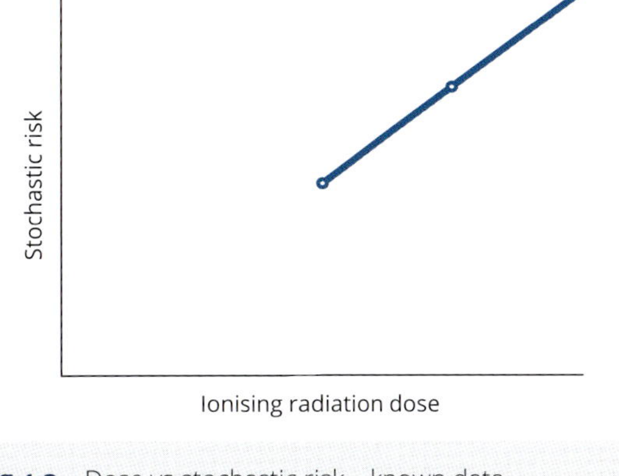

Fig 4-3 Dose vs stochastic risk—known data.

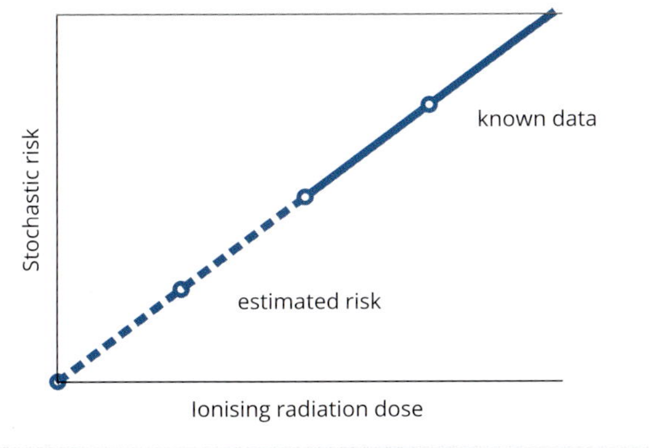

Fig 4-4 Dose vs stochastic risk—linear no threshold model.

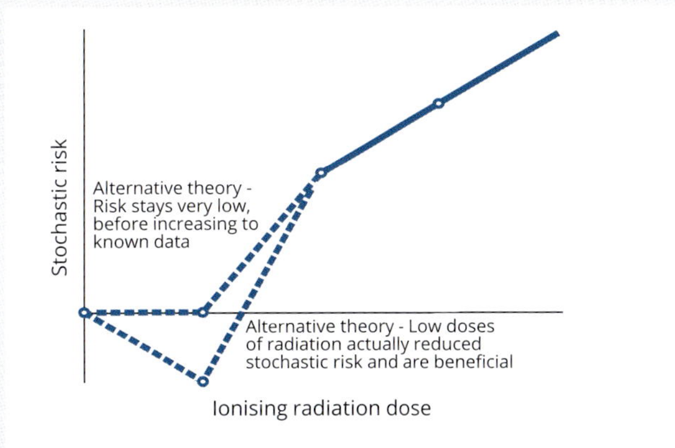

Fig 4-5 Dose vs stochastic risk—alternative theories.

Estimating risk

The risk of cancer induction from having a radiographic exam cannot be accurately determined. It is estimated from the known exposures of victims of atomic bombs, nuclear power plant explosions, and other such accidents.

As such, these doses were quite high and generally whole body doses (Fig 4-3); however, there is a clear pattern when all the data is plotted on a graph that demonstrates a linear relationship between higher doses and fatal cancer induction.

There is some controversy about the relationship when the doses are lower, such as in diagnostic radiology. The likely answer is that the linear relationship continues to zero, and this is the model used when risk is estimated (Fig 4-4).

Interestingly, one of the other schools of thought is that a small amount of radiation could be actually beneficial and that the risk declines at first, before increasing. Alternatively, the risk may be very low at low doses before increasing up towards the known data at higher doses (Fig 4-5).

These alternative theories are backed up when we look at the different natural background doses that people receive in different areas of the UK, and the fact that the cancer incidence is no higher in the areas with significantly higher natural background doses.

This having been said, it is widely accepted by physicists and radiologists that the risk of fatal cancer induction is approximately 1:20 000 per mSv, and the number of fatal cancers attributed to medical and dental exposures in the UK is estimated at 700 per annum (of which 10 are dental radiographic exposures).

To most patients, the units Gray and Sievert discussed in the preceding section are of little use when describing risk. Therefore, Table 4-2 includes the doses of various dental radiological exams, some technical data, and the 'real world' equivalents.

It is a great credit to the dental profession that the doses are very low for dental radiographic exams. It

Table 4-2 Doses of radiographic exams, data, and 'real world' equivalents (DPT = dental panoramic tomography).

Radiographic exam	Effective dose μSv	Equivalent to a single periapical exam	Equivalent hours of aeroplane travel	Equivalent number of days background radiation	Estimated risk of fatal malignancy to child <16	Estimated risk of fatal malignancy to adult 18–65
Periapical radiograph	1	1	0.25	0.2	2 000 000	4 000 000
Eating a banana	0.1	1/10th	0.025	0.0	n/a	n/a
Dentition-only DPT	10	10	2.5	1.8	<1 000 000	<2 000 000
Full DPT	22	22	5.5	4.0	1 000 000	2 000 000
Average small-volume CBCT	50	50	12.5	9.1	250 000	500 000
CT head	2000	2000	500	365.0	5000	10 000
Yearly UK average background radiation	2700	540	675	365	n/a	n/a

Notes
- Periapical radiograph taken with rectangular collimation, 70kV, 200 mm fsd and fast film/detector plate (source: Guidelines on Radiological Standards for Primary Dental Care, 1994).
- Annual natural background estimated at 2700 μSv.
- Aeroplane travel estimated to give 4 μSv per hour.
- Risk of malignancy is calculated from National Radiological Protection Board (NRPB) booklet Guidelines on patient dose to promote the optimisation of protection for diagnostic medical exposures, 1999.
- Banana equivalent dose widely regarded as 0.1 μSv. Radioactivity comes from small amounts of radioactive potassium (^{40} K) in the potassium-rich banana.

is important to prolong this trend of maintaining low doses when using higher radiation dose techniques such as CBCT.

Dose-reducing measures

Justification

Before exposing a patient to CBCT, one should always ask—is this scan justified? Have I checked the relevant guidelines and selection criteria? Will this scan add important information to the clinical picture? Could the information be gained by other low-dose techniques or non-ionising imaging? If you accept referrals from other healthcare professionals, bear in mind that you as the operator of the CBCT machine are responsible for correct justification of the scan.

For the full recommended uses of CBCT you are recommend to refer to the SEDENTEXCT guidelines, which are authorised by the European Union and endorsed by the British Society of Dental and Maxillofacial Radiology, and represent the most complete guidelines on the use of CBCT. The European Society of Endodontology has also provided guidance on the use of CBCT in endodontics (European Society of Endodontology, 2014). Both these guidance documents are available to download for free on the internet.

Ensure patient is set up correctly

Perhaps the most obvious dose-saving technique is the reduction (or elimination) of incorrect scans. This can be achieved by setting up the scanner and associated hardware and software correctly, ensuring that the manufacturers' positioning instructions and patient immobilisation measures are used (Fig 4-6).

Raise kV and reduce mA

Raising the kV results in a reduction in dose by the methods explained in Table 4-3.

Dose-reduction feature

Some scanners incorporate a dose reduction (DR) program. This can be useful in cases where high-definition detail is not required. It should be noted that actual readings for DR programs are measured during quality assurance (QA) to ensure the dose reduction

Table 4-3 The effects of raising kV.

Increasing kV	Knock-on effect
Decreased photoelectric absorption—photoelectric absorption is inversely proportional to photon energy cube	Reduced contrast
Higher kV means the beam is more penetrating, so more of it passes through the patient and hits the detector	Reduces patient dose—with higher kV, the mA can be reduced in order to keep the same detector dose

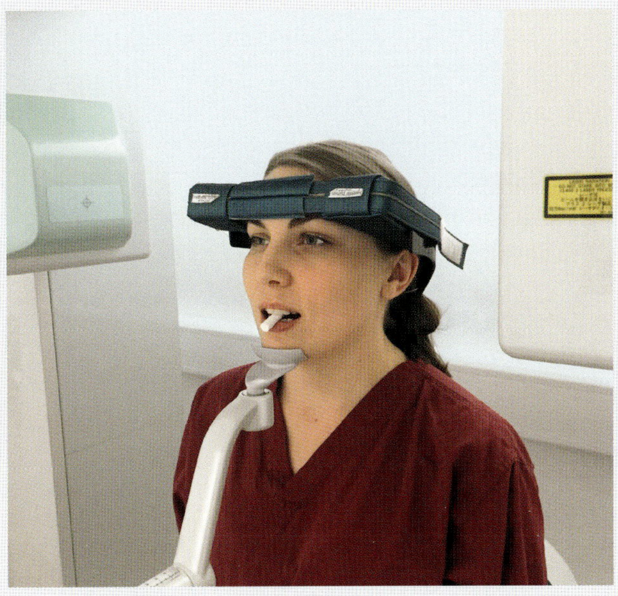

Fig 4-6 Immobilisation devices in use (note head support, chin rest, and that the teeth are apart).

program does that. The exact method by which each machine achieves its DR function is not always known, as manufacturers are often not forthcoming. Medical physics experts and the users of the specific machine, however, should have thorough knowledge of how and when to use this feature.

Larger voxels

This is often adjustable, but may or may not be present on every machine. Larger voxels should give reduced dose at the expense of lower spatial resolution. The authors know of one machine where the increase in voxel size is reconstructive only, and the scanner still gives the same tube output; thus, there is no benefit to the patient and the images are lower resolution. The doses should be assessed during QA.

Low mA

This may be achieved by raising the kV (see earlier in this chapter). Protocols for scans may give guidelines for mA figures. Children and thin or frail people should have reduced mA.

Correct filtering

Machines should have the statutory minimum amount of beam filtering (2.5 mm aluminium equivalent) but may have adjustable filtration. Filtering aims to remove the lower-energy X-ray photons from the beam—these photons are always absorbed by the patient, so contribute nothing to the image but increase the patient dose. Filtering effectively removes the lower-energy photons, leaving only the high-energy ones; this increases transmission and therefore results in a lower image contrast.

mA modulation

By altering the mA during a scan, the dose can be reduced. If the tissue is less attenuating, the machine automatically reduces the mA; when a thicker part of the patient is scanned, the machine can increase the mA back to the maximum value.

Physical collimation

Physical collimation will reduce the beam size and therefore reduce the dose. It also has the added effect of reducing scatter and therefore improving the image. Machines that use a fixed beam size and electronic collimation will not reduce the dose to the patient. This will be highlighted in QA.

180-degree views

If the CBCT scanner can reconstruct from 180-degree views, it can reduce the radiation dose dramatically. It would seem logical that a 180-degree view is half the dose of a 360-degree one—however, due to scanner geometry and reconstruction techniques, this is not always the case. 180-degree reconstructed images are significantly noisier than 360-degree reconstructions—this is partly due to the smaller overall number of photons recorded and thus worse signal-to-noise ratio (SNR), and partly due to the reconstruction process.

Pulsed beam

This feature is available on some machines and reduces the acquisition time by turning off the beam during the rotation between the individual projections. The scan time, however, will remain the same.

Average dose for CBCT scanners

For small-volume CBCT, the dose varies between scanners. There may be discrepancy between the manufacturer-quoted figures and those from independent sources. Some scanners are able to achieve around 20 to 40 μSv for a small-volume CBCT scan with acceptable contrast and spatial resolution for use in endodontics. The relative risk and comparison to plain film methods is found in the earlier section, 'Estimating risk'.

The dose will vary depending on the specific ares of the jaws being scanned, and therefore adjacent radiosensitive anatomy being irradiated.

The radiation doses are specific to each scanner, and there can be up to a 16-fold difference in radiation dose between different CBCT scanners (Pauwels et al, 2012).

Artefacts in CBCT

An artefact is a visible error in the volume data, which is not present in the visualised object. Every CBCT scan will have some degree of volume data error but they are not always visible. These artefacts include but are not limited to:

- beam geometry
- noise (quantum, structural and electronic)
- hardware inconsistencies
- reconstruction algorithms.

The following section describes what artefacts may look like, what they are called, how they come about, and how they can be minimised or eliminated.

Extinction artefacts

Also known as zero artefacts, these occur when a structure blocks all of the X-ray photons and the area of the detector records a zero reading for the projection. A similar problem is seen in underexposing computed radiography plates when too low an exposure is used. Common structures that cause this are gold crowns and titanium implants, which are sufficiently attenuating. Increasing the kV can eliminate this—which will make the X-ray photons more penetrating, and thus more likely to pass through the material and record on the dose receptor.

Beam-hardening artefacts

As described in Chapter 2, the X-ray beam is polychromatic—it is made up of X-ray photons of varying energy. The lower-energy photons will be stopped more easily, leaving only higher-energy photons. This is the principle behind filtering the beam; the aluminium-added filtration removes the lower-energy photons (which would only contribute to dose and not the image), leaving only the mid- to higher-energy photons. When a particular projection line is effectively heavily filtered by, for example, dental amalgam, the average energy in that particular line is very high; when this is back projected, a streak appears. Beam-hardening artefacts are very common due to the radiopaque nature of dental restorations (Fig 4-7). They can be reduced in the scan by trying to exclude beam-hardening areas from the scan volume. When imaging the mandible, try to miss the maxilla restorations, and ensure that the occlusal plane is parallel to the floor, as this will result in all the streaks lying in the same plane, so as not to degrade the whole scan.

Partial volume effect

If there is a high-contrast object that is smaller than the size of the pixels in the detector, the small object will effectively fill the pixel and appear larger than it actually is. A good example of this would be a small fragment of gutta-percha, which if smaller than the voxel size of the scan will appear larger than it actually is. Conversely, if there is a low-contrast object smaller than the detector pixel size, then it may not be seen at all, as the attenuation is averaged over a large area and thus contrast is reduced (Fig 4-8).

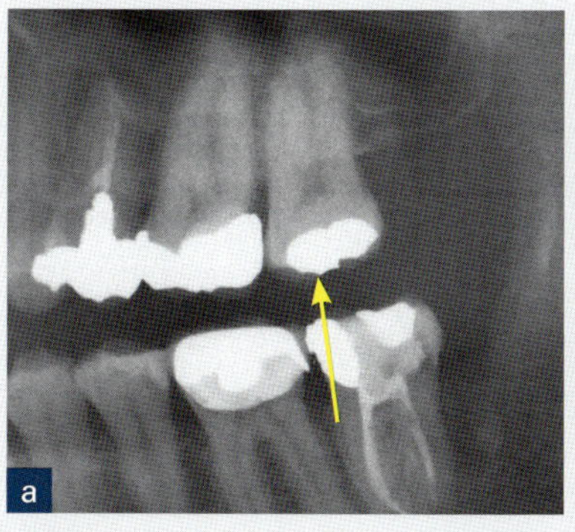

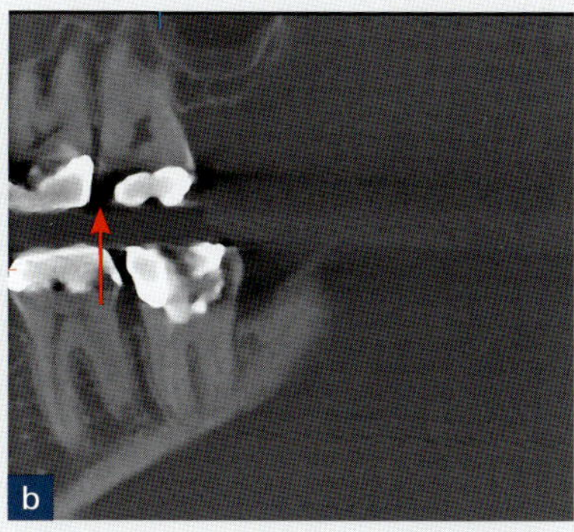

Fig 4-7 (a) Periapical radiograph, and (b) sagittal CBCT image of the same anatomy reveals an extensive beam-hardening artefact, which makes evaluating the metal margin with CBCT difficult. Note on the CBCT scan that the mesial wall of UR7 appears to be absent, possibly carious (red arrow); however, periapical radiograph (yellow arrow) reveals healthy tooth structure.

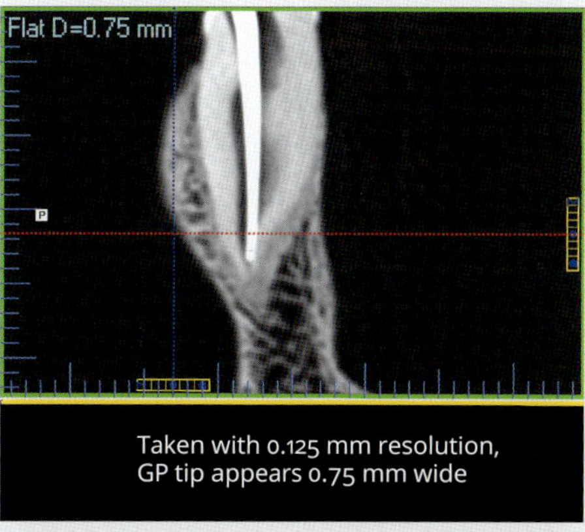

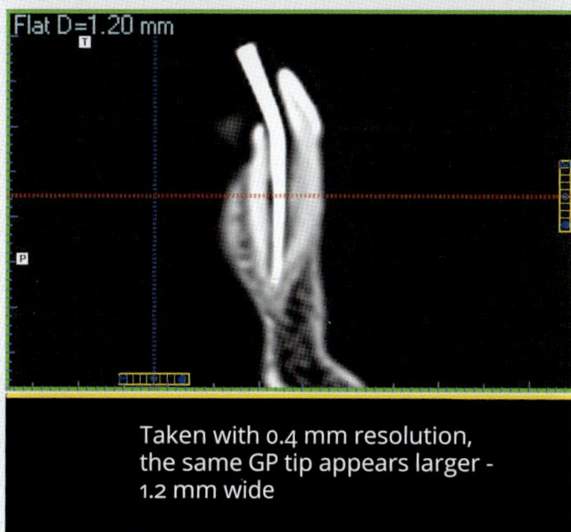

Fig 4-8 Partial volume effect.

Partial volume effects are therefore minimised by reducing the voxel size.

Aliasing artefacts

In all imaging methods, the subject must be sampled a certain number of times to ensure accurate and correct reproduction. A good example of this is if you video record a fast-moving object, such as an aeroplane propeller or a car wheel; as the speed increases after a certain point, the wheel or propeller will appear to reverse-spin slowly. This is because the frame capture rate of the camera is slower than the time taken for the wheel or propeller to rotate.

In CBCT, the sampling frequency required is the pixel size of the detector. As the X-ray beam is cone-shaped and divergent, it is not difficult to see how the parts of the object furthest from the source may be undersampled.

An aliasing artefact is therefore most visible at the peripheries of the scanned object, and is known as a Moiré pattern (Fig 4-9). Moiré patterns are inherent to the CBCT geometry and cannot be removed. Fortunately, they are only a problem at the peripheries, and for small-volume CBCT they will rarely be visible.

Ring artefacts

Ring artefacts are due to inconsistencies in the detector plate; this may be a particular area or pixel that is defective and either records no data, or over-records. It is rare to see this in CBCT due to QA programs, which can quickly and easily highlight detector faults. If ring artefacts are detected, then the scanner may need recalibrating or servicing (Fig 4-10).

Motion artefacts

These have been discussed under 'Movement unsharpness'; the two are interchangeable (Figs 4-11 and 4-12).

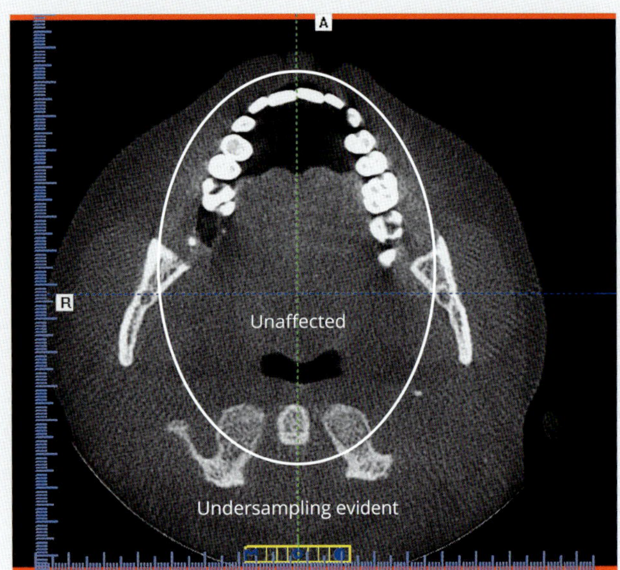

Fig 4-9 Aliasing artefact. Undersampled artefact can be seen manifesting as curved spindle lines. It is most evident at the peripheries of the scan—the central area is unaffected.

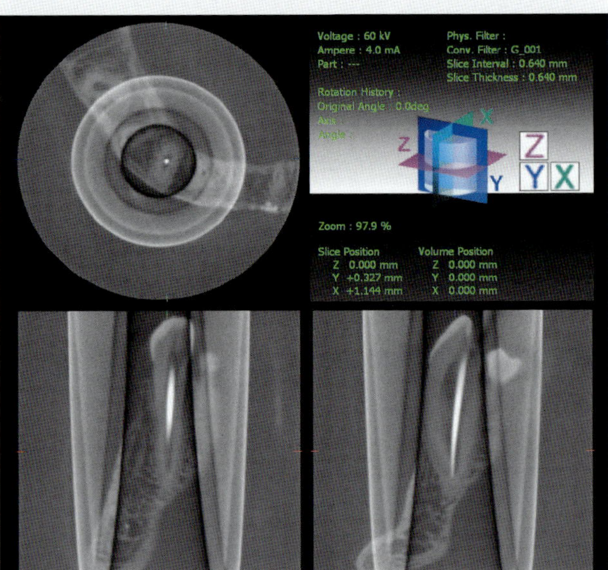

Fig 4-10 Ring artefact. A fault on the detector plate has caused a ring—this will always appear around the centre of rotation as the fault is on the detector plate, so does not move.

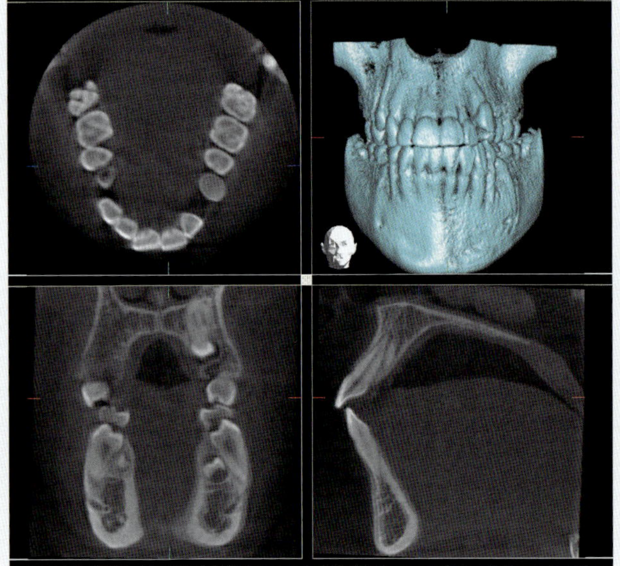

Fig 4-11 Motion artefact. Note that there are two cortices for the lower labial plate.

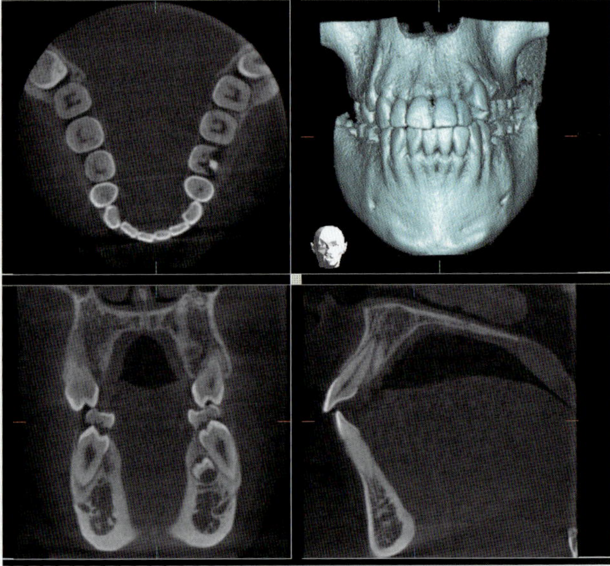

Fig 4-12 Motion artefact reduced when reconstructed from 180 degrees of data.

Noise

Noise degrades the image by mottling the picture and reducing contrast resolution and sharpness. The methods by which noise are produced have been described in Chapters 2 and 3. Quantum noise is minimised by increasing the number of photons detected at the image receptor (increase mA or kV). Electronic noise can be minimised by using better hardware. Structural noise can be reduced by regular QA (Figs 4-13 and 4-14).

Summary of artefacts

Artefacts exist on CBCT due to problems with scanning the patient, the detector, and the inherent geometry. While not all artefacts can be removed, with increasing computing power a larger number of them can be

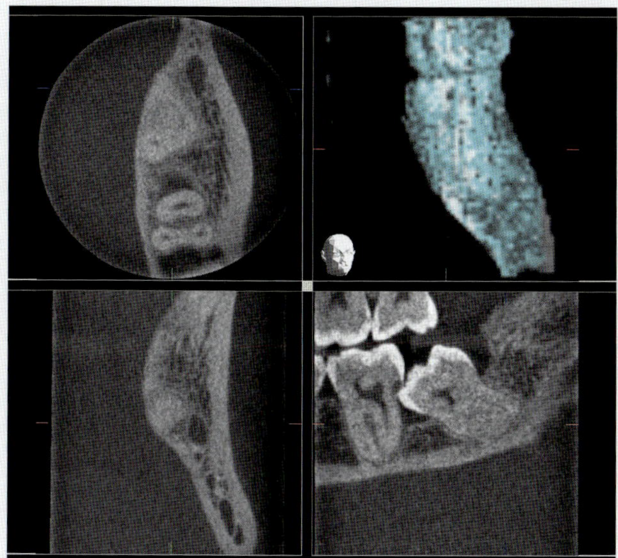

Fig 4-13 Quantum noise. Notice how contrast and spatial resolution suffer. In this application (pre-extraction of wisdom tooth), the noisy image is still diagnostic; however, if looking for microfractures, the whole scan has a mottled grey 'fog', which decreases both contrast and spatial resolution.

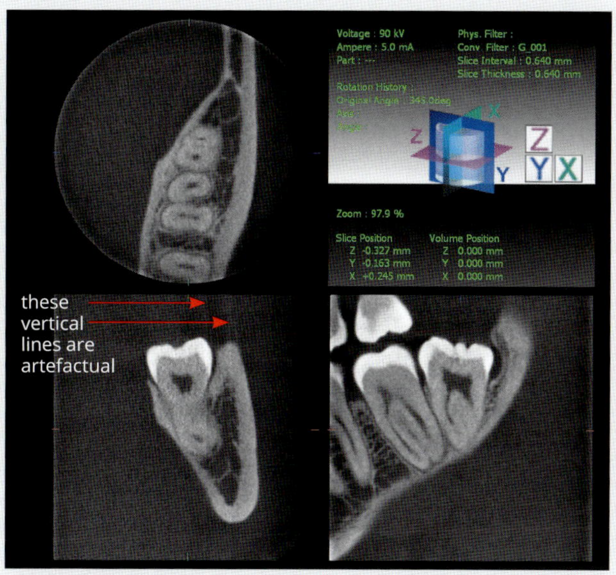

Fig 4-14 Structural noise.

reduced. A good knowledge of different artefacts, how they are caused, and what they look like is essential for CBCT interpretation.

Viewing and storing images

PACS

PACS stands for 'picture archiving and communication systems'. Practices that use digital radiography will have some form of PACS already; however, this may not be compatible with CBCT. Fortunately, CBCT machines come with generally very good software.

PACS can be linked to other software programs to streamline workflow—for example, it could be linked to a patient information database or reporting software. If you are carrying out few CBCT scans, this may be unnecessary; however, great care must be taken to ensure that manually entered data is correct on all systems.

DICOM

The scans will normally be saved in a Digital Imaging and Communications in Medicine (DICOM) format, which is a set of standards to ensure scans are correctly labelled. DICOM files include a huge amount of information, as well as the scan, including:

- patient details (name, DOB, hospital number, etc)
- scan parameters (kV, mA, scan time, acquisition time, scan volume)
- general factors (time, date, hospital).

Viewing monitor

A good-quality viewing monitor and good viewing conditions are essential. If the CBCT machine is set up correctly and taking excellent-quality images but the viewing screen is poor quality, then useful information is lost and the scan will be less helpful. The Royal College of Radiologists (RCR) recommends that specialist medical viewing monitors are used for primary diagnosis; it is then acceptable to use an 'off the shelf' PC monitor for secondary viewing (e.g. in the dental surgery).

The RCR viewing monitor criteria are outlined in Table 4-4.

A good-quality off the shelf monitor can provide dentists with acceptable results when viewing dental plain films; however, for CBCT, a higher-quality monitor is recommended.

Table 4-4 Viewing monitor requirements.

	Minimum	Recommended
Screen resolution (native pixel array)	≥ 1280 × 1024 (~1.3 megapixels)	≥ 1500 × 2000 (~3 megapixels)
Screen size (diagonal)	≥ 17′	≥ 20′
Maximum luminance	> 170 cd/m²	≥ 500 cd/m²
Luminance contrast ratio	≥ 250:1	≥ 500:1
Greyscale calibration	Within 10% GSDF	Calibrated to GSDF
Greyscale bit depth	8 bit greyscale (24 bit colour)	≥ 10 bit greyscale
Video display interface	Digital (e.g. VGI, HDMI, displayport)	Digital
Pixel defects	Class 2—two parts per million	Class 1—no defects

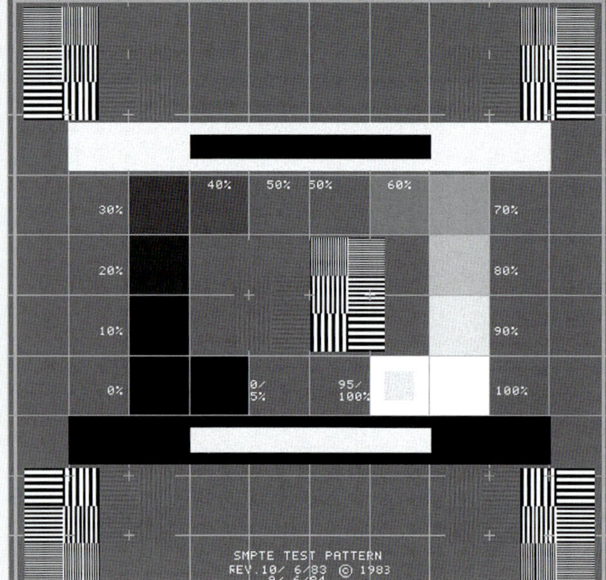

Fig 4-15 SMPTE test pattern.

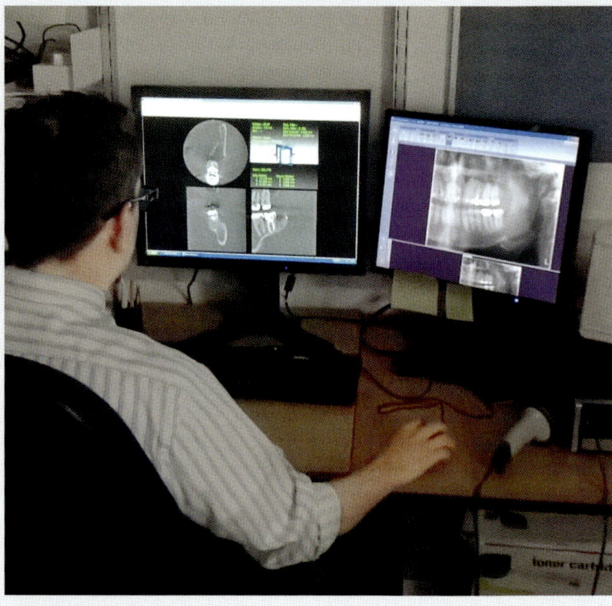

Fig 4-16 Viewing area. This should have: no overhead lights or windows to cause reflection; large, specialist medical monitors; darkened area, but not pitch black; ergonomic use of computer and mouse.

To check the viewing performance of your monitors, you might choose to download the SMPTE test pattern, which should be used on monitors on which scans are viewed (Fig 4-15). The smaller 5% and 95% contrast squares within the 0% and 100% should be visible on a well-adjusted, high-quality monitor, as should all the line patterns in the corners and in the centre.

Lighting conditions

Viewing the images in a darkened environment is also important—in a dental surgery, there is far too much light to examine the scan correctly. Showing patients selected images in surgery can be an excellent tool to aid explanation of treatment, but these conditions are not ideal for reporting. Studies have shown that dimmed lighting in the region of <300 lumens offers the ideal viewing conditions to enable the most information to be gleaned (Fig 4-16).

Storage of images

It is essential that data protection is adhered to when using CBCT; the computers should all be password protected and any data taken off the main hub PC should be encrypted—this should be either on an encrypted USB or encrypted files 'burned' onto CD. Email is generally not safe for transferring patient scans unless both the sender and recipient are using a secure email system.

Training requirements

While there is legislation in the form of IRR99 and IRMER2000 covering the use of radiation for medical exposures, the authors have included some guidelines for training in the use, justification and reporting of CBCTs.

Dentists who wish to request CBCTs should attend a 'level 1' CBCT training course lasting no less than 12 hours of practical or theoretical training.

Dentists who wish to justify and report CBCTs should have completed the 'level 1' course and no less than an additional 12 hours of theoretical training and 12 hours of practical training.

This chapter will offer dentists a sound basis of the knowledge and understanding component of 'level 1'—however, regulations and laws regarding X-ray and CBCT use in your country should also be read and understood. The authors would strongly recommend reading the European Academy of DentoMaxilloFacial Radiology Guidelines (Brown et al, 2014) on training (from which the above is adapted), and completion of extra training. National certification in the UK has been considered but is currently not required.

CBCT-specific regulations

UK legislation regarding X-ray use is covered extensively in other texts; however, in two areas the regulations and guidelines differ slightly from the rest of dental radiography.

In the case of equipment failure and overexposure, the Health and Safety Executive (HSE) must be notified if the dose to the patient is 10 times than intended. For the rest of dental radiography, the figure is 20 times. Any overexposure, however, should be investigated locally.

All radiographic exams are required to be graded for quality. At least 95% of CBCTs should be grade 1—diagnostically acceptable. A maximum of 5% can be grade 2—diagnostically unacceptable.

Assessment of images

The entire volume of data must be assessed in each of the three planes. The root(s) of each tooth should be uprighted before it is viewed.

It is essential that CBCT users should have appropriate training. A radiological report from a specialist must be sought if the interpretation of the scan is beyond the competence of the clinician who has prescribed and/or taken the scan.

Further reading

Allisy-Roberts P, Williams J. Farr's Physics for Medical Imaging, ed 2. London, UK: Elsevier, 2007.

Brown J, Jacobs R, Jäghagen EL, et al. Basic training requirements for the use of dental CBCT by dentists: a position paper prepared by the European Academy of DentoMaxilloFacial Radiology. Dentomaxillofac Radiol 2014;43:20130291.

European Society of Endodontology, Patel S, Durack C, et al. European Society of Endodontology position statement: the use of CBCT in Endodontics. Int Endod J 2014;47:502–504.

Holroyd JR, Gulson AD. The Radiation Protection Implications of the use of Cone Beam Computed Tomography in Dentistry – What You Need to Know. HPA guidance document, 2009.

NRPB guidelines. Dental practitioners: safe use of x-ray equipment. Public Health England, 2001.

Pauwels R, Beinsberger J, Collaert B, et al. Effective dose range for dental cone beam computed tomography scanners. Eur J Radiol 2012;81:267–271.

Shaw C. Cone Beam Computed Tomography. New York, NY: CRC Press, 2014.

Wall B, Haylock R, Jansen J, Hillier M, Hart D, Shrimpton P. Radiation risks from medical X-ray examinations as a function of the age and sex of the patient. HPA-CRCE-028. Chilton: HPA, 2011.

Whaites E, Drage N. Essentials of Dental Radiography and Radiology, ed 5. London, UK: Churchill Livingstone, 2013.

Chapter 5

Dentoalveolar Anatomy

Cindy Verdegaal, Hagay Shemesh

Introduction

Cone beam computed tomography (CBCT) is most suitable for the imaging of bony structures, like the mandible and the maxillary bones. However, soft tissue differentiation is impossible because the quantum of radiation applied is insufficient to distinguish between the different soft tissue structures.

The anatomical structures in any desired plane may be viewed on a CBCT scan. Reconstructed images are usually displayed in the coronal, sagittal and axial planes (Fig 5-1).

The anatomy of the maxilla and palatine bone

Two maxillary bones, one left and one right, form the maxilla and the central portion of the facial skeleton. All facial bones except the mandible articulate with the maxilla. Sutures connect the different bone structures and should be distinguished from possible fracture lines on CBCT scans. The left and right palatine processes of the maxillary bones are fused at the median palatine suture (Fig 5-2). The horizontal plate of the palatine bone is located posterior to the palatine processes and is fused by the transverse palatine suture. Together they form the hard palate, the bony roof of the oral cavity.

The horizontal plate of the palatine bone completes the posterior portion of the hard palate. The superior plate of the palatine bone forms part of the walls of the nasal cavity. The major palatine foramen containing the descending palatine vessels and major palatine nerve is located on either side of the horizontal plate of the palatine bone. This foramen is usually located in line with the upper third (wisdom) molar. It is visualised on a CBCT scan as a round/oval-shaped radiolucency (Fig 5-3).

Immediately inferior to the nose, the two maxillary bones meet and form the anterior nasal spine at their junction (Fig 5-4). This pronounced cephalometric landmark is located above and anterior to the maxillary incisors. It is clearly seen in a sagittal reconstruction.

Posterior to the roof tip of the incisor teeth is the incisive foramen. It is a funnel-shaped radiolucency in the median palatine structure (Fig 5-5). The orifices of the left and right incisive canals are located in this opening. The incisive canals run in a vertical direction parallel to the buccal surface of the anterior maxilla. They contain the terminal branch of the descending palatine artery and the nasopalatine nerve.

When united, the posterior border of the left and right palatine bones at the median palatine structure form the posterior nasal spine—a sharp, pointed process located distally from the maxillary molar teeth (Figs 5-4 and 5-5).

The frontal process of the maxillary bone forms the inferior wall of the orbit and contains the infraorbital foramen. The foramen allows the infraorbital nerve and artery to reach the face from the infraorbital canal. The lateral wall of the orbit is shaped by the zygomatic bone (Fig 5-6).

The frontal processes of the maxillary bones extend superiorly to the frontal bone, forming part of the lateral aspects of the bridge of the nose. This feature cannot be distinguished in a small field of view (FOV) CBCT scan of the dentoalveolar area and is therefore not described further.

The regions that flank the nasal cavity laterally contain the medial border of the maxillary sinuses. The latter extend from the orbits to the maxillary teeth. The maxillary bones articulate laterally with the zygomatic bones and their zygomatic processes (Fig 5-7).

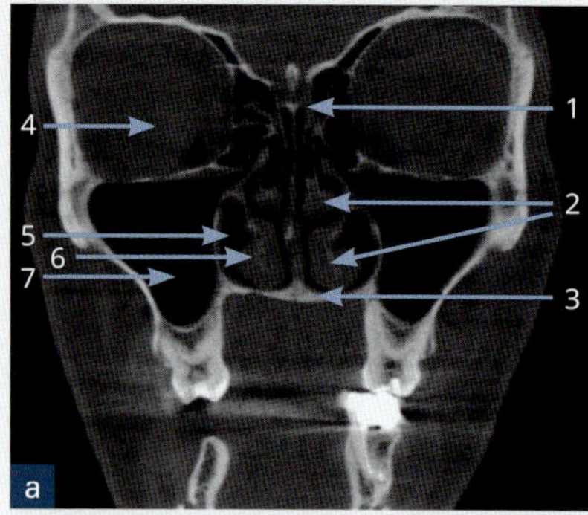

Fig 5-1 Overview of the mandible and maxilla: (a) coronal, (b to d) axial, (e to g) sagittal views.
1: ethmoid bone, 2: middle and inferior nasal turbinate, 3: palatine bone, 4: orbit, 5: inferior nasal meatus, 6: inferior nasal turbinate, 7: maxillary sinus, 8: nasal bone, 9: mandibular ramus, 10: odontoid peg of C2, 11: C1 vertebrae, 12: incisive foramen, 13: frontal bone, 14: frontal sinus, 15: posterior ethmoid cells, 16: sphenoid sinus, 17: clivus bone, 18: vomer, 19: body of the mandible, 20: condylar head, 21: external auditory meatus.

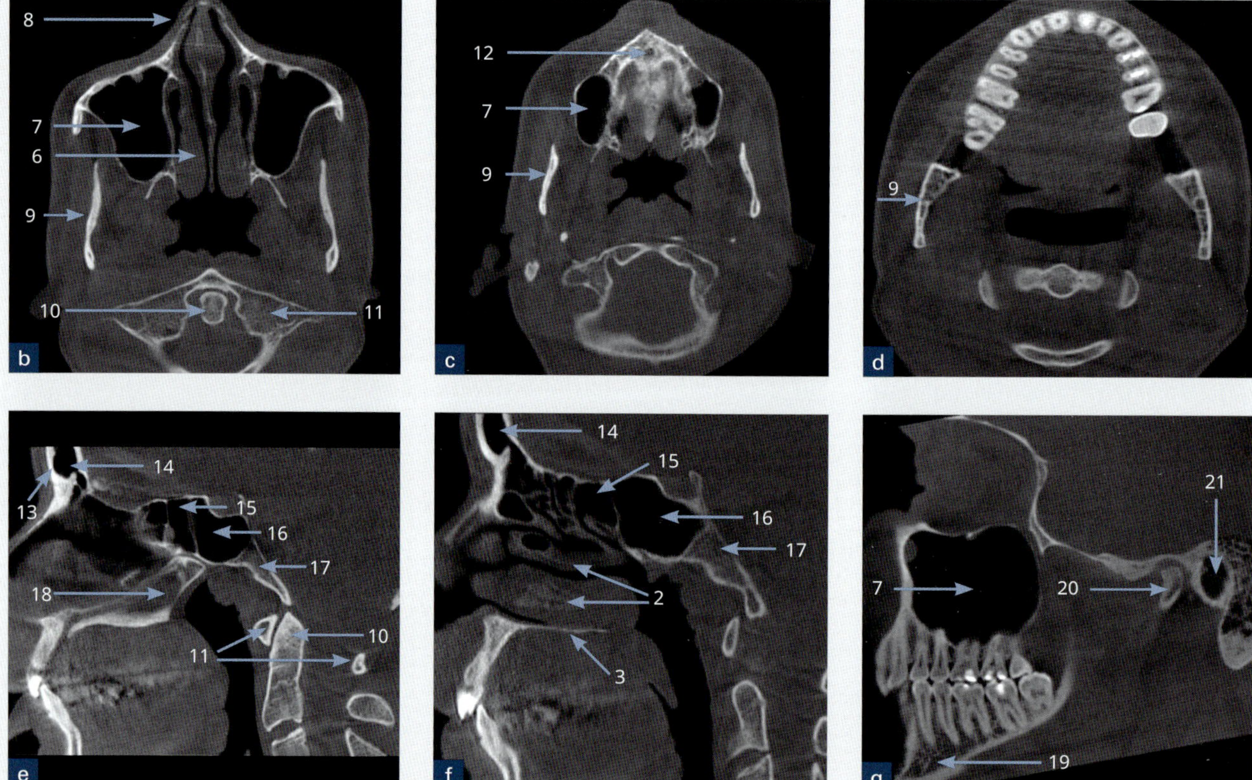

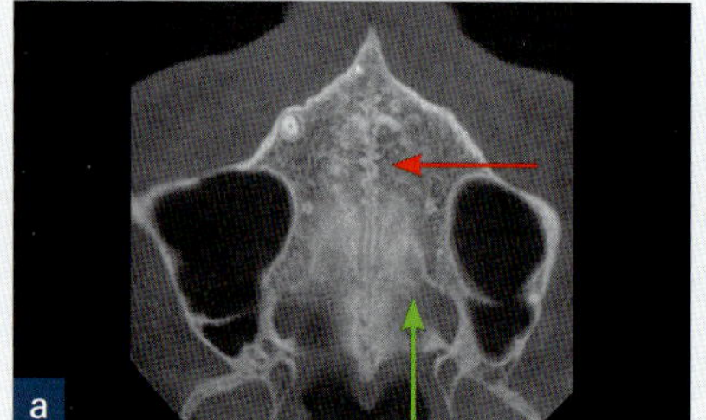

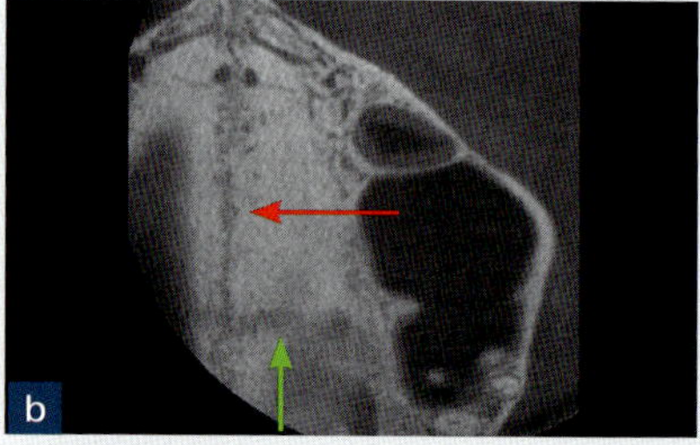

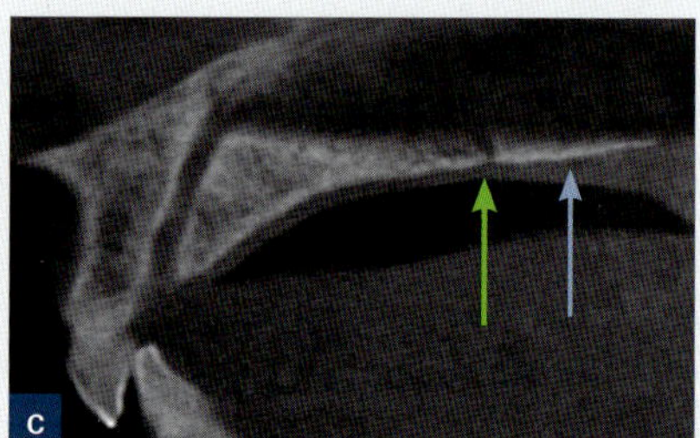

Fig 5-2 Overview of palatal structures: (a to b) axial, (c) sagittal views. The right and left palatine processes are fused and form the median palatine suture (red arrow). These processes are either irregular radiopaque lines, separated by a radiolucent line, or can have a radiolucent appearance only. The green arrow shows the transverse palatine suture. The blue arrow points at the horizontal plate of the palatine bone.

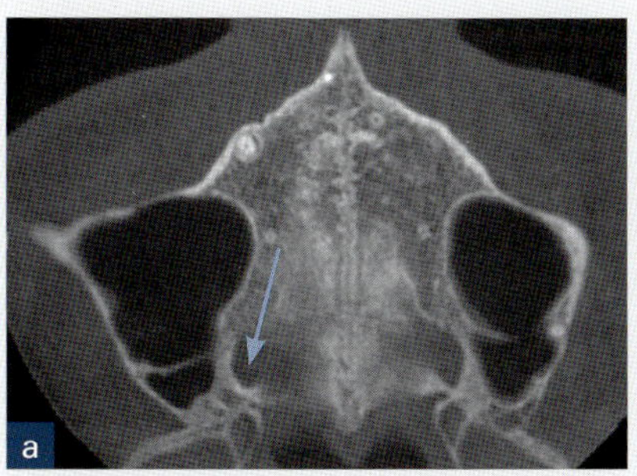

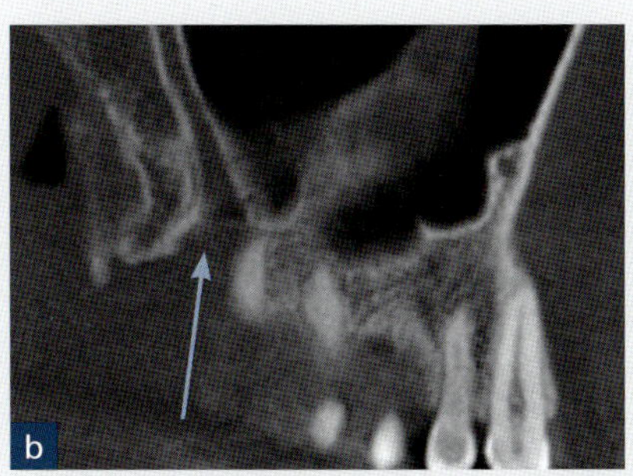

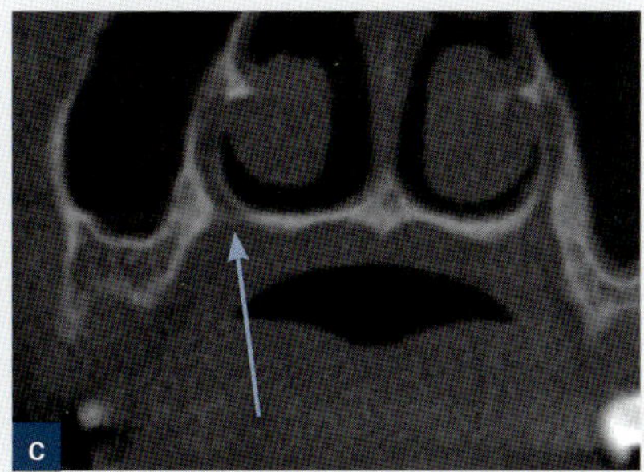

Fig 5-3 Overview of the maxilla: (a) axial, (b) sagittal, (c) coronal views. The blue arrow reveals the foramen of the major palatine canal.

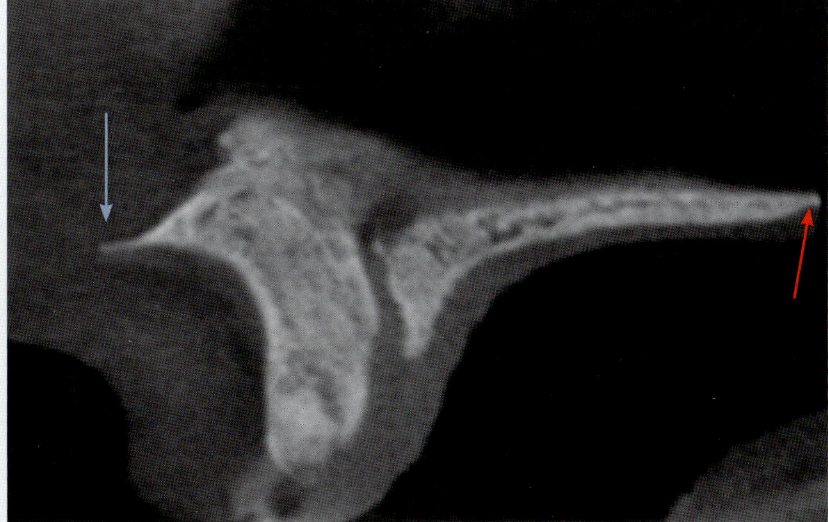

Fig 5-4 Sagittal view of the anterior nasal spine (blue arrow) and the posterior nasal spine (red arrow).

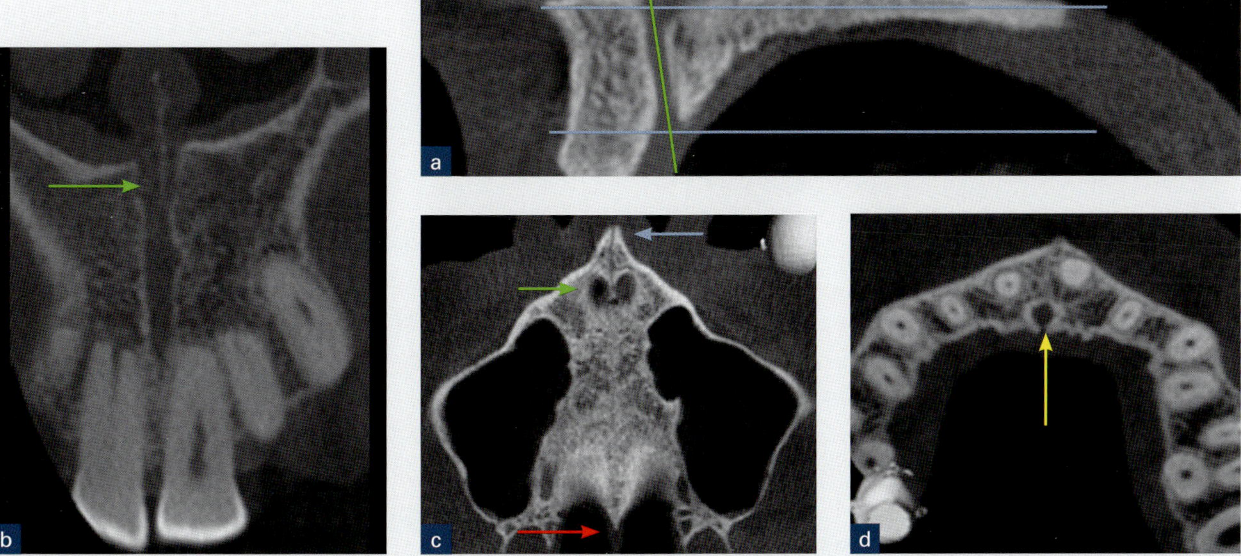

Fig 5-5 (a to d) Cross-sections demonstrated by the blue lines; the incisive canals are shown by the green arrow. The incisive canals run through the palatine processes of the maxillary bones and are fused at the incisive foramen (yellow arrow). In the axial slide, the blue arrow shows the anterior nasal spine and the red arrow shows the posterior nasal spine.

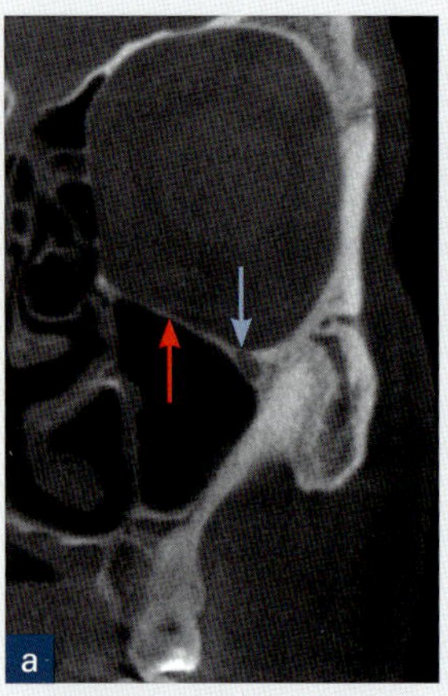

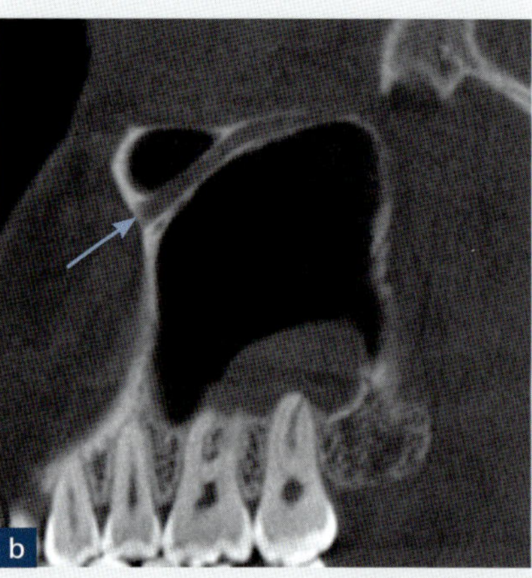

Fig 5-6 Overview of the maxilla: (a) coronal, (b) sagittal views. The blue arrow pointing at the round radiolucency in the (a) coronal plane shows the infraorbital foramen. The sagittal plane (b) demonstrates the infraorbital canal. The red arrow shows the frontal process of the maxillary bone.

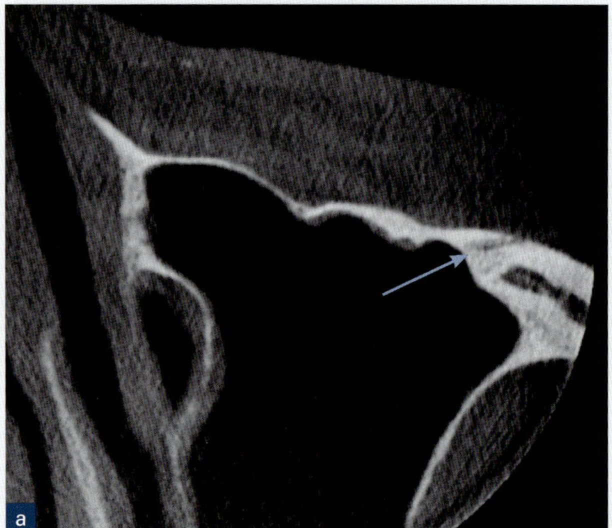

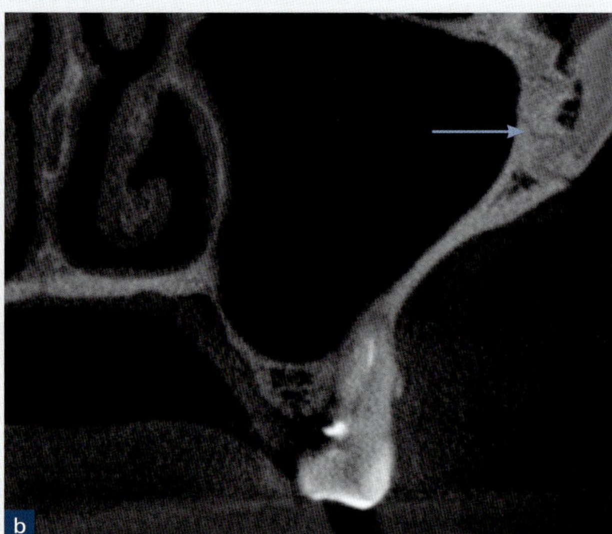

Fig 5-7 (a) Axial, (b) coronal views. The blue arrow points at the radiolucent line that demonstrates the connection between the zygomatic process of the maxillary bone and the zygomatic arch.

The anatomy of the nose and nasal cavity

The nose consists mostly of cartilage, which is not clearly seen on a CBCT scan. The bony part of the nose consists of two thin, rectangular nasal bones fused medially, forming the nasal bridge. They vary in size and form, articulating with the frontal bone superiorly, the maxillary bones laterally, and the ethmoid bone posteriorly (Fig 5-8).

The ethmoid bone forms the roof of the nasal cavity. The palatine processes of the maxillary and palatine bones form the floor. The superior and middle conchae of the ethmoid bone, the perpendicular plates of the palatine bone, and the inferior nasal conchae shape the lateral walls. The depressions of the conchae on the lateral walls are the superior, middle, and inferior meatuses. The nasal conchae form a long, narrow and curled bone shelf that protrudes into the breathing passage of the nose. The airways are clearly visible on a CBCT scan as black radiolucent structures (Fig 5-9).

The nasal septum divides the nasal cavity into right and left sections. The vomer is the bony inferior part of the septum. The superior, less-dense part is formed by the perpendicular plate of the ethmoid bone (Fig 5-10).

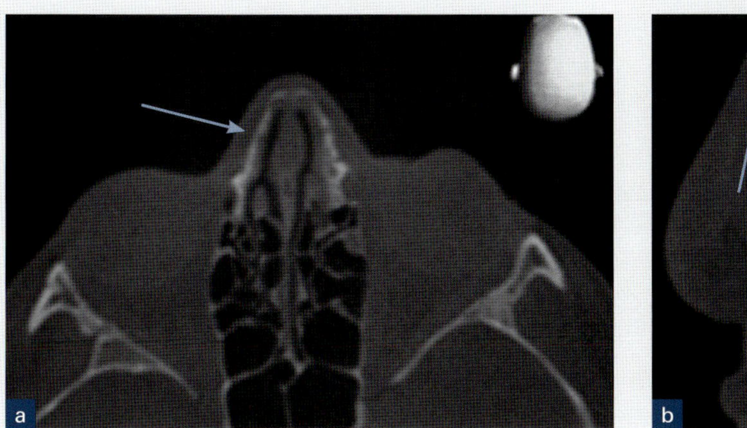
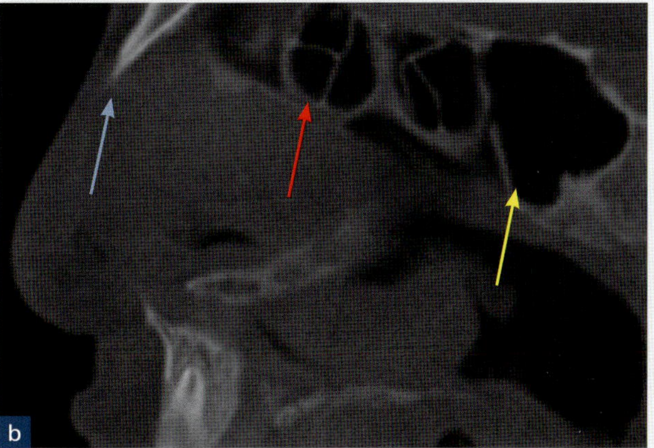

Fig 5-8 Overview of nose and nasal cavity: (a) axial, (b) sagittal views. The blue arrow shows the nasal bone (a). The red arrow shows the ethmoid bone, while the yellow arrow shows the sphenoid bone (b).

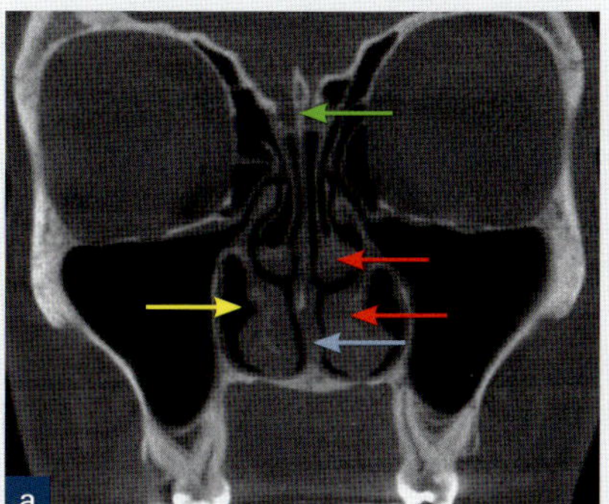
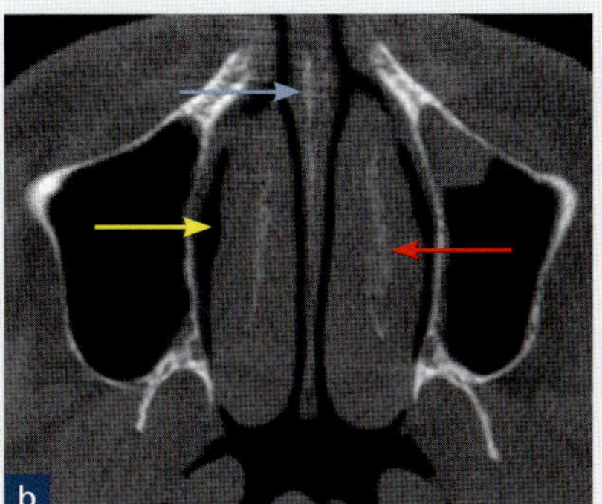
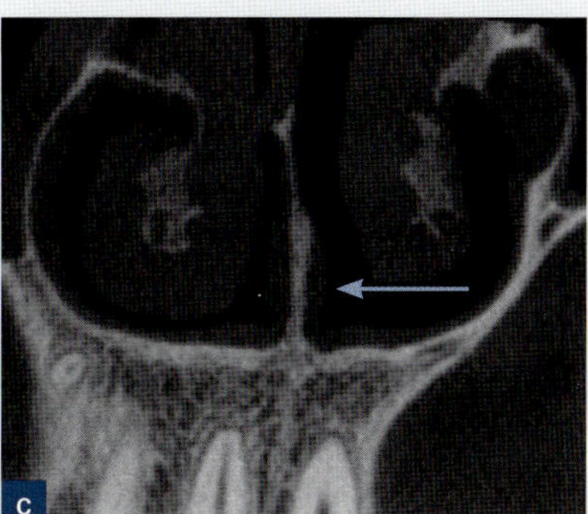

Fig 5-9 In the (a) coronal plane, the ethmoid bone is shown by the green arrow and the middle and inferior nasal conchae by the red arrows; the yellow arrow shows the inferior nasal meatus. In the (b) axial slide, the red arrow shows the inferior nasal conchae, the yellow arrow the inferior nasal meatus, and the blue arrow (in b and c) the vomer bone.

The anatomy of the maxillary sinus

The maxillary sinus is a membrane-lined air space surrounded by maxillary bone. It extends from the orbit to the maxillary teeth and from the nasal cavity to the zygomatic processes (Fig 5-9). The lumen of the sinus cavity enlarges during adolescence until the end of physical growth. Further enlargement is seen after tooth loss (Sharan and Madjar, 2008).

The floor of the maxillary sinus is in close relationship with the root tips of the maxillary premolars and molar teeth. The thickness of the cortical and cancellous bone of the maxillary alveolar ridge can be accurately determined on a CBCT scan, as well as the inclination of roots in relation to the surrounding jaw.

The mesiobuccal root of the maxillary second molar is usually in closest contact with the sinus floor (Jung et al, 2012; Erberhardt et al, 1992; Ok et al, 2014). With a thinner bone layer between the root tip and the floor of the sinus, it is more likely that the root tip will protrude into the sinus. The position and rotation of the tooth in the alveolar bone and the location of the maxillary sinus floor influence the anatomical relationship between the roots and maxillary sinus. The measured distance between the root tip and the sinus floor depends on the reconstructed

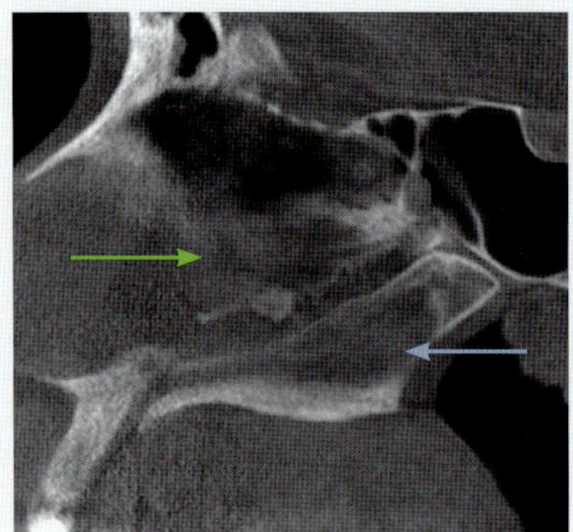

Fig 5-10 Sagittal view of the maxilla showing the vomer by the blue arrow; the perpendicular plate of the ethmoid bone by the green arrow.

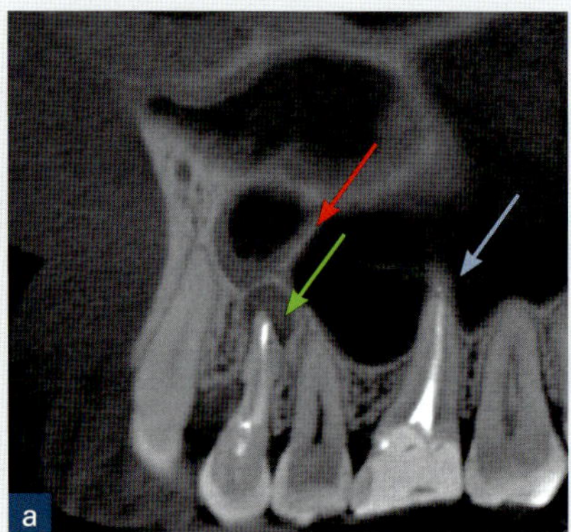

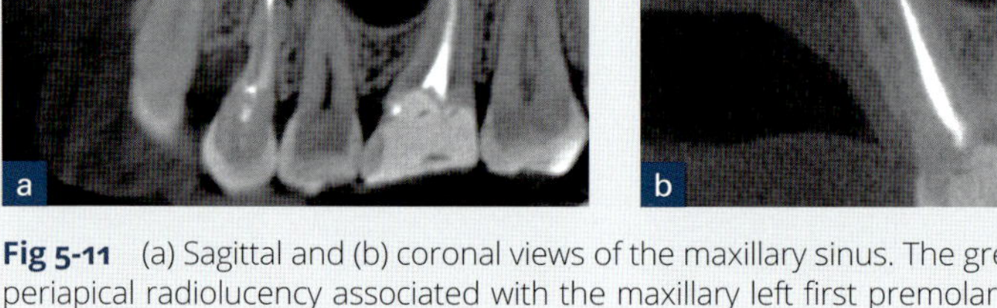

Fig 5-11 (a) Sagittal and (b) coronal views of the maxillary sinus. The green arrow shows periapical radiolucency associated with the maxillary left first premolar. The blue arrow shows the mesiobuccal root, with extruded root-filling material in the left and right image of the maxillary left first molar tooth. The red arrow shows septa in the maxillary sinus.

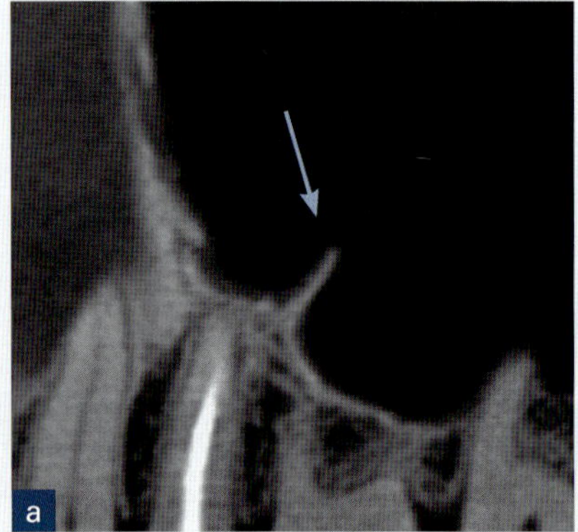

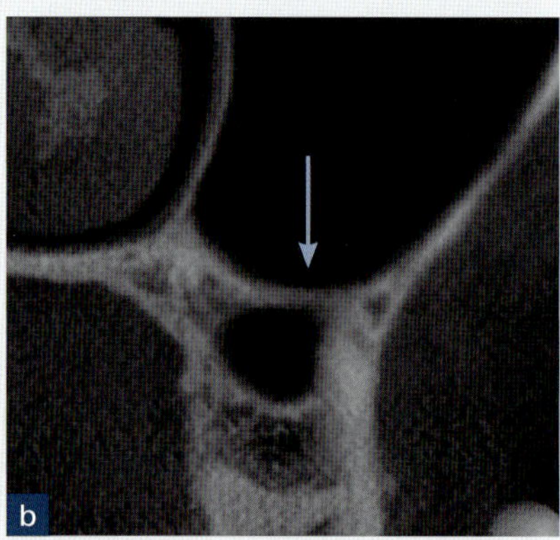

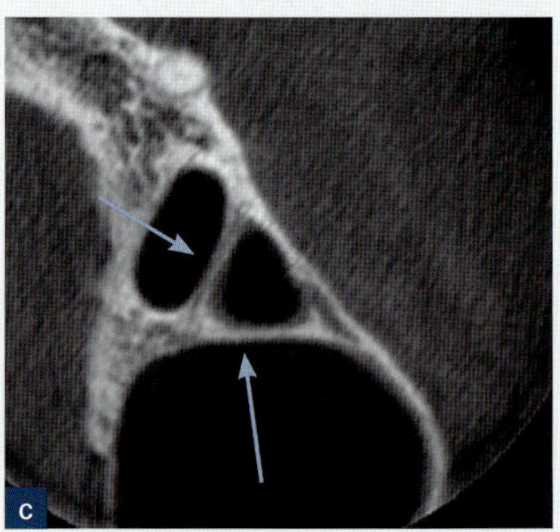

Fig 5-12 (a to c) Septa in the left maxillary sinus.

CBCT plane. Higher values are obtained in coronal sections compared to sagittal planes (von Arx et al, 2014). This can result in the overestimation of the bone thickness, with a higher risk of complications (extrusion of irrigants or filling material, and perforation during endodontic microsurgery) (Fig 5-11).

The presence of septa in the maxillary sinus is a common occurrence; they are most commonly located in the molar region. A recent study evaluating the maxillary sinus anatomy by CBCT revealed the presence of septa in 47% of patients, and 33.2% of sinuses (Neugebauer et al, 2010) (Fig 5-12).

Mild mucosal thickening of the maxillary sinus of up to 2 mm is considered a normal radiographic finding (Rak et al, 1991). Mucosal thickening of more than 2 mm is reported to indicate maxillary sinusitis (Vallo et al, 2010; Lu et al, 2012) (Fig 5-13). Thickening increases with associated apical periodontitis, age and male gender (Shanbdag et al, 2013) (Fig 5-14).

The anatomy of the alveolar bone

The maxilla houses the maxillary teeth in the alveolar process of the maxillary bone. The process can be divided into the alveolar bone proper and the supporting alveolar bone.

The supporting alveolar bone consists of cortical bone plates and cancellous bone. The cortical plates are thick, compact bone plates on the palatal and buccal side of the alveolar process, which consist of lamellar compact bone. The alternating pattern of the fibres' orientation within the lamellar provides strength to the bone.

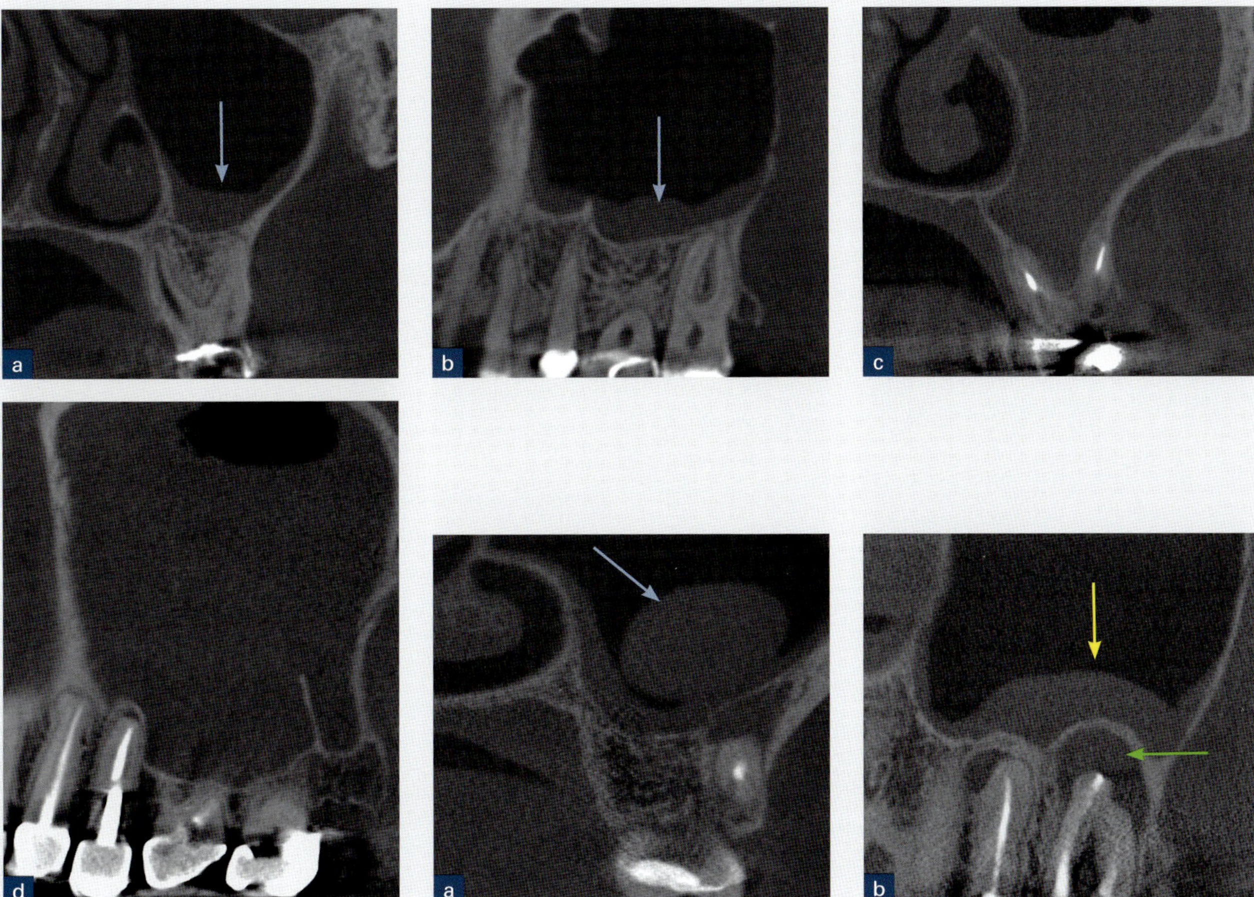

Fig 5-13 Mucosal thickening in the left maxillary sinus. (a and b) Coronal and sagittal images of mild mucosal thickening. (c and d) Maxillary sinusitis.

Fig 5-14 (a) A massive polyp on the left maxillary sinus floor is shown by the blue arrrow. (b) Mucosal thickening (yellow arrow) with an associated apical periodontitis of tooth 26, shown by the green arrow.

The lamellae of the cancellous bone form a trabecular pattern, which has a great variation in form, shape, size and thickness, from cylindrical rods to wide, uneven, irregular sheets of bone. Trabeculae do not pass from one cortical plate to the opposite plate, but fuse and interconnect with marrow spaces in between. The maxillary bone contains more trabeculae and is of a smaller size compared to other bones (Fig 5-15).

The alveolar bone proper is the lining of the tooth socket adjacent to the periodontal ligament. It is a compact bone that contains numerous holes where the Volkmann canals pass from the alveolar bone to the periodontal ligament. The fibres from the ligament are inserted into the alveolar bone. This makes this bone less compact than the cortical bone, but still much more dense than the cancellous bone on a CBCT image. The radiopaque line on radiographs surrounding the periodontal ligament space is termed the lamina dura, and consists of cortical bone (Fig 5-16).

The anatomy of the maxillary teeth

The enamel is the most radiopaque dental tissue. Dentine contains less hydroxyapatite and is therefore less radiopaque than the surrounding enamel. The pulp tissue will appear more radiolucent.

Calcifications of pulp tissue are a common occurrence. Pulp calcifications may complicate and block access to the root canals and are therefore of clinical significance. The exact location of calcifications within the pulp tissue can be determined on CBCT as a radiopaque appearance in the pulp chamber or root canal (Fig 5-17).

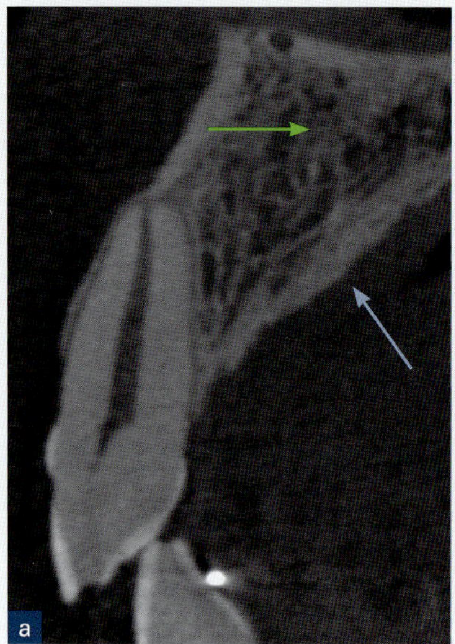

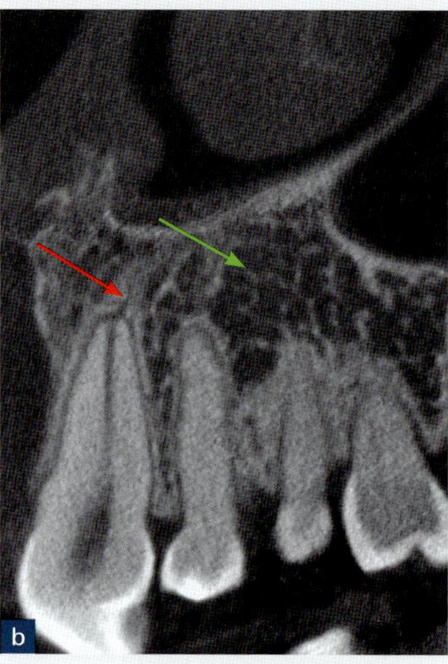

Fig 5-15 (a) The green arrow shows the trabecular pattern of the cancellous bone. The blue arrow shows the palatal cortical bone. The red arrow (b) shows a nutrient canal of tooth 21.

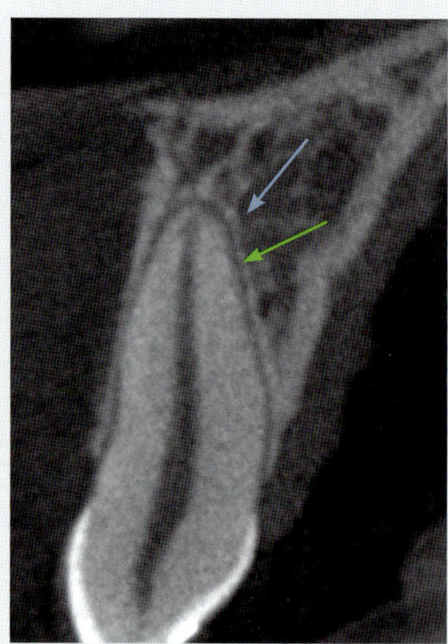

Fig 5-16 The image shows the alveolar bone proper (blue arrow) adjacent to the radiopaque lamina dura (green arrow). The enamel shows the highest radiopacity.

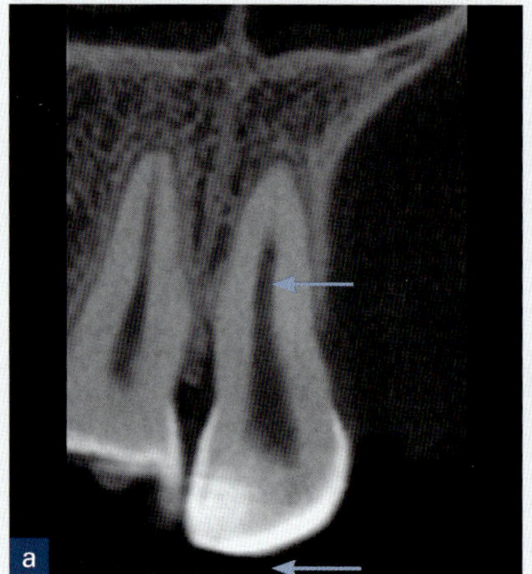

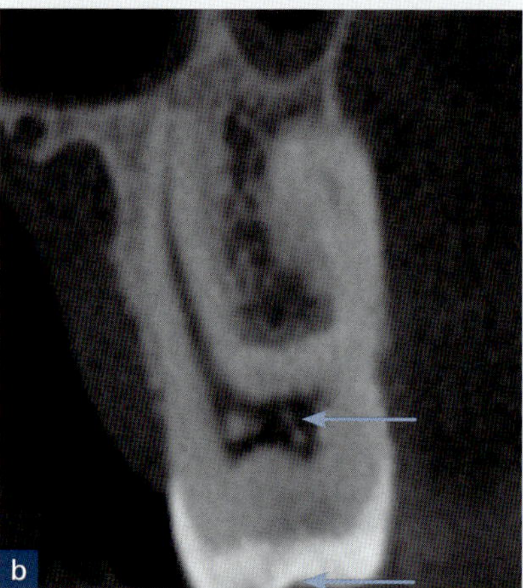

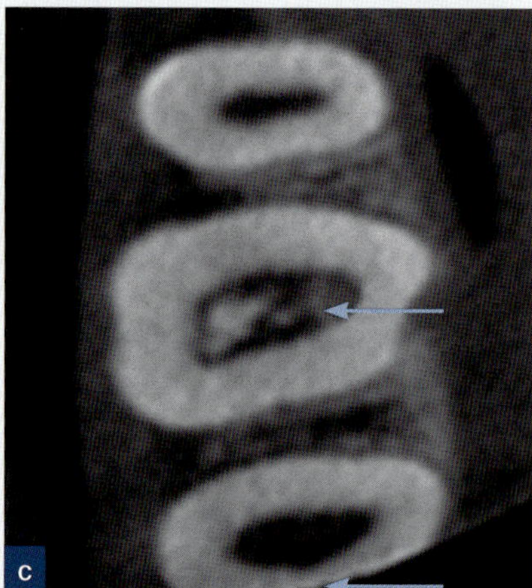

Fig 5-17 (a to c) Radiographic images of teeth to locate calcifications and pulp stones (blue arrows).

The anatomy of the mandible

The mandible (or jawbone) is the largest and strongest bone of the facial skeleton. Two anatomical structures in the mandible are of special importance during non-surgical and surgical endodontic treatment—namely, the mandibular canal and the mental foramen. The anatomy of the mandible is simpler compared to the maxilla, as less anatomical structures superimpose and there are no sinuses.

In the midline on the mandible's anterior surface is a faint ridge, the mandibular symphysis, where the bone was formed by fusion of the right and left processes during the development stage. Like other symphyses in the body, this is a midline articulation where the bones are joined by fibrocartilage and fuse in early childhood. The mandible's structure and the interrelationships between its different parts change with age. The important changes are listed in Table 5-1.

The mandible is divided into two parts: the mandibular ramus and the mandible body (Fig 5-18). The significance of the mandibular ramus in endodontics is limited. However, it is of relevance for temporomandibular joint disorders, surgery after maxillofacial trau-

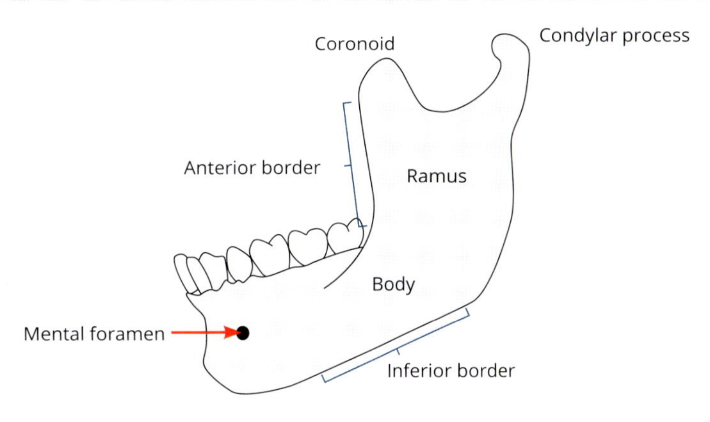

Fig 5-18 Schematic presentation of the mandible.

Table 5-1 Structural changes in the mandible with age.

	Mandibular canal	Mental foramen	Angle	Condyle location	General remarks
At birth	Large, wide canal located near the lower border of the bone	Opens beneath the socket of the first deciduous tooth	Obtuse ≈ 175 degrees	Nearly in line with the body of the mandible and lower than the coronoid	
After birth	Canal moves slightly above the mylohyoid line	Opens below the second premolar	Less obtuse ≤ 140 degrees	Coronoid usually above the level of the condyle	Body becomes elongated to provide space for the three permanent teeth developed in this part
Adulthood	Canal is parallel to the mylohyoid line	Opens midway between the upper and lower borders of the mandible	Ramus is almost vertical ≈ 120 degrees Sigmoid notch becomes deeper	Condyle is higher than the coronoid	The alveolar and sub-alveolar portions of the body of the mandible are usually of equal depth
Old age	Becomes narrow, located close to the alveolar border	Opens close to the alveolar border, from the mandibular canal	≈ 140 degrees	Condyle is bent backwards	Bone becomes greatly reduced in volume due to the loss of teeth and consequent resorption of the alveolar processes and sockets

ma, or bone harvesting for grafting of bone defects. The following description focuses on the body of the mandible.

The external surface of the mandible is marked in the median line by a faint ridge, indicating the symphysis of the two pieces of bone from which it is composed at an early period of life. This ridge divides below and encloses a triangular eminence, the mental protuberance, and the mental tubercle. On either side of the symphysis, just below the incisor teeth, is a depression, the incisive fossa, where the mentalis and a small portion of the orbicularis oris muscles originate.

Below the second premolar tooth, on either side, midway between the upper and lower borders of the body, is the mental foramen, for the passage of the mental vessels and nerve. Running posteriorly and superiorly from each mental tubercle is a faint ridge, the oblique line, which is continuous with the anterior border of the ramus; it affords attachment to important masticatory muscles.

The internal (lingual) surface of the body of the mandible is concave. Near the lower part of the symphysis are the mental spines, where the genioglossus muscle originates. In some cases, the mental spines

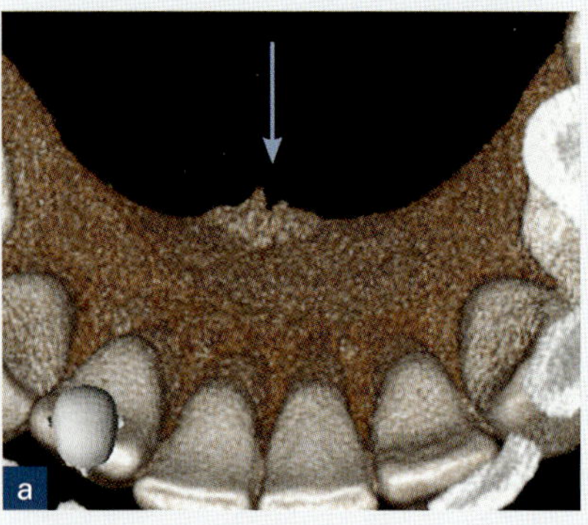
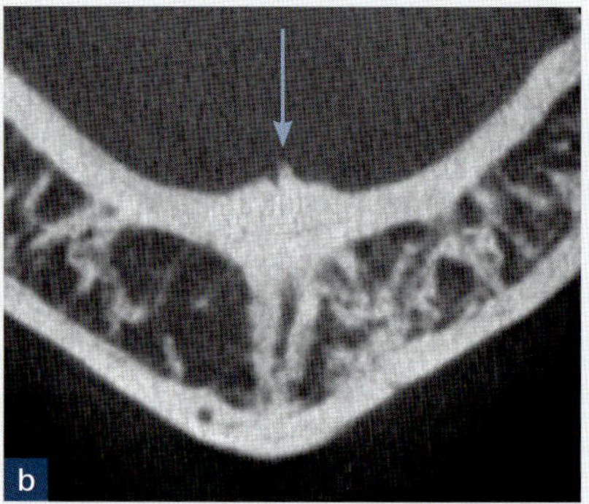
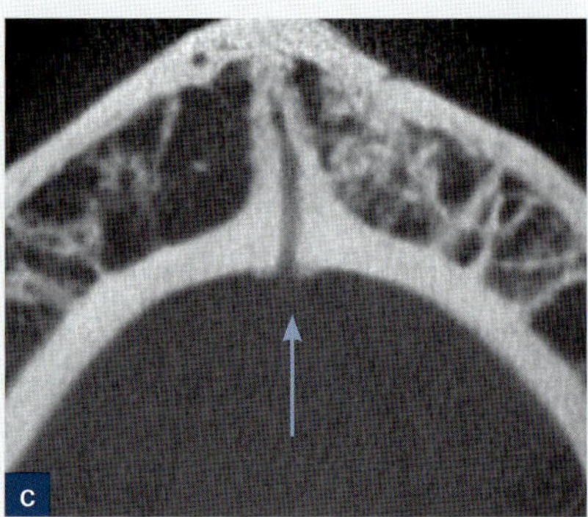

Fig 5-19 (a to c) Axial views of internal aspect of the mandible. The blue arrow shows the mental spine, the symphysis, and the lingual foramen.

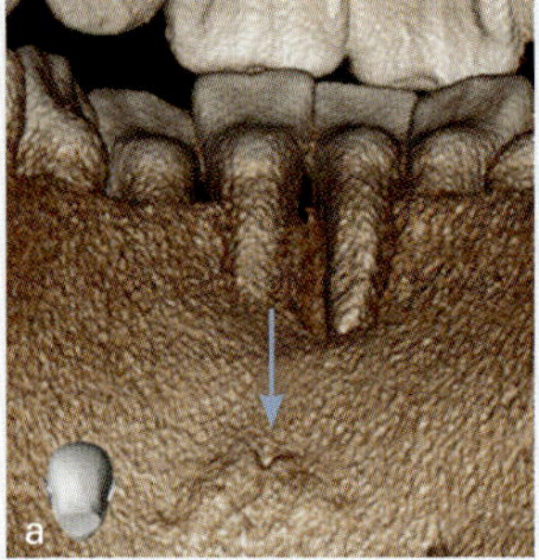
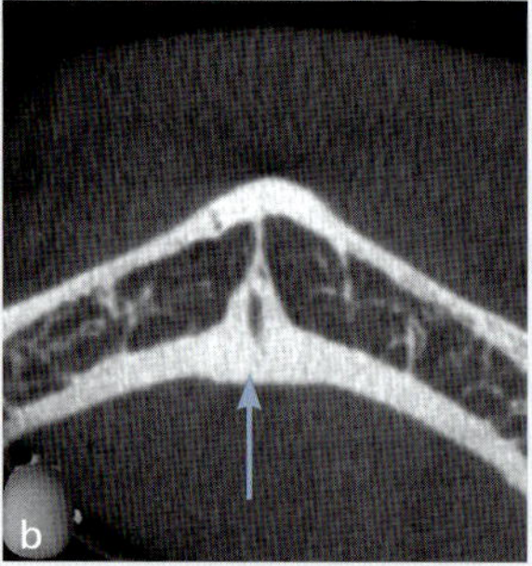
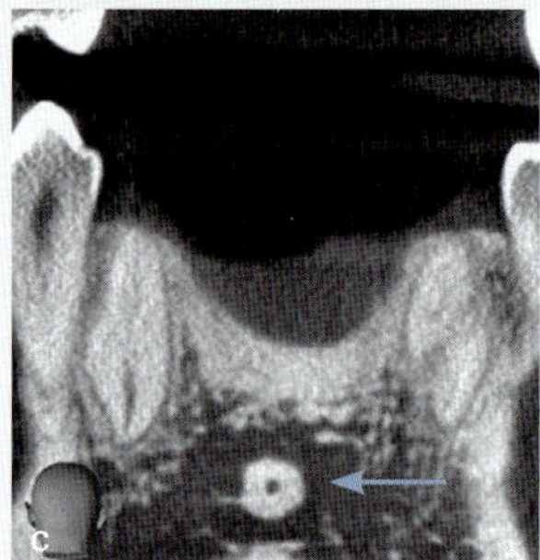
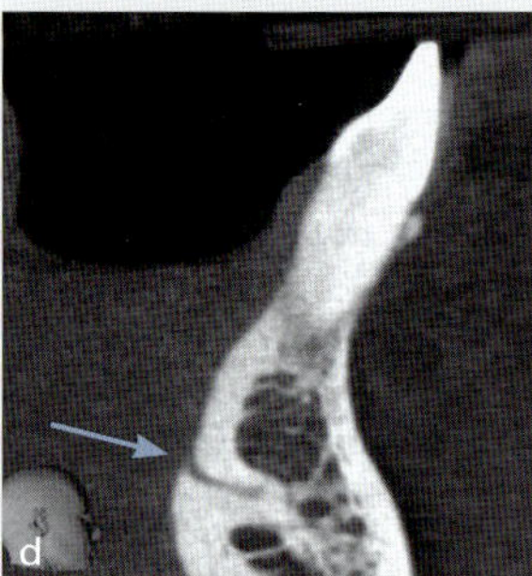

Fig 5-20 (a) Reconstructed 3D image of lingual aspect of the mandible reveals the lingual foramen (blue arrow); (b) axial, (c) coronal and (d) sagittal views.

fuse to form a single eminence, or may be absent (Fig 5-19).

The sublingual artery is one of the major branches of the lingual artery; it enters the bones through the lingual foramen on the lingual surface of the mandible (Fig 5-20). The lingual foramen is often found around the mandibular incisors and premolars and is anatomically important when performing apical surgery on the anterior of the mandible. Confirming the location of the lingual foramens through CBCT images is required, since it is not easy to locate them on either panoramic or standard radiographs.

The anatomy of the mandibular canal

The mandibular canal contains the inferior alveolar nerve, artery, and vein. It runs obliquely downward and forward in the ramus, and then horizontally forward in the body, where it runs under the alveoli. When inferior to the mandibular premolars, the main branch exits buccally via the mental foramen, giving off a small canal known as the mandibular incisive canal, which run to the sockets containing the incisor teeth.

Localisation of the mandibular canal might be difficult on panoramic radiographs because the mandibular ramus region would overlap with the opposite side of the mandible and the pharynx.

The mandibular canal may run close to the apices of the second premolar and molar teeth (Fig 5-21) (Sato et al, 2005; Kovisto et al, 2011). The inferior alveolar nerve may be damaged due to the extrusion of disinfection solutions and/or root canal filling material from the root canal directly into the mandibular canal (Pogrel, 2007; Gambarini et al, 2011).

Age and gender have been shown to influence the distance of tooth apices to the mandibular canal; females tend to have a shorter distance (Sato et al, 2005), and the distance increases with age (Kovisto et al, 2011).

The mandibular canal may be divided into two or three lumens by a thin septum. These bifid or trifid anatomical forms were thought to be extremely rare when panoramic radiographs were inspected, but are now known to be present in more than 20% of the population (Rashsuren et al, 2014) (Fig 5-22).

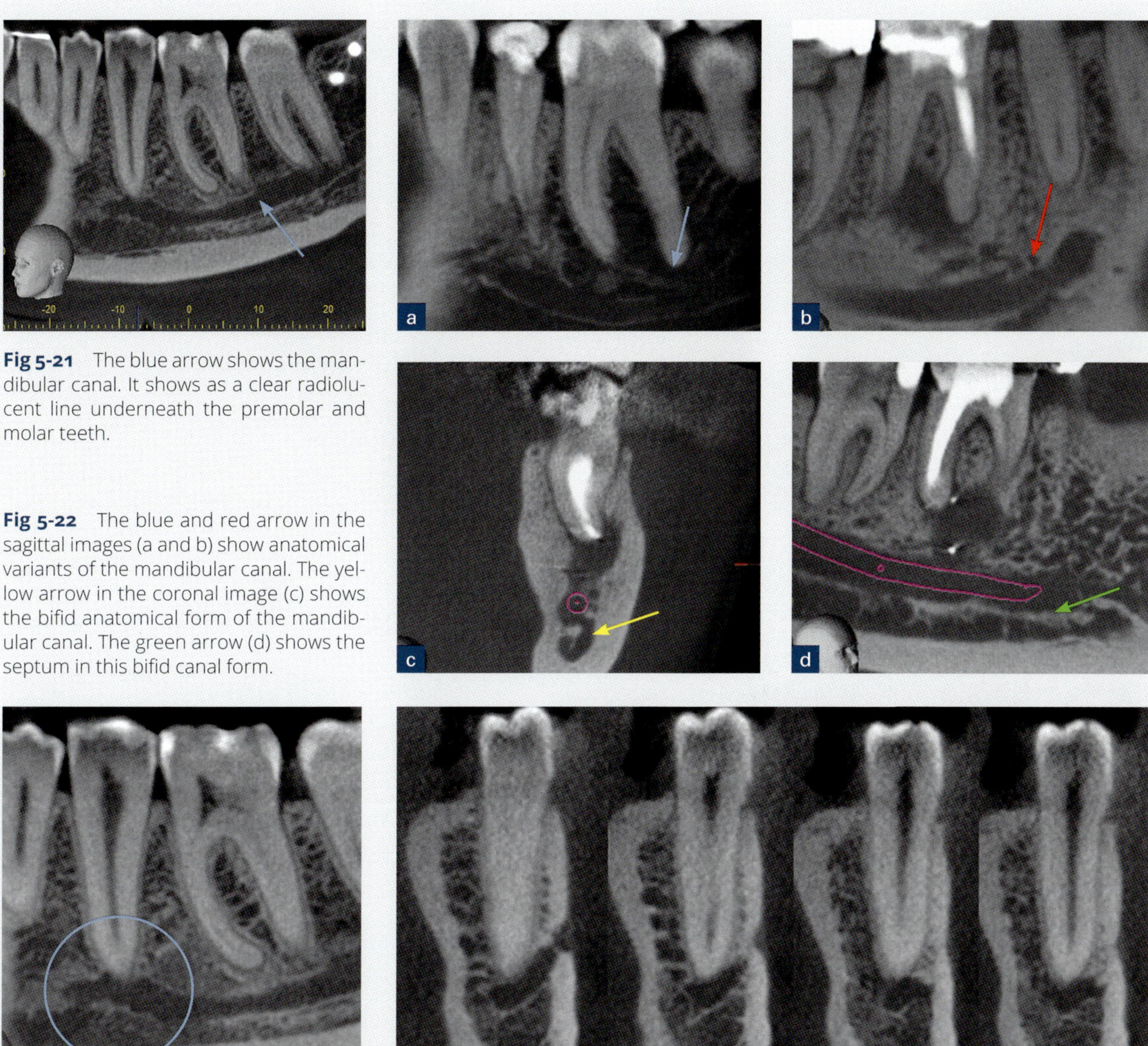

Fig 5-21 The blue arrow shows the mandibular canal. It shows as a clear radiolucent line underneath the premolar and molar teeth.

Fig 5-22 The blue and red arrow in the sagittal images (a and b) show anatomical variants of the mandibular canal. The yellow arrow in the coronal image (c) shows the bifid anatomical form of the mandibular canal. The green arrow (d) shows the septum in this bifid canal form.

Fig 5-23 The blue ring in the (a) sagittal image shows the location of the mental formen. The coronal images (b) show from distal to mesial how the inferior alveolar nerve runs through the mental foramen into the cortical and cancellous bone.

The anatomy of the mental foramen

The final portion of the inferior alveolar nerve passes below the inferior border and the anterior wall of the mental foramen and, after giving off a small incisive branch, curves back to enter the foramen and emerges at the soft tissues as the mental nerve (Fig 5-23). This anatomical feature is also known as an 'anterior loop' of the inferior alveolar nerve (Fig 5-24) (Vujanovic-Eskenazi et al, 2015). Special care should be taken during root canal therapy of second premolars, which are usually in close proximity to the mental foramen (Ngeow, 2010).

The mandibular alveolar bone

The tooth-bearing part of the mandible has similar features to the maxillary alveolar bone. Neurovascular channels may also be seen on a CBCT scan (Fig 5-25).

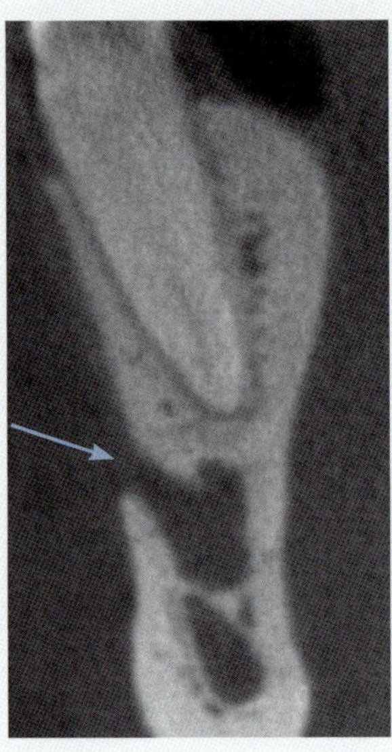

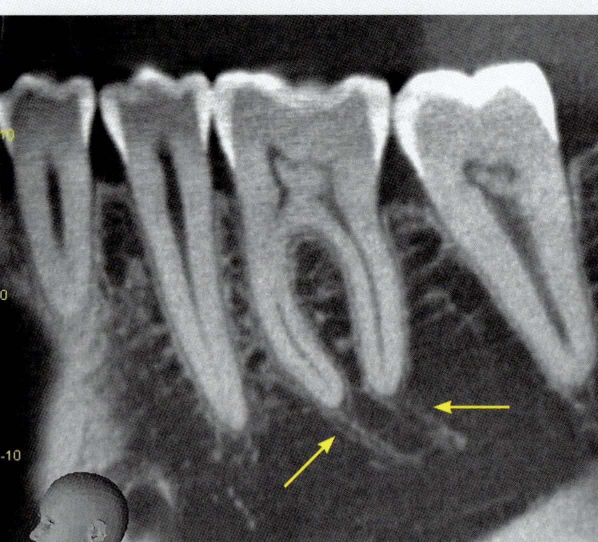

Fig 5-24 Coronal view in mandibular premolar region with mental foramen indicated (blue arrow).

Fig 5-25 Neurovascular canals extending from the apices of the mandibular molar (yellow arrows).

Conclusions

Many anatomical features may be distinguished on CBCT scans because of their ability to demonstrate three-dimensional structures and minimise superimposition of adjacent structures. The clinician should be familiar with these anatomical features in order to differentiate between normal and pathological anatomical features.

References

von Arx T, Fodich I, Bornstein MM. Proximity of premolar roots to maxillary sinus: a radiographic survey using cone beam computed tomography. J Endod 2014;40:1541–1548.

Eberhardt JA, Torabinejad M, Christiansen EL. A computed tomographic study of the distances between the maxillary sinus floor and the apices of the maxillary posterior teeth. Oral Surg Oral Med Oral Pathol 1992;73:345–346.

Gambarini G, Plotino G, Grande NM, et al. Differential diagnosis of endodontic-related inferior alveolar nerve paraesthesia with cone beam computed tomography: a case report. Int Endod J 2011;44:176–181.

Jung YH, Cho BH. Assessment of the relationship between the maxillary molars and adjacent structures using cone beam computed tomography. Imaging Sci Dent 2012;42:219–224.

Kovisto T, Ahmad M, Bowles WR. Proximity of the mandibular canal to the tooth apex. J Endod 2011;37:311–315.

Lu Y, Liu Z, Zhang L, et al. Associations between maxillary sinus mucosal thickening and apical periodontitis using cone beam computed tomography scanning: a retrospective study. J Endod 2012;38:1069–1074.

Neugebauer J, Ritter L, Mischkowski RA, et al. Evaluation of maxillary sinus anatomy by cone-beam CT prior to sinus floor elevation. Int J Oral Maxillofac Implants 2010;25:258–265.

Ngeow WC. Is there a "safety zone" in the mandibular premolar region where damage to the mental nerve can be avoided if periapical extrusion occurs? J Can Dent Assoc 2010;76:a61.

Ok E, Güngör E, Colak M, Altunsoy M, Nur GB, Ağlarci OS. Evaluation of the relationship between the maxillary posterior teeth and the sinus floor using cone beam computed tomography. Surg Radiol Anat 2014;36:907–914.

Pogrel MA. Damage to the inferior alveolar nerve as the result of root canal therapy. J Am Dent Assoc 2007;138:65–69.

Rak KM, Newell JD 2nd, Yakes WF, Damiano MA, Luethke JM. Paranasal sinuses on MR images of the brain: significance of mucosal thickening. AJR Am J Roentgenol 1991;156:381–384.

Rashsuren O, Choi JW, Han WJ, Kim EK. Assessment of bifid and trifid mandibular canals using cone-beam computed tomography. Imaging Sci Dent 2014;44:229–236.

Sato I, Ueno R, Kawai T, Yosue T. Rare courses of the mandibular canal in the molar regions of the human mandible: a cadaveric study. Okajimas Folia Anat Jpn 2005;82:95–101.

Shanbdag S, Karnik P, Shirke P, Shanbdag V. Association between periapical lesions and maxillary sinus mucosal thickening: a retrospective cone beam computed tomography study. J Endod 2013;39:853–857.

Sharan A, Madjar D. Maxillary sinus pneumatization following extractions: a radiographic study. Int J Oral Maxillofac Implants 2008;23:48–56.

Vallo J, Suominen-Taipale L, Huumonen S, Soikkonen K, Norblad A. Prevalence of mucosal abnormalities of the maxillary sinus and their relationship to dental disease in panoramic radiography: results from the Health 2000 Health Examination Survey. Oral Surg Oral Med Oral Pathol Oral Radiol Endod 2010;109:e80–87.

Vujanovic-Eskenazi A, Valero-James JM, Sánchez-Garcés MA, Gay-Escoda C. A retrospective radiographic evaluation of the anterior loop of the mental nerve: comparison between panoramic radiography and cone beam computerized tomography. Med Oral Patol Oral Cir Bucal 2015;20:e239–245.

Chapter 6

Assessment of Root Canal Anatomy

Francesca Abella, Shalini Kanagasingam

Introduction

Anatomical variations exist with each tooth type and may be a result of differences in ethnic background, age and gender of the population being investigated (Cleghorn et al, 2006). Variations in canal number, configuration, curvature, and presence of accessory roots may pose both diagnostic and clinical challenges (Kulild and Peters, 1990; Vertucci, 2005). An awareness and understanding of root canal anatomy is essential to facilitate endodontic risk assessment and treatment planning.

At present, conventional periapical radiography is regarded as the best clinical practice for preoperative assessment of root canal anatomy (European Society of Endodontology, 2006). However, two-dimensional imaging only permits visualisation of the dentition in the mesiodistal plane. The buccolingual plane (i.e. the third dimension) may not be fully appreciated (Patel, 2009). The diagnostic yield of conventional radiography may be improved by taking additional radiographic views with changes in horizontal angulation (parallax principle) (Vertucci, 2005; Davies et al, 2015). However, even parallax periapical radiographs do not always provide sufficient information on root canal anatomy (Khedmat et al, 2010; Soares de Toubes et al, 2012).

Cone beam computed tomography (CBCT) overcomes these limitations by enabling visualisation of the third dimension, while at the same time eliminating superimposition of overlying dentoalveolar anatomy. The information from a CBCT scan provides the clinician with a more in-depth understanding of the true morphology of root canal systems, including anatomic aberrations (Abella et al, 2011; Zhang et al, 2011). Several studies have concluded that CBCT increases the detection of root canals compared to single and parallax periapical radiography (Cheung et al, 2013; Davies et al, 2015). A recent study demonstrated that both charge-coupled devices (CCDs) and photostimulable phosphor (PSP) plates missed one or more root canals in 40% of anterior and posterior teeth when compared to CBCT (Matherne et al, 2008).

An *in vitro* study by Neelakantan et al (2010) concluded that CBCT analysis of the anatomy and morphology of root canal systems is as accurate as the modified canal staining and clearing technique. Michetti et al (2010) found that there is a high correlation between the information provided by CBCT image reconstructions and histologic examination, which was used as the reference standard.

CBCT has been reported to have comparable accuracy to microcomputed tomography in the analysis of internal and external root geometry (Domark et al, 2013; Paes da Silva Ramos Fernandes et al, 2014). Current evidence appears to validate the reliability and accuracy of CBCT as a tool to assess root canal anatomy.

Complex anatomy

Incisor and canine teeth

CBCT assessment of maxillary central and lateral incisors in a Turkish population reported the prevalence of a supplemental canal in between 0.3% and 3.2% of the study sample. In the same study maxillary canines were shown to have a second canal in 3% of male and 1% of female subjects (Altunsoy et al, 2014). This study also reported a significantly higher prevalence of two canals in maxillary anterior teeth in males.

Mandibular incisors have been shown to exhibit complex anatomy, with the incidence of a supplemental canal in these teeth reported to be as high as 40% (Benjamin and Dawson, 1974). Common variations include oval and flattened canals, which have been

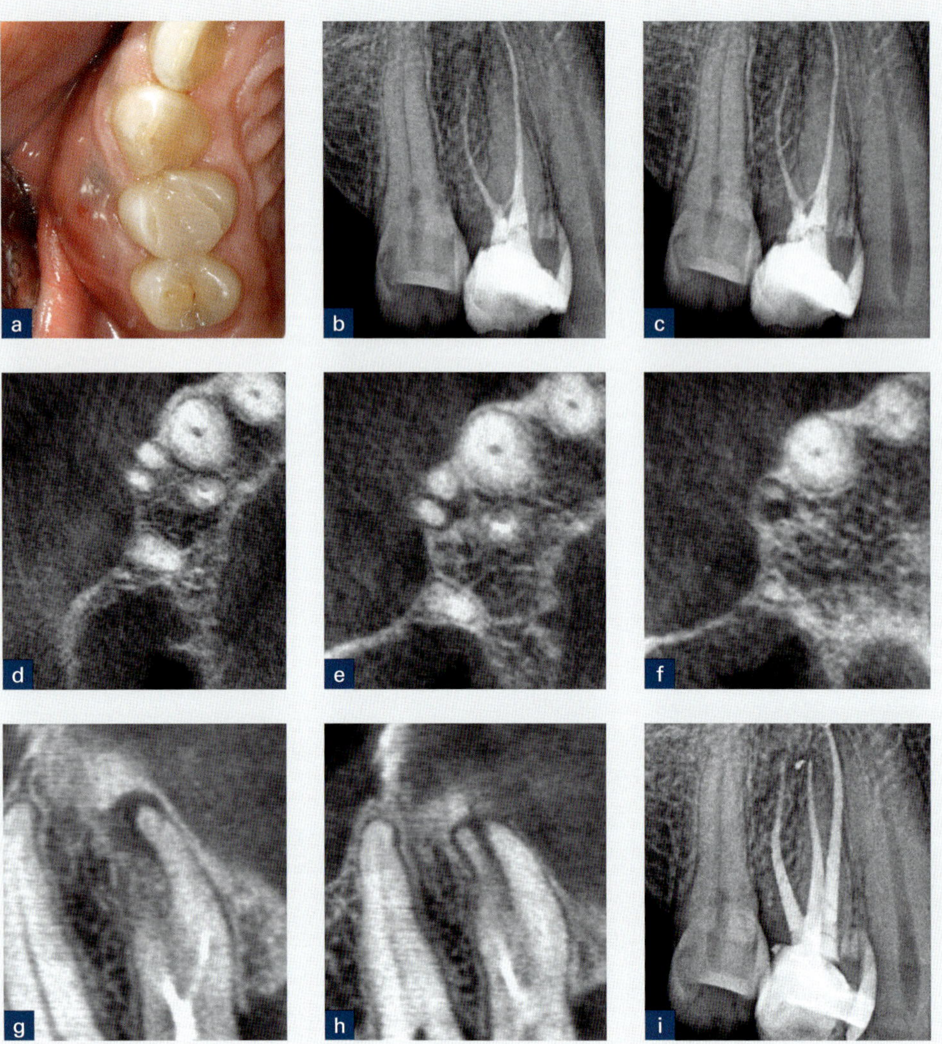

Fig 6-1 (a) Preoperative intraoral photograph of symptomatic right maxillary first premolar, which had been previously root canal treated. (b and c) Two periapical radiographs with differing horizontal beam angles showed that the buccal and palatal canals had been root filled. CBCT axial (d to f) and sagittal (g and h) views revealed the presence of an untreated third root, the mesiobuccal root, associated with a periapical lesion. The mesiobuccal canal was located, guided by the CBCT images. (i) Non-surgical root canal re-treatment was performed and all three canals were obturated to working length, verified by the postoperative periapical radiograph.

reported to be more difficult to disinfect and obturate (Wu et al, 2000). A recent study concluded that CBCT was significantly better than conventional radiography at identifying canals with oval-shaped cross-sections (Paes da Silva Ramos Fernandes et al, 2014).

CBCT studies of mandibular incisor teeth in Chinese and Turkish populations found a higher incidence of a second canal in mandibular lateral incisors compared to central incisors and canines (Altunsoy et al, 2014; Lin et al, 2014; Han et al, 2014).

CBCT also revealed that many of these teeth exhibit bifurcations at the middle third root region (Lin et al, 2014).

Premolar teeth

The assessment of root morphology of maxillary first premolars using CBCT has revealed that the predominant form is a single root with two canals that exit the root apex separately. The next most prevalent configuration is two canals coronally, which join at the apex to form a single canal. The incidence of three roots or three canals is 1% (Tian et al, 2012) (Fig 6-1).

CBCT scans of mandibular first and second premolars showed that 100% and 99%, respectively, were single rooted (Park et al, 2013a). The reported prevalence of one, two and three root canals in mandibular premolar teeth was found to be 87%, 11.2% and 0%, respectively (Yu et al, 2012). An unusual C-shaped canal configuration was seen in 1% of the study sample. In contrast, the ability of conventional radiography to accurately assess the root canal anatomy and morphology of premolar teeth appears to be poor. Khedmat et al (2010) reported that periapical radiographs failed to identify more than 70% of premolar teeth with two or

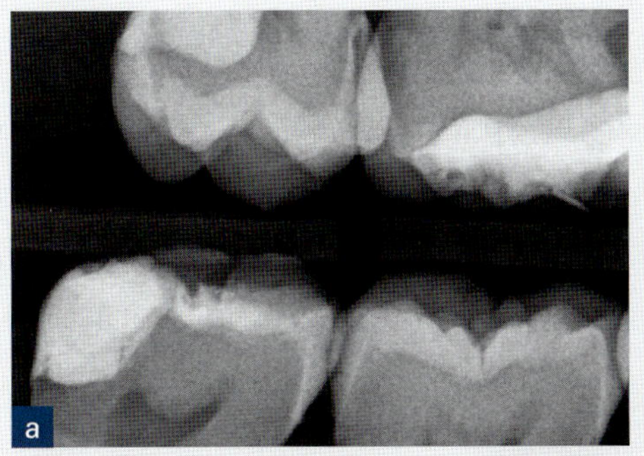

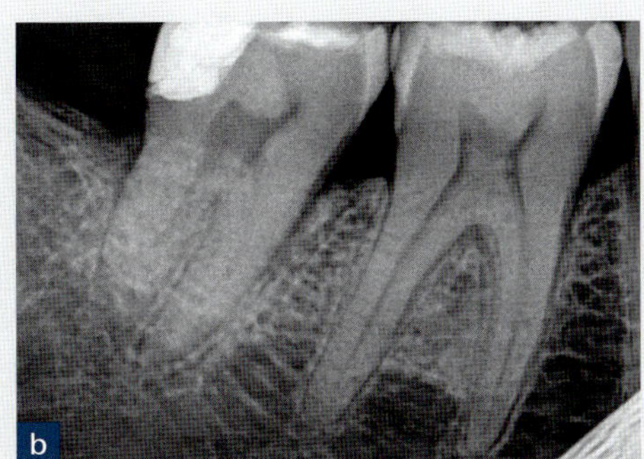

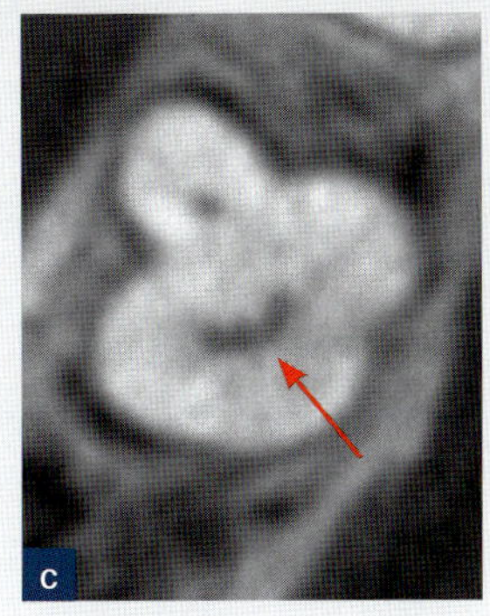

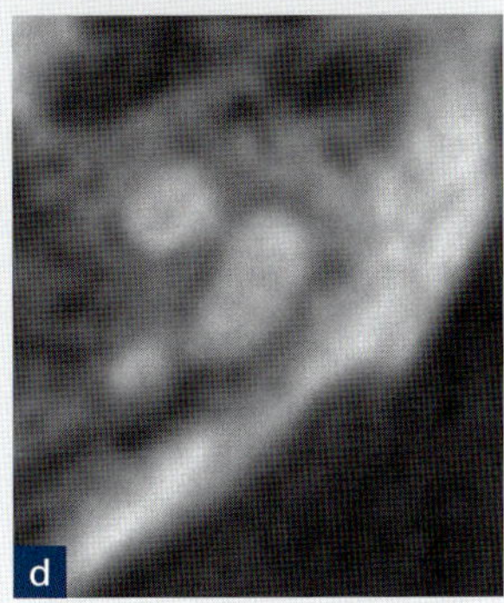

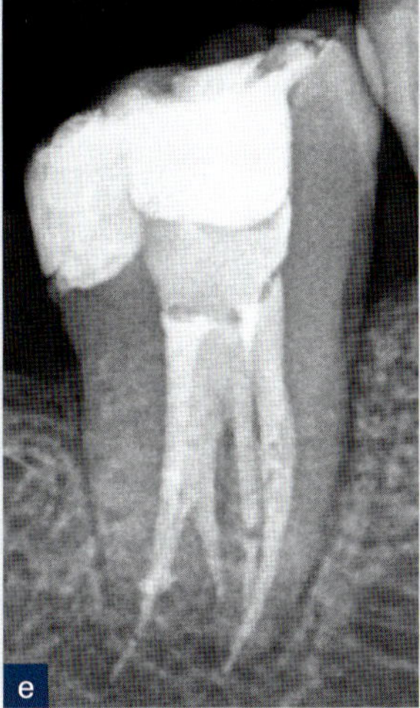

Fig 6-2 (a and b) Bitewing and periapical radiographs of the mandibular right second molar. Due to the buccolingual beam direction of the X-ray, no abnormal anatomy was detected, with the tooth exhibiting separate mesial and distal roots. (c and d) The axial CBCT views demonstrated a C-shaped cross-section as a result of incomplete fusion of the mesial and distal roots. (e) Post-obturation radiograph.

more root canals, compared to the reference standard of cross-sectioning the teeth. The authors found that additional buccolingual periapical views may not identify complex anatomy in mandibular premolars.

Molar teeth

The complexity of the root canal anatomy of maxillary molar teeth has been extensively reported (Kulild and Peters, 1990; Baratto Filho et al, 2009). Although *in vitro* studies have reported that more than 70% of maxillary first molars have a second mesiobuccal (MB2) canal (Görduysus et al, 2001; Barton et al, 2003), parallax periapical radiography has been shown to be unreliable in detecting additional canals in maxillary molar teeth (Barton et al, 2003; Davies et al, 2015). In contrast, the use of CBCT resulted in the detection of more MB2 canals, with reported incidence as high as 91% (Kim et al, 2012; Reis et al, 2013). Bilateral symmetry of mesiobuccal roots has been shown to be in the range of 66% to 88% (Kim et al, 2012; Guo et al, 2014).

The reported incidence of MB2 canals in maxillary second molars, assessed using CBCT, is relatively high, ranging between 34% and 42% (Lee et al, 2011; Kim et al, 2012). Kim et al (2012) reported that fused roots occur more frequently in maxillary second molars, with an incidence of 11% (Kim et al, 2012). The same study identified supplemental canals in 1% of distobuccal roots of maxillary first molars and in 2% of palatal roots of second molars.

Mandibular first molar teeth display several anatomical variations. The major variant in this tooth type is the occurrence of a supplemental distolingual root, which has a reported frequency of between 14% and 29% (Abella et al, 2012; Zhang et al, 2011). Tu et al (2007, 2009) demonstrated that CBCT identifies more of these additional roots compared to conventional periapical radiography. Some mandibular first molar teeth also exhibit an isthmus between the mesiobuccal and mesiolingual canals, which can be instrumented to length (Karapinar-Kazandag et al, 2010). This is known as an accessory mesial canal, an anatomical feature that has been identified by CBCT in between 3% and 27% of Chinese and Brazillian populations, respectively (Wang et al, 2010; Soares de Toubes et al, 2012). The *in vitro* study by Soares de Toubes et al (2012) showed good agreement between CBCT and the dental operating microscope in the detection of accessory mesial canals, compared to parallax digital radiography, which was deemed unreliable for detecting these additional canals.

Mandibular molars with C-shaped canal configurations present distinct endodontic treatment challenges (Fig 6-2). Typically, this canal configuration is

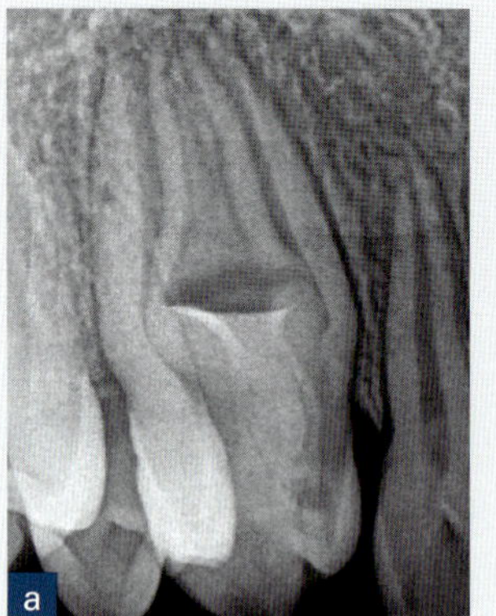

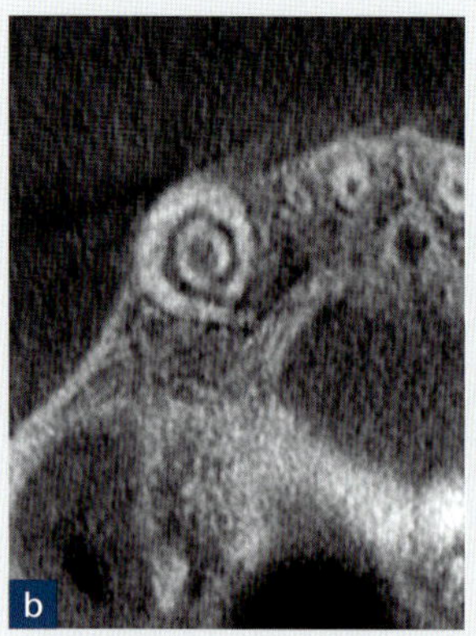

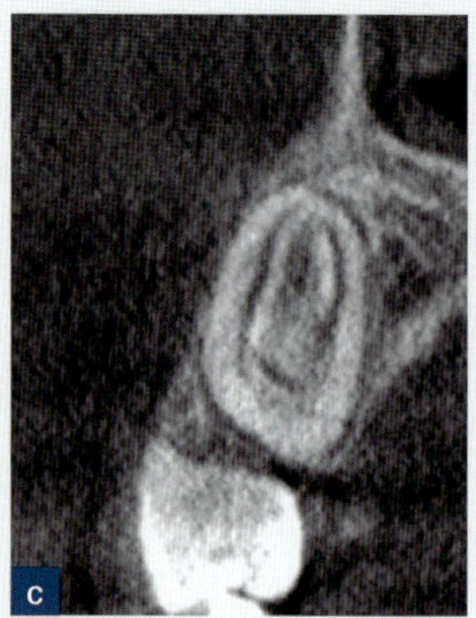

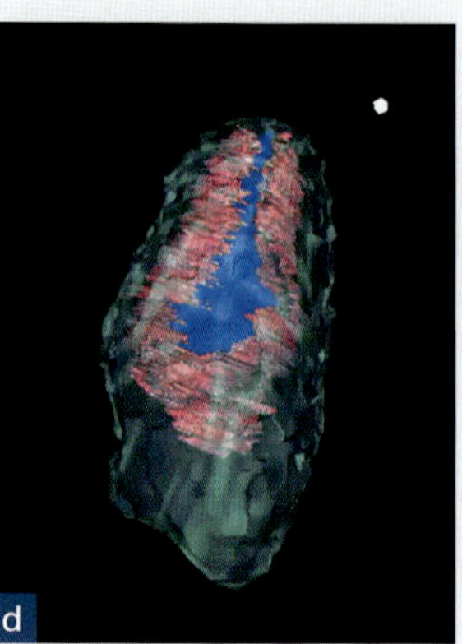

Fig 6-3 (a) Periapical radiograph showing a dens invaginatus of a maxillary right canine. (b and c) CBCT slices were used to reconstruct a three-dimensional (3D) image, which (d) showed no apparent communication between the invagination (blue) and the root canal space (red).

found in teeth with fusion of roots either on the buccal or lingual aspect. The incidence of C-shaped canal systems appears to be dependant on the race of the group under examination and was found to be as low as 3% in an American population, and as high as 31% in Chinese and Korean populations (Yang et al, 1988; Seo et al, 2004).

Zheng et al (2011) examined the root morphology and root canal anatomy of mandibular second molar teeth in a Chinese population using CBCT. They reported that 39% of mandibular second molars had fused roots, and 39% had C-shaped anatomy. The authors also noted that the 'continuous' and 'semi-colon' categories of C-shaped canals have a tendency to divide into multiple canals in the middle and apical regions. C-shaped mandibular molars occurred bilaterally in 81% of the patients studied (Zheng et al, 2011).

Anomalous tooth forms

Genetic, traumatic and environmental factors may cause aberrations in tooth dimension, morphology, position and structure (Brook, 1975). A detailed radiographic examination is essential to determine the existence and nature of the dental anomalies.

Dens invaginatus

Dens invaginatus is a developmental anomaly resulting from epithelial invagination of the crown of the developing tooth before mineralisation. Its prevalence has been reported to be between 0.3% and 10% of teeth, with the maxillary lateral incisor being most commonly affected (Alani and Bishop, 2008). Morphologic variations can range from a minor enamel-lined invagination, to extensive invagination with penetration of the root and communication with the periodontal ligament laterally or at the apical foramen (Oehlers, 1957).

Reconstruction of CBCT data permits a visual and geometrically accurate appreciation of the course of the invagination and how it relates to the main canal(s) of the tooth (Patel, 2010; Nosrat and Schneider, 2015) (Fig 6-3). Case reports have shown how the assessment of CBCT data can allow successful planning of access strategies to the coronal and apical portions of the infected root canal system in cases of dens invaginatus (Durack and Patel, 2011; Capar et al, 2015) (Fig 6-4).

Kfir et al (2013) presented an innovative therapeutic approach by producing precise three-dimensional (3D) models of a tooth with dens invaginatus. These models facilitated the treatment planning process and the trial runs of different treatment techniques prior to clinical implementation. In addition, the authors enhanced the CBCT images with a dynamic 3D video, which clearly illustrated the apical exit of the invagination, its size, and its relationship to the apical foramen of the main root canal.

Taurodontism

Taurodontism is a developmental dental anomaly characterised by vertically enlarged pulp chambers, apical displacement of pulp floors and short roots (Gomes et al, 2012). Taurodontism can occur in between 2.5%

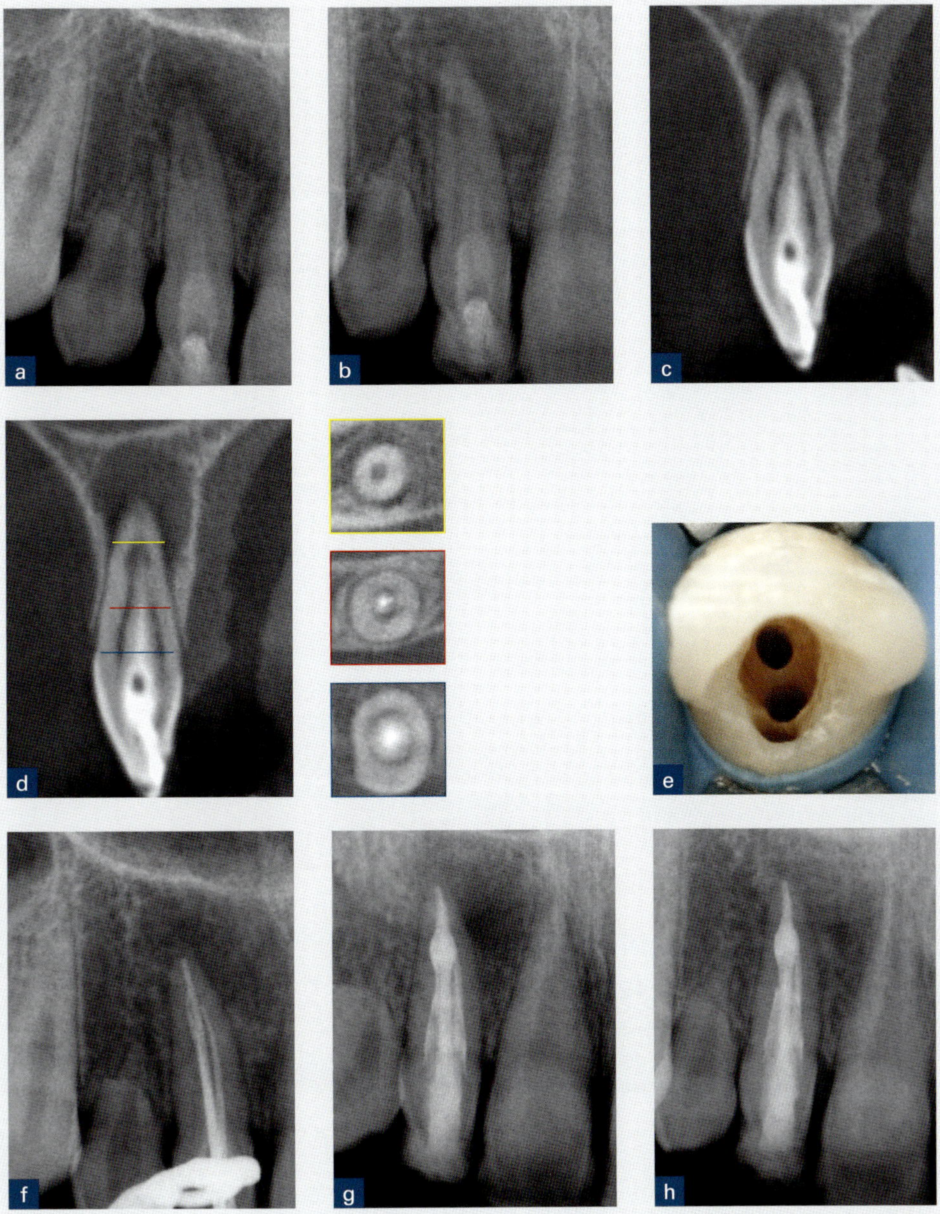

Fig 6-4 (a) Diagnostic periapical radiograph of the invaginated tooth 12. (b) Parallax radiograph. (c) Sagittal reformatted slice of the invaginated tooth. (d) Axial slices at various points denoted on the sagittal section (colour-coded). (e) Access cavity revealing the opening of the invagination (central canal entrance) and the palatal and labial channels created to gain access to the root canal system. (f) Master gutta-percha point radiograph. (g) Post-treatment radiograph. (h) 1-year follow-up revealing complete healing of the periapical radiolucency (courtesy of Durack C, Patel S. The use of cone beam computed tomography in the management of dens invaginatus affecting a strategic tooth in a patient affected by hypodontia: a case report. Int Endod J 2011;44:474–483.

and 3.5% of chromosomally normal Caucasians, but is more commonly associated with syndromic patients (Marques-da-Silva et al, 2010). This anomalous tooth form presents challenges for the location of the root entrances, and exhibits variability in the number of root canals, with some reports describing the existence of up to six canals (Sert and Bayirli, 2004). Extreme variations in root canal anatomy among taurodonts, including maxillary and mandibular hypertaurodonts with C-shaped canals, have been identified using CBCT (Fig 6-5) (Radwan and Kim, 2014).

Fused teeth

Fusion is defined as the union of two or more separately developing tooth germs at the dentinal level during odontogenesis, resulting in the formation of a single large tooth. The prevalence of tooth fusion is estimated to be between 0.5% and 2.5% in the primary dentition, with a lower occurrence in the permanent dentition (Hülsmann et al, 1997). Depending on the stage of development at which fusion occurs, pulp chambers and root canals may be joined or separated (Fig 6-6).

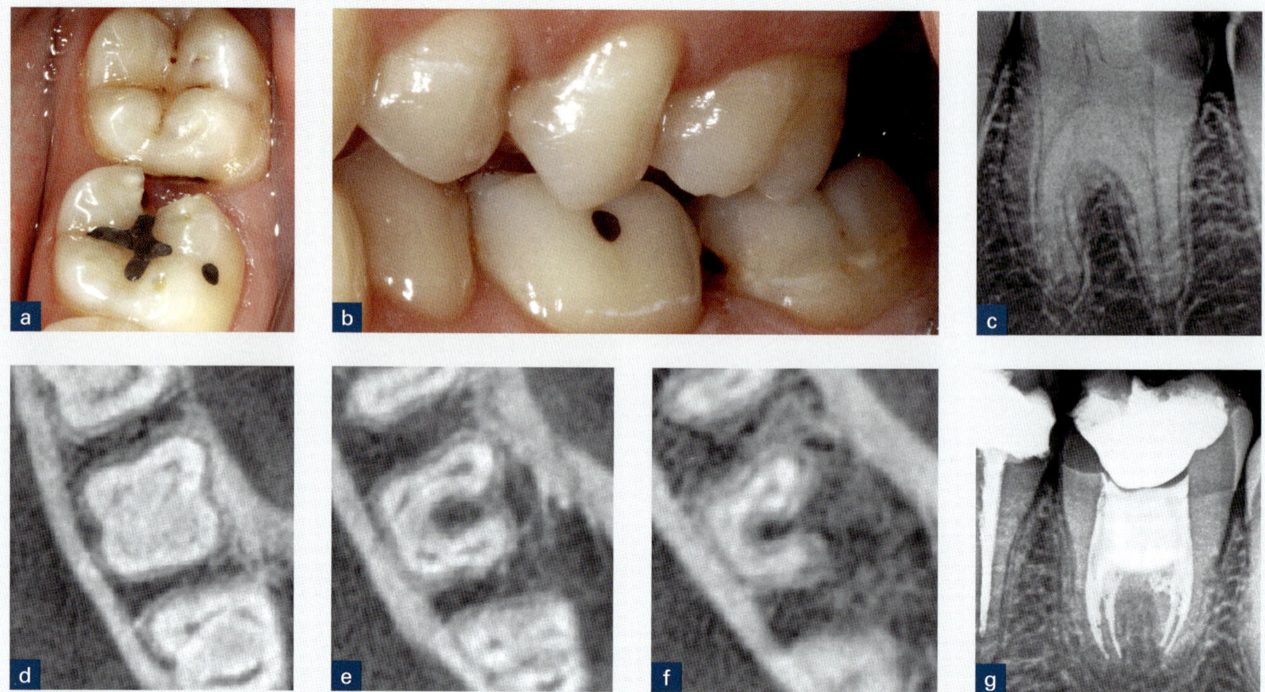

Fig 6-5 (a and b) Intraoral photographs of a carious mandibular left first molar. (c) Periapical radiograph reveals taurodont anatomy. (d to f) CBCT axial views reveal a C-shaped canal anatomy. (g) Guided by the CBCT images, obturation was carried out for all canals.

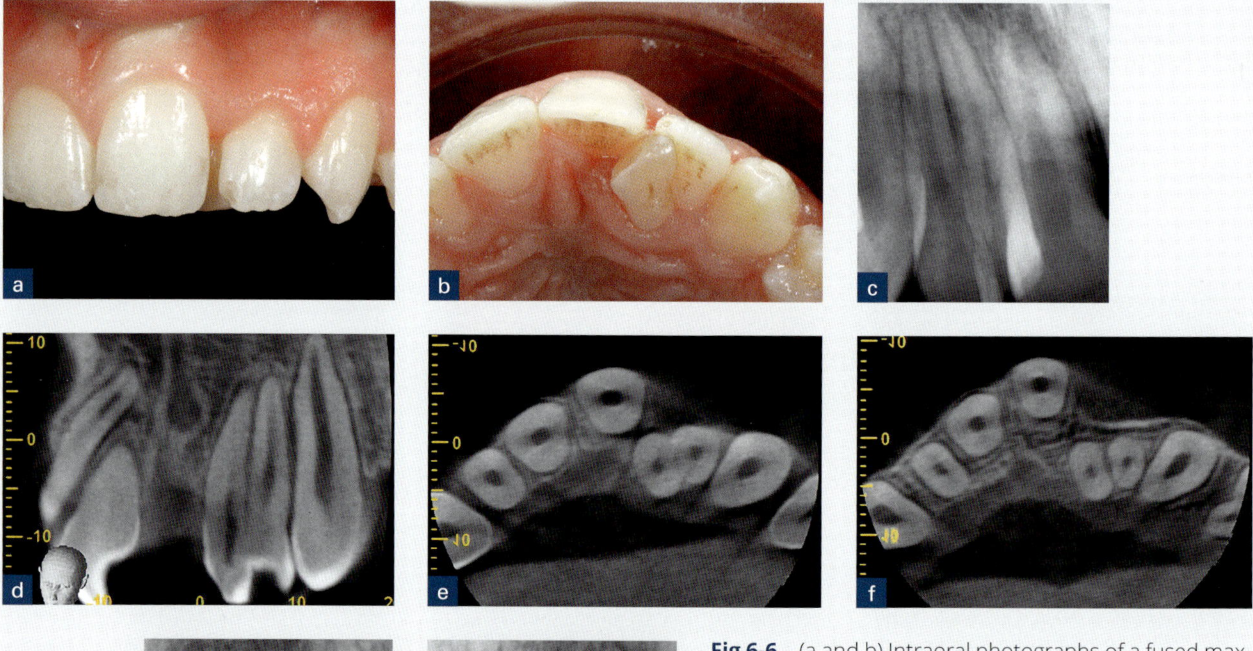

Fig 6-6 (a and b) Intraoral photographs of a fused maxillary left lateral (second incisor) tooth. (c) Periapical radiographs of the same tooth. The palatal portion of the fused tooth was to be surgically removed. (d) Coronal and (e and f) axial reconstructed images confirm no fusion in the apical half, and that the pulp chambers are completely separate, therefore root canal treatment was not required. (g) A post-treatment radiograph after the palatal portion of the tooth was removed. (h) 1-year follow-up radiograph—note the bony infill.

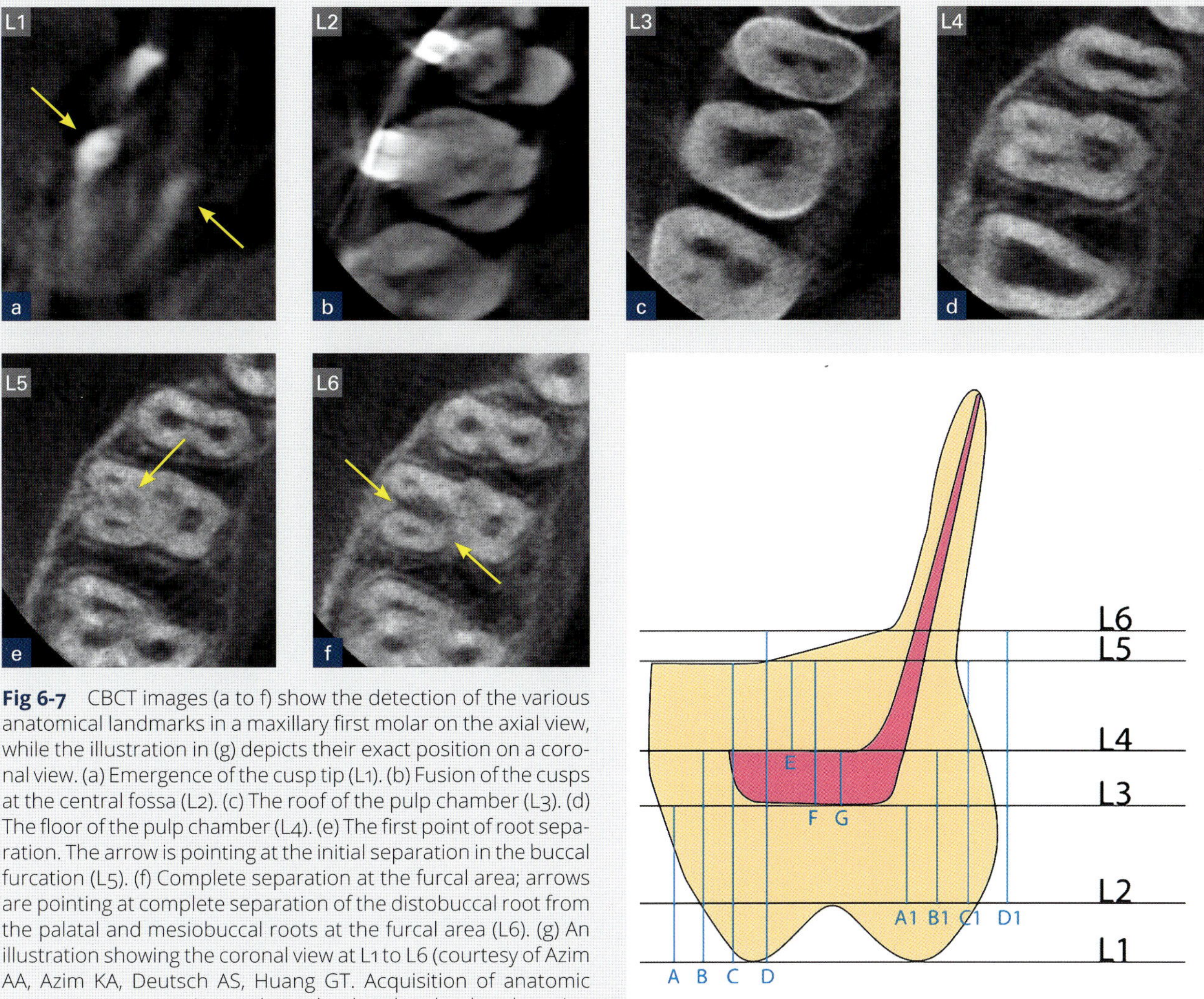

Fig 6-7 CBCT images (a to f) show the detection of the various anatomical landmarks in a maxillary first molar on the axial view, while the illustration in (g) depicts their exact position on a coronal view. (a) Emergence of the cusp tip (L1). (b) Fusion of the cusps at the central fossa (L2). (c) The roof of the pulp chamber (L3). (d) The floor of the pulp chamber (L4). (e) The first point of root separation. The arrow is pointing at the initial separation in the buccal furcation (L5). (f) Complete separation at the furcal area; arrows are pointing at complete separation of the distobuccal root from the palatal and mesiobuccal roots at the furcal area (L6). (g) An illustration showing the coronal view at L1 to L6 (courtesy of Azim AA, Azim KA, Deutsch AS, Huang GT. Acquisition of anatomic parameters concerning molar pulp chamber landmarks using cone-beam computed tomography. J Endod 2014;40:1298–1302).

Song et al (2010) reported on the use of CBCT in the endodontic management of a supernumerary tooth fused to a right maxillary first molar. The information obtained from the CBCT examination facilitated the endodontic treatment of the infected supernumerary tooth and the repair of the communication with the molar tooth, which continued to remain vital and symptom-free following treatment.

Pulp chamber parameters

It has been shown that CBCT imaging can be used to measure pulp chamber parameters and volumetric changes (Azim et al, 2014; Venkatesh et al, 2014). By identifying CBCT coronal view landmarks (e.g. cusp tip, central fossa, pulp chamber roof, furcation, etc), investigators were able to measure the average depth of access preparation in maxillary and mandibular molars (Fig 6-7). They concluded that access preparation should not extend beyond 6.0 mm from the central fossa, or 7.0 mm from the cusp tip, to reach the pulp chamber (Azim et al, 2014). A separate study used CBCT data, which were reconstructed with surface and volume rendering software, to calculate volumetric changes in the pulp cavity during orthodontic treatment. Investigators were able to show that applying orthodontic force had a degenerative effect, which produced a significant decrease in the size of the pulp chamber (Venkatesh et al, 2014).

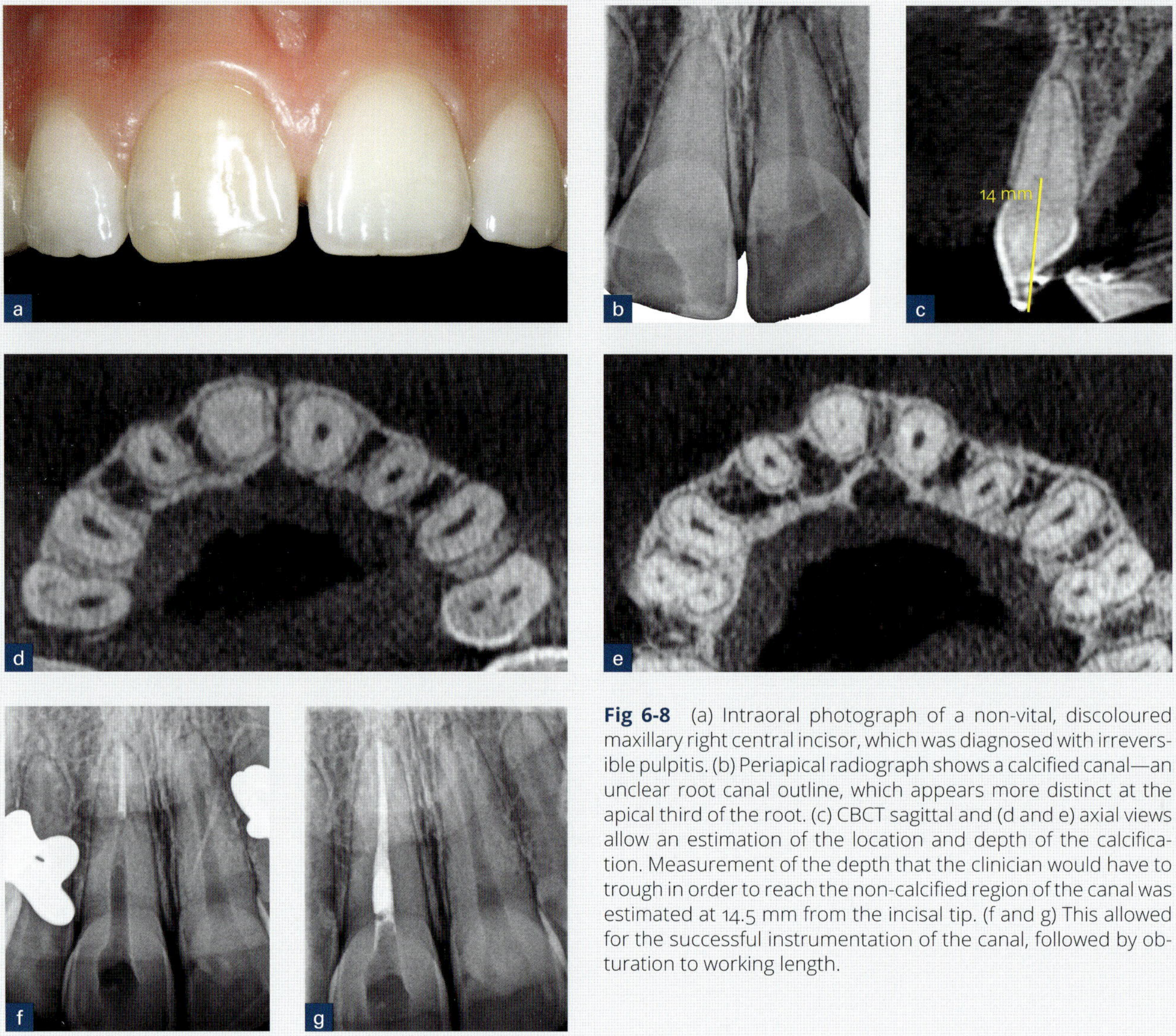

Fig 6-8 (a) Intraoral photograph of a non-vital, discoloured maxillary right central incisor, which was diagnosed with irreversible pulpitis. (b) Periapical radiograph shows a calcified canal—an unclear root canal outline, which appears more distinct at the apical third of the root. (c) CBCT sagittal and (d and e) axial views allow an estimation of the location and depth of the calcification. Measurement of the depth that the clinician would have to trough in order to reach the non-calcified region of the canal was estimated at 14.5 mm from the incisal tip. (f and g) This allowed for the successful instrumentation of the canal, followed by obturation to working length.

Root length and curvature

Information regarding root canal length and curvature is essential to facilitate root canal instrumentation to the appropriate length and to minimise treatment aberrations. A prospective, controlled clinical study examined endodontic working-length measurements in patients with pre-existing CBCT scans and reported a high correlation between the working lengths determined using CBCT and electronic apex locators (Jeger et al, 2012).

Ex vivo human cadaver studies have confirmed the accuracy and reliability of CBCT measurement of root length compared to reference standard, which involved extraction and direct measurement of working length with endodontic files (Liang et al, 2013, Metska et al, 2014). Furthermore, CBCT measurements of the working lengths of posterior teeth are significantly more accurate than those obtained using periapical radiography (Metska et al, 2014). In cases of calcified canals, information from CBCT allows conservative removal of tooth structure to aid with their location. The CBCT measurement tool is useful in these cases to provide an approximation of the distance and direction for continued dentine removal in order to locate the root canal (Fig 6-8). CBCT imaging has also been shown to be able to locate the position of the apical foramen (Jeger et al, 2012; Liang et al, 2013) , as well as recreating the root canal anatomy system (Fig 6-9).

Estrela et al (2008) presented a simple and reliable method for assessing the severity of the radius of

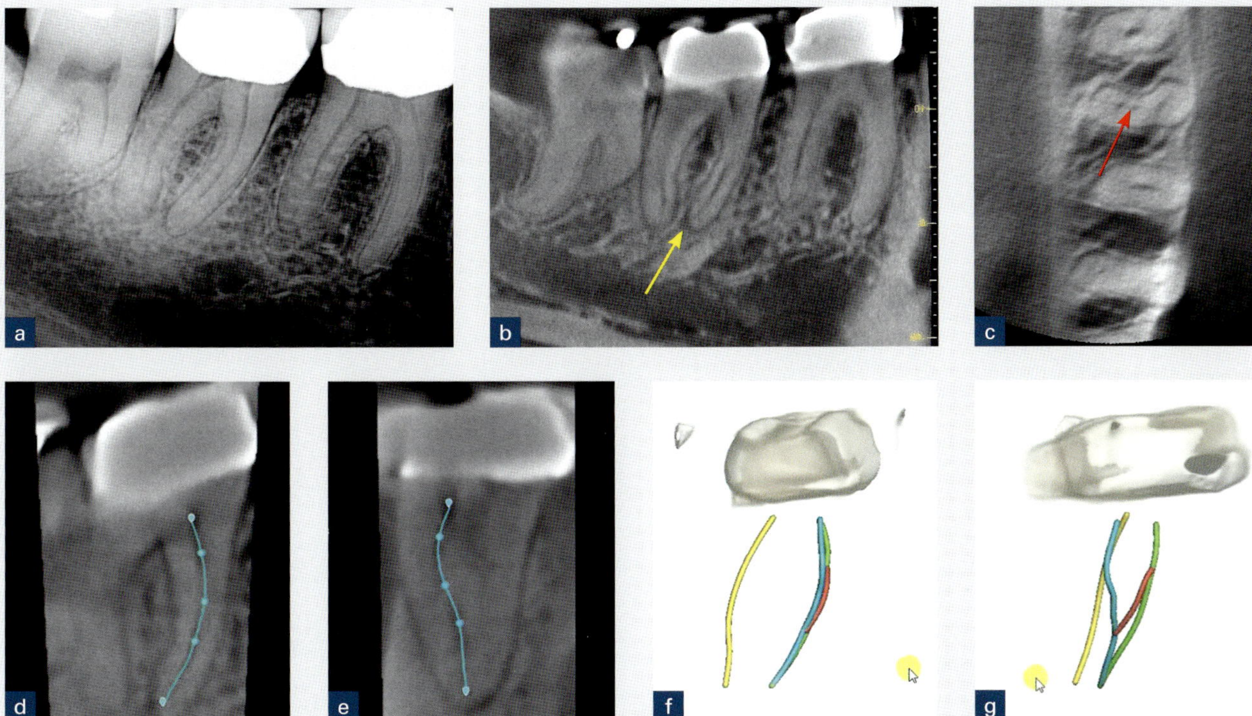

Fig 6-9 (a) A periapical radiograph of the mandibular right first and second molar teeth. (b) A CBCT reconstructed sagittal view confirms the presence of a periapical radiolucency associated with the distal root of the second molar tooth (yellow arrow). (c) The reconstructed axial view reveals a third, mid-mesial root canal (red arrow). (d and e) The DICOM data is imported into 3D Endo software (Dentsply, Ballaigues, Switzerland), which allows the clinician to trace each canal in the (d) sagittal and (e) coronal views. (f and g) Once all the root canals have been traced, the root canal anatomy can be assessed in real-time in 3D. This gives the clinician a real appreciation of the anatomy of the tooth, which is especially relevant for inexperienced clinicians. Note how the mid-mesial canal (red) branches off the mesiolingual canal (green) and joins the mesiobuccal canal (blue).

curvature of root canals using CBCT, based on three mathematical points. Park et al (2013b) employed sophisticated mathematical modelling software and CBCT scans to calculate points of maximum curvature, or points of maximum abruptness of curvature. Analysis of the transverse and sagittal CBCT slices enabled the determination of the mesiodistal and labiolingual direction of curvature (Fig 6-10). The authors concluded that the curvature of the maxillary lateral incisor root canals was mainly oriented in the distopalatal direction, with the point of maximum curvature located 0.5 mm from the root apex.

Conclusion

The ability to identify the location of all root canals and to recognise their anatomical and morphological features and/or aberrations is essential to improve the outcome of endodontic treatment (Baratto Filho et al, 2009; Khedmat et al, 2010).

Periapical radiography is an integral part of endodontic diagnosis and is essential for the assessment of root canal anatomy. However, the diagnostic yield of this imaging modality is limited by it being two-dimensional in nature. Sufficient appreciation of teeth with complex root canal anatomy may not be possible from a periapical radiograph, although the parallax technique may provide additional information in certain cases (Klein et al, 1997). However, as described in this chapter, CBCT may reveal additional information about the root canal and root anatomy, which may ultimately influence the management of teeth with complex anatomy.

CBCT is associated with a higher ionising radiation dose to the patient. Each CBCT examination must therefore be justified (ICRP, 2007; Patel and Horner, 2009). In order to minimise unnecessary exposure of patients to ionising radiation, the use of CBCT should

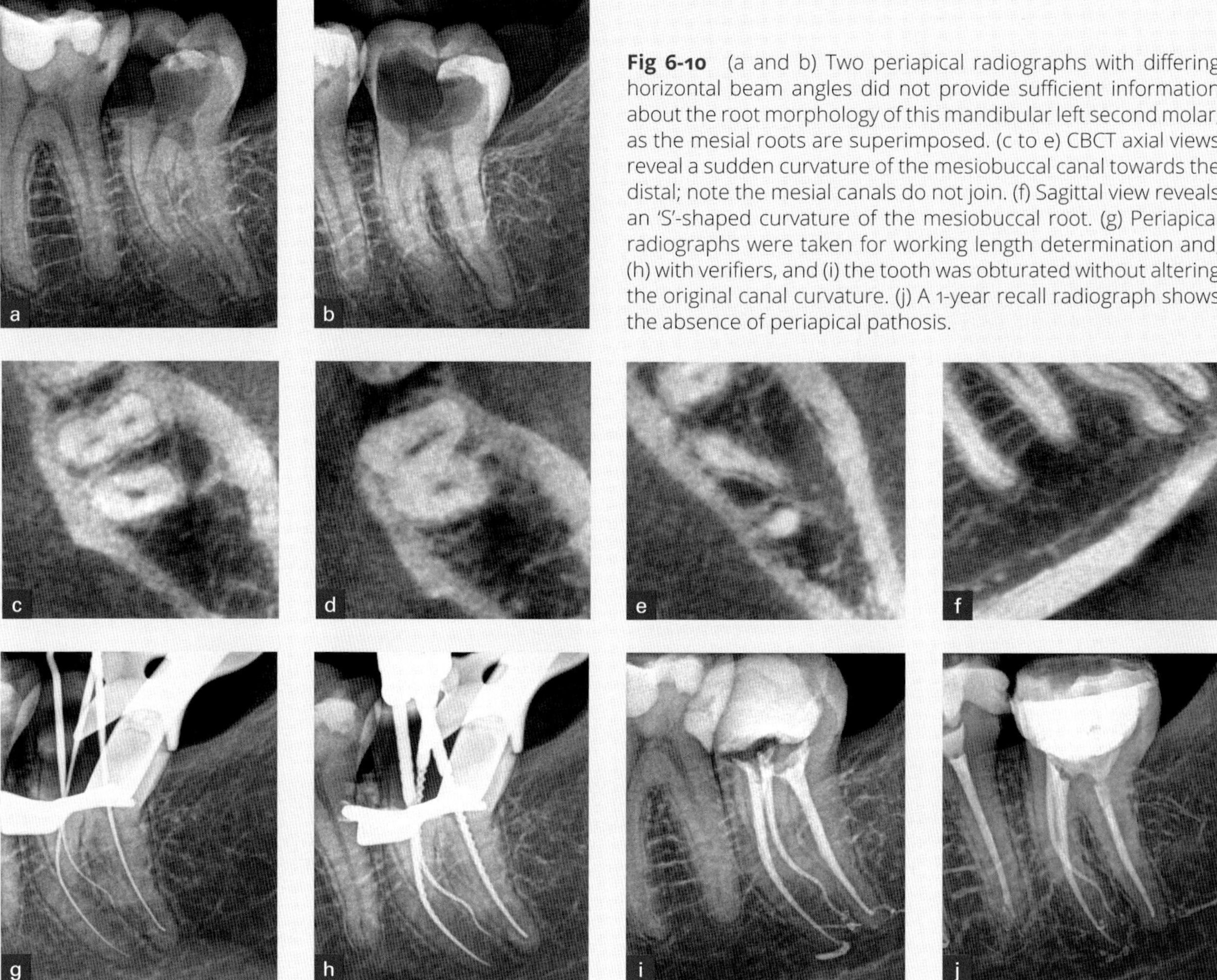

Fig 6-10 (a and b) Two periapical radiographs with differing horizontal beam angles did not provide sufficient information about the root morphology of this mandibular left second molar, as the mesial roots are superimposed. (c to e) CBCT axial views reveal a sudden curvature of the mesiobuccal canal towards the distal; note the mesial canals do not join. (f) Sagittal view reveals an 'S'-shaped curvature of the mesiobuccal root. (g) Periapical radiographs were taken for working length determination and, (h) with verifiers, and (i) the tooth was obturated without altering the original canal curvature. (j) A 1-year recall radiograph shows the absence of periapical pathosis.

only be used for the assessment of complex root canal anatomy, morphology, and anomalous tooth forms where conventional radiographs and clinical examination do not provide sufficient information to facilitate predictable endodontic treatment (European Society of Endodontology CBCT position statement, 2014).

Clinicians must be aware of the inherent limitations of CBCT (see Chapter 4). Due to their relatively low resolution, CBCT scans are unlikely to detect sclerosed or accessory canals (European Society of Endodontology CBCT position statement, 2014). Existing root canal filling materials may introduce artefacts, which may impair the detection of supplemental canals in re-treatment cases and also possibly mimic fracture lines and/or supplemental canals (Soğur et al, 2007; Huybrechts et al, 2009; Patel, 2009; Vizzotto et al, 2013), potentially leading to misdiagnoses.

References

Abella F, Mercadé M, Durán-Sindreu F, Roig M. Managing severe curvature of radix entomolaris: three-dimensional analysis with cone beam computed tomography. Int Endod J 2011;44:876–885.

Abella F, Patel S, Durán-Sindreu F, Mercadé M, Roig M. Mandibular first molars with disto-lingual roots: review and clinical management. Int Endod J 2012;45:963–978.

Alani A, Bishop K. Dens invaginatus. Part 1: classification, prevalence and aetiology. Int Endod J 2008;41:1123–1136.

Altunsoy M, Ok E, Nur BG, Ağlarci AS, Güngör E, Colak M. A cone-beam computed tomography study of the root canal morphology of anterior teeth in a Turkish population. Eur J Dent 2014;8:302–306.

Azim AA, Azim KA, Deutsch As, Huang GT. Acquisition of anatomic parameters concerning molar pulp chamber landmarks using cone-beam computed tomography. J Endod 2014;40:1298–1302.

Baratto Filho F, Zaitter S, Haragushiku GA, de Campos EA, Abuabara A, Correr GM. Analysis of the internal anatomy of maxillary first molars by using different methods. J Endod 2009;35:337–342.

Barton DJ, Clark SJ, Eleazer PD, Scheetz JP, Farman AG. Tuned-aperture computed tomography versus parallax analog and digital radiographic images in detecting second mesiobuccal canals in maxillary first molars. Oral Surg Oral Med Oral Pathol Oral Radiol Endod 2003;96:223–228.

Benjamin KA, Dawson J. Incidence of two root canals in human mandibular incisor teeth. Oral Surg Oral Med Oral Pathol 1974;38:122–126.Brook AH. Variables and criteria in prevalence studies of dental anomalies of number, form and size. Community Dent Oral Epidemiol 1975;6:288–293.

Brook AH. Variables and criteria in prevalence studies of dental anomalies of number, form and size. Community Dent Oral Epidemiol 1975;6:288–293.

Capar AD, Ertas H, Arslan H, Ertas AT. A retrospective comparative study of cone-beam computed tomography versus rendered panoramic images in identifying the presence, types, and characteristics of dens invaginatus in a Turkish population. J Endod 2015;41:473–478.

Cheung GS, Wei WL, McGrath C. Agreement between periapical radiographs and cone-beam computed tomography for assessment of periapical status of root filled molar teeth. Int Endod J 2013;46:889–895.

Cleghorn BM, Christie WH, Dong CC. Root and root canal morphology of the human permanent maxillary first molar: a literature review. J Endod 2006:32:813–821.

Davies A, Mannocci F, Mitchell P, Andiappan M, Patel S. The detection of periapical pathoses in root filled teeth using single and parallax periapical radiographs versus cone beam computed tomography - a clinical study. Int Endod J 2015;48:582–592.

Domark JD, Hatton JF, Benison RP, Hildebort CF. An ex vivo comparison of digital radiography, cone beam and micro computed tomography in the detection of the number of canals in the mesiobuccal roots of maxillary molars. J Endod 2013;39:901–905.

Durack C, Patel S. The use of cone beam computed tomography in the management of dens invaginatus affecting a strategic tooth in a patient affected by hypodontia: a case report. Int Endod J 2011;44:474–483.

Estrela C, Bueno MR, Sousa-Neto MD, Pécora JD. Method for determination of root curvature radius using cone-beam computed tomography images. Braz Dent J 2008;19:114–118.

European Society of Endodontology. Quality guidelines for endodontic treatment: consensus report of the European Society of Endodontology. Int Endod J 2006;39:921–930.

European Society of Endodontology, Patel S, Durack C, et al. European Society of Endodontology position statement: the use of CBCT in Endodontics. Int Endod J 2014;47:502–504.

Gomes RR, Habckost CD, Junqueira LG, et al. Taurodontism in Brazilian patients with tooth agenesis and first and second-degree relatives: a case-control study. Arch Oral Biol 2012;57:1062–1069.

Görduysus MO, Görduysus M, Friedman S. Operating microscope improves negotiation of second mesiobuccal canals in maxillary molars. J Endod 2001;27:683–686.

Guo J, Vahidnia A, Sedghizadeh P, Enciso R. Evaluation of root and canal morphology of maxillary permanent first molars in a North American population by cone-beam computed tomography. J Endod 2014;40:635–639.

Han T, Ma Y, Yang L, Chen X, Zhang X, Wang Y. A study of the root canal morphology of mandibular anterior teeth using cone-beam computed tomography in a Chinese subpopulation. J Endod 2014;40:1309–1314.

Hülsmann M, Bahr R, Grohmann U. Hemisection and vital treatment of a fused tooth—literature review and case report. Endod Dent Traumatol 1997;13:253–258.

Huybrechts B, Bud M, Bergmans L, Lambrechts P, Jacobs R. Void detection in root fillings using intraoral analogue, intraoral digital and cone beam CT images. Int Endod J 2009;42:675–685.

ICRP Publication 103. The 2007 Recommendations of the International Commission on Radiological Protection. Ann ICRP 2007;37:1–332.

Jeger FB, Janner SF, Bornstein MM, Lussi A. Endodontic working length measurement with preexisting cone-beam computed tomography scanning: a prospective, controlled clinical study. J Endod 2012;38:884–888.

Karapinar-Kazandag M, Basrani BR, Friedman S. The operating microscope enhances detection and negotiation of accessory mesial canals in mandibular molars. J Endod 2010;36:1289–1294.

Kfir A, Telishevsky-Strauss Y, Leitner A, Metzger Z. The diagnosis and conservative treatment of a complex type 3 dens invaginatus using cone beam computed tomography (CBCT) and 3D plastic models. Int Endod J 2013;46:275–288.

Khedmat S, Assadian H, Saravani AA. Root canal morphology of the mandibular first premolars in an Iranian population using cross-sections and radiography. J Endod 2010;36:214–217.

Kim Y, Lee SJ, Woo J. Morphology of maxillary first and second molars analyzed by cone-beam computed tomography in a Korean population: variations in the number of roots and canals and the incidence of fusion. J Endod 2012;38:1063–1068.

Klein RMF, Blake SA, Nattress BR, Hirschmann PN. Evaluation of X-ray beam angulation for successful twin canal identification in mandibular incisors. Int Endod J 1997;30:58–63.

Kulild JC, Peters DD. Incidence and configuration of canal systems in the mesiobuccal root of maxillary first and second molars. J Endod 1990;16:311–317.

Lee JH, Kim KD, Lee JK, et al. Mesiobuccal root canal anatomy of Korean maxillary first and second molars by cone-beam computed tomography. Oral Surg Oral Med Oral Pathol Oral Radiol Endod 2011;111:785–791.

Liang YH, Jiang L, Chen C, et al. The validity of cone-beam computed tomography in measuring root canal length using a gold standard. J Endod 2013;39:1607–1610.

Lin Z, Hu Q, Wang T, et al. Use of CBCT to investigate the root canal morphology of mandibular incisors. Surg Radiol Anat 2014;36:877–882.

Marques-da-Silva B, Baratto Filho F, Abuabara A, Moura P, Losso EM, Moro A. Multiple taurodontism: the challenge of endodontic treatment. J Oral Sci 2010;52:653–658.

Matherne RP, Angelopoulus C, Kulild JC, Tira D. Use of cone-beam computed tomography to identify root canal systems in vitro. J Endod 2008;34:87–89.

Metska ME, Liem VML, Parsa A, Koolstra JH, Wesselink PR, Ozok AR. Cone-beam computed tomographic scans in comparison with periapical radiographs for root canal length measurement: an in situ study. J Endod 2014;40:1206–1209.

Michetti J, Maret D, Mallet JP, Diemer F. Validation of cone beam computed tomography as a tool to explore root canal anatomy. J Endod 2010;36:1187–1190.

Neelakantan P, Subbarao C, Subbarao VC. Comparative evaluation of modified canal staining and clearing technique, cone-beam computed tomography, peripheral quantitative computed tomography, spiral computed tomography, and plain and contrast medium-enhanced digital radiography in studying root canal morphology. J Endod 2010;36:1547–1551.

Nosrat A, Schneider SC. Endodontic management of a maxillary lateral incisor with four root canals and a dens invaginatus tract. J Endod 2015;41:1167–1171.

Oehlers FA. Dens invaginatus (dilated composite odontome). I. Variations of the invagination process and associated anterior crown forms. Oral Surg Oral Med Oral Pathol 1957;10:1204–1218.

Paes da Silva Ramos Fernandes LM, Rice D, Ordinola-Zapata R, et al. Detection of various anatomic patterns of root canals in mandibular incisors using digital periapical radiography, 3 cone-beam computed tomographic scanners, and micro-computed tomographic imaging. J Endod 2014;40:42–45.

Park JB, Kim N, Park S, Kim Y, Ko Y. Evaluation of root anatomy of permanent premolars and molars in a Korean population with cone-beam computed tomography. Eur J Dent 2013a;7:94–101.

Park PS, Kim KD, Perinpanayagam H, et al. Three-dimensional analysis of root canal curvature and direction of maxillary lateral incisors by using cone-beam computed tomography. J Endod 2013b;39:1124–1129.

Patel S. New dimensions in endodontic imaging: part 2. Cone beam computed tomography. Int Endod J 2009;42:463–475.

Patel S. The use of cone beam computed tomography in the conservative management of dens invaginatus: a case report. Int Endod J 2010;43:707–713.

Patel S, Horner K. The use of cone-beam computed tomography in endodontics. Int Endod J 2009;42:755–756.

Radwan A, Kim SG. Treatment of a hypertaurodontic maxillary second molar in a patient with 10 taurodonts: a case report. J Endod 2014;40:140–144.

Reis AG, Grazziotin-Soares R, Barletta FB, Fontanella VR, Mahl CR. Second canal in mesiobuccal root of maxillary molars is correlated with root third and patient age: a cone-beam computed tomographic study. J Endod 2013;39:588–592.

Seo MS, Park DS. C-shaped root canals of mandibular second molars in a Korean population: clinical observation and in vitro analysis. Int Endod J 2004;37:139–144.

Sert S, Bayirli GS. Evaluation of root canal configurations of the mandibular and maxillary permanent teeth by gender in the Turkish population. J Endod 2004;30:391–398.

Soares de Toubes KM, Ilma de Souza Côrtes M, de Abreu Valadares MA, Fonseca LC, Nunes E, Silveira, FF. Comparative analysis of accessory mesial canal identification in mandibular first molars by using four different diagnostic methods. J Endod 2012;38:436–441.

Song CK, Chang HS, Min KS. Endodontic management of supernumerary tooth fused with maxillary first molar by using cone-beam computed tomography. J Endod 2010;36:1901–1904.

Soğur E, Baksi BG, Gröndahl HG. Imaging of root canal fillings: a comparison of subjective image quality between limited cone-beam CT, storage phosphor and film radiography. Int Endod J 2007;40:179–185.

Tian YY, Guo B, Zhang R, et al. Root and canal morphology of maxillary first premolars in a Chinese subpopulation evaluated using cone-beam computed tomography. Int Endod J 2012;45:996–1003.

Tu MG, Huang HL, Hsue SS, et al. Detection of permanent three-rooted mandibular first molars by cone-beam computed tomography imaging in Taiwanese individuals. J Endod 2009;35:503–507.

Tu MG, Tsai CC, Jou MJ, et al. Prevalence of three-rooted mandibular first molars among Taiwanese individuals. J Endod 2007;33:1163–1166.

Venkatesh SM, Ajmera S, Ganeshkar SV. Volumetric pulp changes after orthodontic treatment determined by cone-beam computed tomography. J Endod 2014;40:1758–1763.

Vertucci FJ. Root canal morphology and its relationship to endodontic procedures. Endod Topics 2005;10:3–29.

Vizzotto MB, Silveira PF, Arús NA, Montagner F, Gomes BP, da Silveira HE. CBCT for the assessment of second mesiobuccal (MB2) canals in maxillary molar teeth: effect of voxel size and presence of root filling. Int Endod J 2013;9:870–876.

Wang Y, Zheng QH, Zhou XD, et al. Evaluation of the root and canal morphology of mandibular first permanent molars in a western Chinese population by cone-beam computed tomography. J Endod 2010;36:1786–1789.

Wu MK, R'oris A, Barkis D, Wesselink PR. Prevalence and extent of long oval canals in the apical third. Oral Surg Oral Med Oral Pathol Oral Radiol Endod 2000;89:739–743.

Yang ZP, Yang SF, Lin YC, Shay JC, Chi CY. C-shaped root canals in mandibular second molars in a Chinese population. Endod Dent Traumatol 1988;4:160–163.

Yu X, Guo B, Li KZ, et al. Cone-beam computed tomography study of root and canal morphology of mandibular premolars in a western Chinese population. BMC Med Imaging 2012;20:12–18.

Zhang R, Wang H, Tian YY, Yu X, Hu T, Dummer PM. Use of cone-beam computed tomography to evaluate root and canal morphology of mandibular molars in Chinese individuals. Int Endod J 2011;44:990–999.

Zheng Q, Zhang L, Zhou X, et al. C-shaped root canal system in mandibular second molars in a Chinese population evaluated by cone-beam computed tomography. Int Endod J 2011;44:857–862.

Chapter 7

Apical Periodontitis

Shanon Patel, Conor Durack

Introduction

Apical periodontitis (AP) is an acute or chronic inflammatory condition occurring around the root of a tooth. It is caused by microbial infection of the root canal space and is characterised by destruction of the periradicular bone (Huumonen and Ørstavik, 2002). Prevalence studies on AP show that, depending on the age and location of the population, up to 80% of individuals may be affected with AP when conventional radiography is used to assess the periapical status of their teeth (Kabak and Abbott, 2005). While acute AP is commonly diagnosed from its clinical presentation, the diagnosis of chronic AP is usually dependent on the presence of radiographic signs of the disease.

The ability of radiographs to accurately detect signs of AP is essential for diagnosis, treatment planning, assessment of outcome, and epidemiological studies. Currently, the accepted reference standard for the radiological detection of AP is periapical radiography (European Society of Endodontology, quality guidelines, 2006). However, several studies have highlighted the limitations of conventional radiography for detecting AP (Bender and Seltzer, 1961a; Patel et al, 2009; Tsai et al, 2013).

Limitations of conventional periapical radiography

In a series of *ex vivo* investigations, Bender and Seltzer (1961a, b) concluded that simulated AP lesions confined to the cancellous bone could not be readily identified on radiographs (Fig 7-1). This was due to the lesions being masked by the overlying denser cortical bone (i.e. anatomical noise); other research groups reported similar results (Pauls and Trott, 1966; Schwartz and Foster, 1971). However, in a post-mortem study using human specimens, Brynolf (1967) found that AP confined to the cancellous bone in the anterior maxilla region could be detected using periapical radiographs. In some instances, it may be possible to detect destruction within the cancellous bone without associated loss of cortical or junctional bone (Shoha et al, 1974).

For AP to be detected radiographically, the bone loss has to reach a 'critical threshold' in relation to the surrounding bone. If the ratio of healthy (mineralised) bone to demineralised bone (i.e. AP) reaches this critical level, then AP will be detected. The ratio will depend on several factors, including: the density of the bone; the nature of cancellous and cortical bone; the X-ray beam angulation; the exposure parameters; and the nature of the lesion (i.e. size and degree of demineralisation). These factors not only vary depending on the position of the lesion within the jaw, but also between the maxilla and mandible, as well as between individuals. For example, the mineral density of the posterior mandible region is higher than the anterior maxilla region. Therefore, a small volume of demineralised bone may be readily identifiable in the anterior maxilla, but not in the more radiodense posterior mandible.

A second angled (parallax) radiograph has been suggested to improve the ability to diagnose periapical lesions (European Society of Endodontology, quality guidelines, 2006; Vertucci and Haddix, 2010). However, there is limited evidence that parallax radiographs do improve the detection of periapical lesions (Soğur et al, 2012). Recently, Davies et al (2015a) compared the ability of single radiographs, two parallax radiographs, and cone beam computed tomography (CBCT) to detect AP *in vivo*, and revealed periapical lesions in 41%, 38% and 68% of radiographic systems, respectively. Using CBCT as a reference standard, these results suggest that there is no increased accuracy in detecting AP

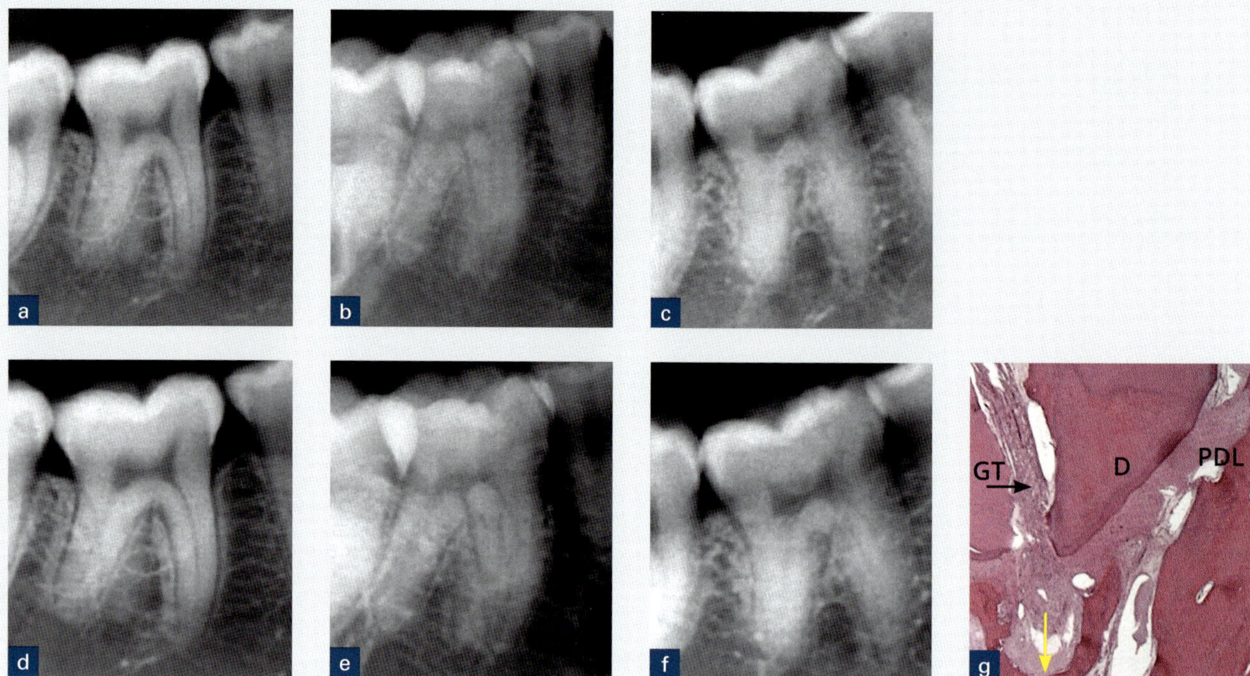

Fig 7-1 Despite the use of parallax radiographs, AP is not readily identifiable regardless of whether a film or digital radiographic system is used. (a) Conventional film-centred view; (b) mesial shift (-10 degrees); (c) distal shift (+10 degrees), as well as (d) digital imaging system centred view; (e) mesial shift and (f) distal shift. None of these images detected an existing periapical lesion associated with the distal root. Histopathological examination of the same distal root (g) showed AP: decalcified root structure with necrotic apical pulp and granulomatous tissues (magnification 4×; H&E staining). Yellow arrow showing area of inflammation with bone resorption, GT = granulomatous tissue, D = dentine, PDL = periodontal ligament (Kanagasingham et al [2016a], submitted for publication, Int Endod J).

with parallax radiographs compared to a single view. However, Kangasingam et al (2016a) found that the combination of two additional (parallax) images, with mesial and distal horizontal angulations, did improve the detection of AP lesions when compared to a single view. In this study, block dissection and histopathological analysis of the periapical tissues in relatively fresh (unpreserved) human cadavers was used as the reference standard (Figs 7-1 and 7-2).

With digital periapical radiographic systems, the image produced is dynamic and can therefore be enhanced (contrast/brightness) to potentially improve its diagnostic yield (Kullendorff et al, 1996). Several well-designed *ex vivo* studies have shown that there is no difference in the ability to detect artificially created periapical lesions using conventional radiographic films and digital sensors (Kullendorff and Nilsson, 1996; Stavropoulos and Wenzel, 2007; Özen et al, 2009). In the abovementioned autopsy study using human cadavers, Kangasingam et al (2016a) also found no statistical difference between the accuracy of parallax digital and conventional (film) periapical radiographs, for assessing AP. However, single digital periapical radiographs were found to be more accurate than single conventional radiographs.

'Enhancing' radiographic images (e.g. colourising and inverting) with software also does not appear to improve the detection of periapical lesions (Barbat and Messer, 1998).

Detection of apical periodontitis

Numerous *ex vivo* studies with reference standards in both animal (Stavropoulos and Wenzel, 2007) and human (Özen et al, 2009; Patel et al, 2009; Tsai et al, 2013) models have conclusively demonstrated that CBCT is a significantly more accurate imaging system than periapical radiography for detecting the presence (sensitivity) of artificially created bone lesions. All *ex vivo* studies have the disadvantage of not truly mimicking the 'real-life' clinical situation. However, the advantage

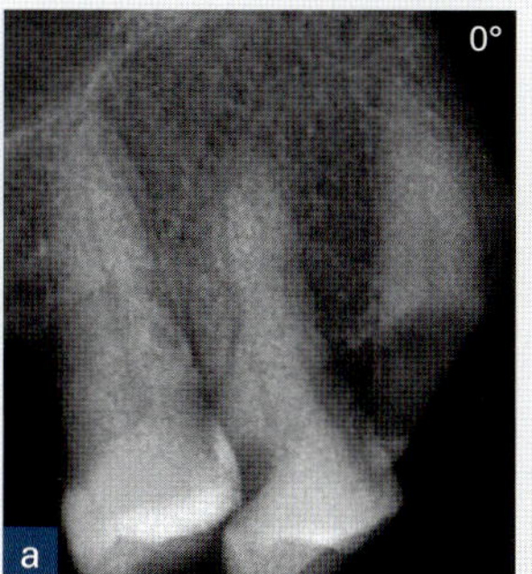

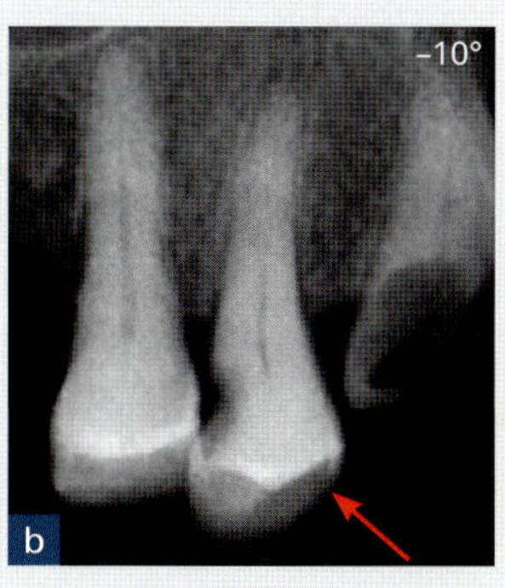

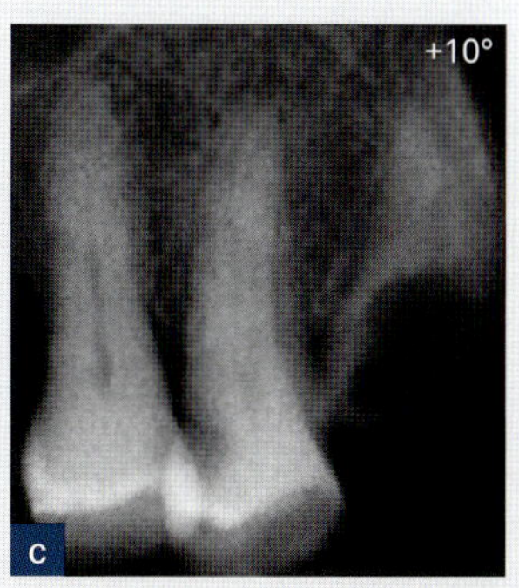

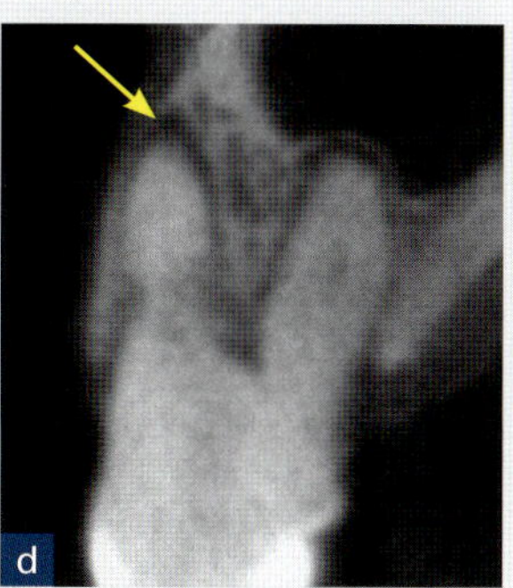

Fig 7-2 Digital periapical radiographs, centred view (a), mesial shift (b) and distal shift (c) do not detect any periapical lesion associated with the maxillary right first premolar. Coronal (d) reconstructed CBCT images shows a periapical radiolucency associated with the buccal (yellow arrow) root. (e) Diagnosis of apical periodontitis (AP) was confirmed from the histopathological examination. The histopathological examination of the specimen with X2 magnification; H&E staining showing: Highly inflammed pulp with granulation tissue at apical area (Kanagasingham et al (2016b) submitted for publication, Int Endod J).

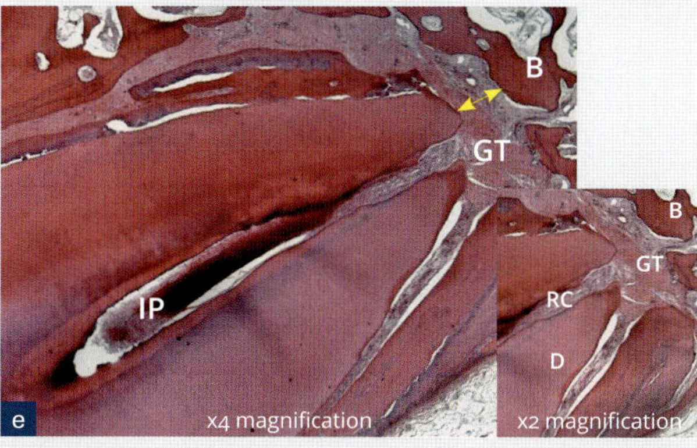

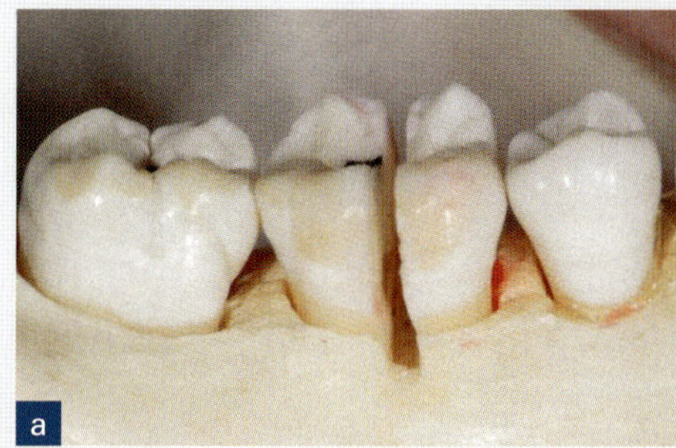

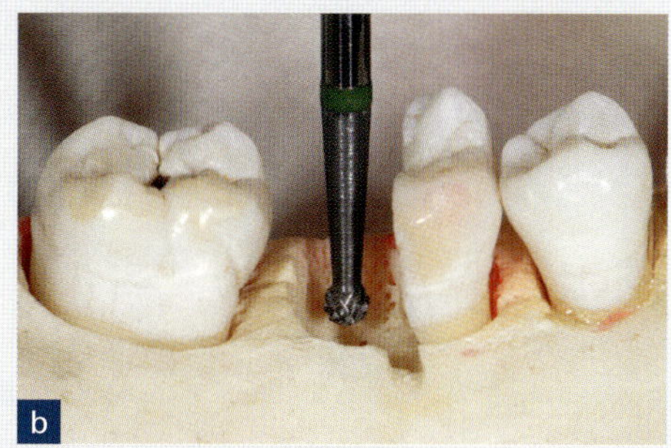

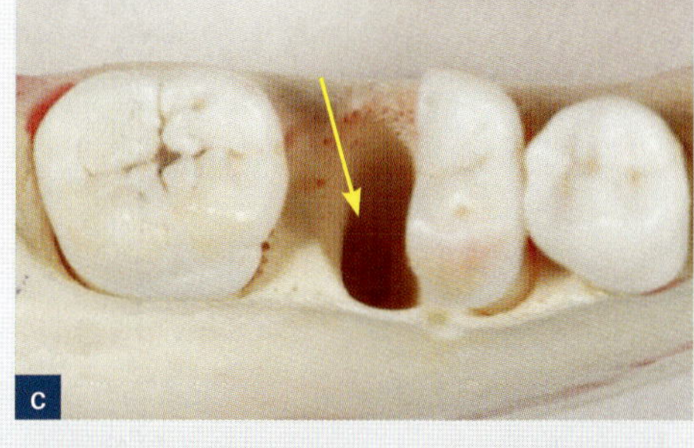

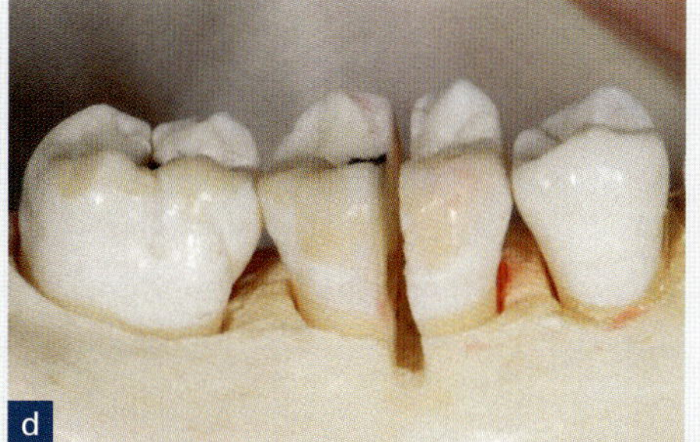

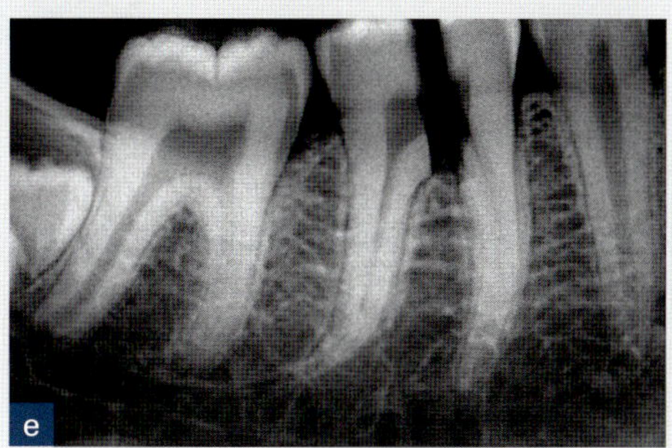

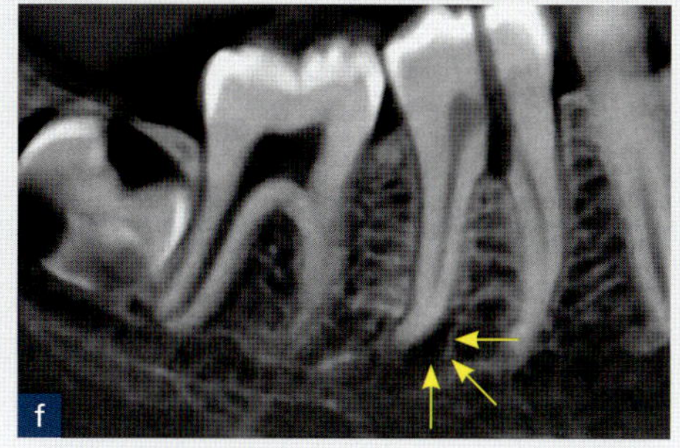

Fig 7-3 (a) A dry human mandible model used to simulate periapical lesion. (b) The distal root of the mandibular first molar has been sectioned; and (c) atraumatically extracted to allow a standardised simulated periapical lesion (yellow arrow) to be created within the cancellous bone with a laboratory bur and handpiece. (d) The distal root has been re-seated. (e) The digital periapical radiograph does not reveal the presence of a 2-mm diameter periapical lesion within the cancellous bone. (f) A reconstructed sagittal CBCT image clearly reveals the simulated periapical lesion (yellow arrows) on the distal root.

of such studies is that standardised periapical defects have been intentionally created, thus giving a reference standard that allows imaging techniques to be assessed with more confidence (Fig 7-3).

In a well-designed animal study using histology as a reference standard, Paula-Silva et al (2009a) reaffirmed that CBCT was a more accurate diagnostic tool than conventional radiography for diagnosing chronic AP. In this study, 83 block dissections of periapical tissues and root tips were histologically assessed in teeth with and without radiographic signs of AP. The specificity and positive predictive value was 1 for radiographs and CBCT, i.e. both imaging systems were accurate in determining when no disease was present. However, the sensitivity for CBCT (<0.91) was much higher than for radiographs (0.77) for detecting existing disease.

Using similar methodology to Brynolf (1967), Kanagasingam et al (2016b) assessed the accuracy of single, parallax digital radiographs and CBCT for diagnosing AP in fresh human cadavers using histology as the reference standard. In total, 86 teeth were assessed (Fig 7-2). The specificity of all the imaging systems was excellent, i.e. all imaging techniques could correctly detect healthy periapical tissues. However, the sensitivity of digital radiographs varied from 0.27 to 0.38, depending on whether a single view or parallax views, respectively, were assessed. This compared to a sensitivity of 0.89 for CBCT. The overall accuracy of the digital radiographic techniques was 0.5 for a single view and 0.58 for parallax views, and there was a significantly higher accuracy (0.92) for CBCT.

Several clinical studies have concluded that the diagnostic accuracy of CBCT in the detection of AP is superior to that of periapical radiography (Low et al, 2008; Patel et al, 2012a). Lofthag-Hansen et al (2007) examined and compared the periapical status of teeth with suspected endodontic disease using CBCT and periapical radiography. The authors reported that 38% more periapical lesions were detected with CBCT. Subsequent studies have reported similar findings (Bornstein et al, 2011; Abella et al, 2012). Patel et al (2012a) compared the prevalence of AP lesions associated with the roots of teeth with primary endodontic disease. CBCT was able to identify lesions of AP in 28% more teeth than periapical radiographs (Fig 7-4). Similar findings have been reported for endodontically treated teeth (Davies et al, 2015a).

Assessment of the outcome of endodontic treatment

It follows that the superior diagnostic accuracy of CBCT over conventional radiography in the detection of AP permits a more accurate and objective assessment of the outcome of endodontic treatment. Liang et al (2011) compared the outcome of endodontic treatment using periapical radiographs and CBCT 2 years after treatment. They found that a favourable outcome was reached in 87% of cases assessed with periapical radiographs, compared to only 74% of cases assessed with CBCT; the 13% difference being attributed to the superior sensitivity of CBCT in detecting AP. Patel et al (2012b) compared the outcome of primary endodontic treatment carried out on 132 teeth 1 year after treatment. The 'healed' rate (absence of radiolucency at review) of the treated teeth was 87% and 62.5% when assessed using periapical radiographs and CBCT, respectively. When more relaxed criteria (i.e. healing and healed) were used to assess outcome, the percentage of teeth demonstrating a reduction in the size of the associated apical radiolucency was 95.1% and 84.7% for conventional radiography and CBCT, respectively. Paula-Silva et al (2009b) assessed the outcome of root canal treatment in dogs and found a 44% lower success rate when the periapical tissues were assessed with CBCT (35%), compared with periapical radiographs (79%).

Davies et al (2015b) reviewed the outcome of secondary (re-treatment) carried out in 98 teeth 1 year after re-treatment with conventional radiographs and CBCT. They found that there was a significantly different success rate between radiographs (93%) and CBCT (77%).

Radiographic appearance of apical periodontitis

Conventional radiography

While long-standing lesions of AP with significant bone destruction are generally readily discernible on conventional radiographs, incipient lesions of AP are often much more difficult to identify. Alterations to structures of the apical periodontium, such as the medullary bone trabeculae, the periodontal ligament (PDL)

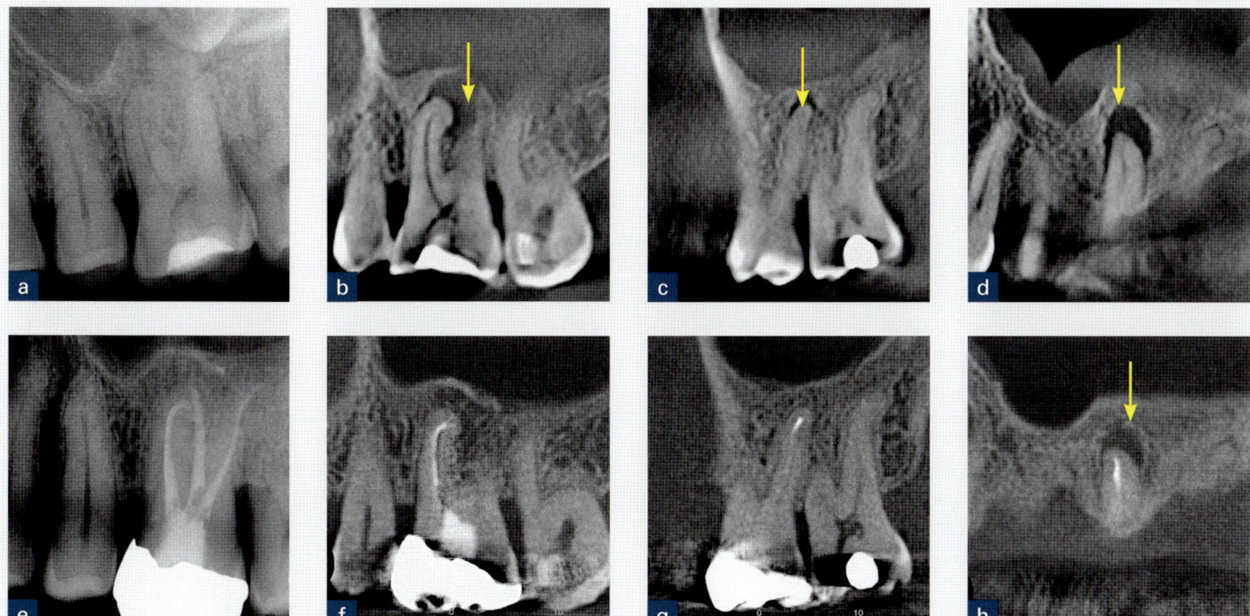

Fig 7-4 A 72-year-old male patient has symptoms of a poorly localised and intermittent dull ache associated with the maxillary left quadrant. Clinical examination is unremarkable, and all maxillary left premolar and molar teeth give a delayed response to sensitivity testing. (a) A periapical radiograph of the maxillary left quadrant reveals sclerosis of the root canals of the maxillary left premolar and molar teeth, although there are no radiographic signs of AP. A CBCT scan was taken to aid diagnosis, and reconstructed coronal images of the (b) mesiobuccal, (c) distobuccal, and (d) palatal canals clearly show signs of AP associated with the maxillary left first molar, while periapical tissues associated with the other teeth appeared normal. A diagnosis of chronic AP was made for this tooth; root canal treatment was carried out in a single visit. A 1-year follow-up radiograph (e) revealed healthy periapical tissues (no change from pre-treatment radiograph), while the 1-year follow-up reconstructed coronal CBCT images revealed complete healing of the pre-treatment periapical lesions on the (f) mesiobuccal and (g) distobuccal roots, and incomplete healing on the (h) palatal root.

space, and the lamina dura may be early indicators of AP (Gröndahl and Huumonen, 2004). As such, an appreciation of the normal radiographic appearance of these structures is essential.

The conventional radiographic appearance of cancellous bone surrounding a healthy tooth varies between the maxilla and mandible. Typically, maxillary alveolar bone trabeculae have a fine, granular appearance, while mandibular alveolar bone trabeculae have a coarser, horizontally striated appearance and are interspersed with comparatively wider marrow spaces. Subtle structural changes in the cancellous bone are generally the earliest signs of AP recognisable on conventional radiographs. These changes include a disruption and disorganisation of the normal trabecular pattern around the apex (or other portal of exit) of the affected tooth. The disorganisation of the affected area may be well defined and easily differentiated from the surrounding bone or, alternatively, the margins of the disorganised area may blend with the surrounding bone such that it is difficult to delineate it from the surrounding healthy tissue, thus making interpretation more challenging (Fig 7-5a and b; Fig 7-6a and b).

Widening of the PDL space associated with the affected tooth may be an early indication of AP. However, endodontic infection is not the sole cause of a widened PDL space, which may also be a feature of tooth mobility, marginal periodontitis, or even neurogenic inflammation (Pope et al, 2014). Furthermore, the specific exposure angle of the radiograph may lead to the appearance of a widened PDL space (Bender et al, 1961a). This should be borne in mind when assessing a tooth for the early signs of AP (Fig 7-7a and b). A widened PDL space specifically associated with AP will be localised to the apex of the tooth (or the affected portal of exit) and the immediately adjacent areas. The PDL space coronal (and/or apical, if for example a lateral canal is involved) to this area will be unaffected, and there will be a marked transition between the affected and unaffected sites.

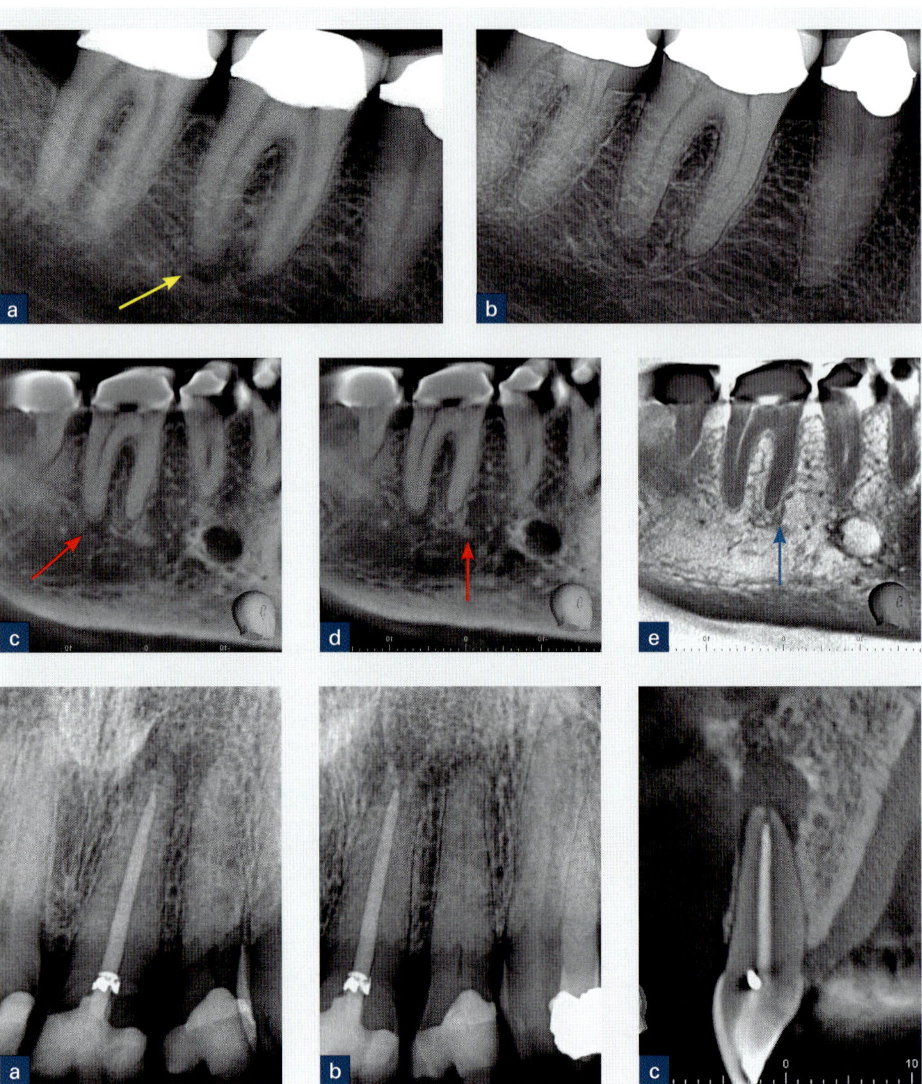

Fig 7-5 A patient with poorly localised pain associated with the mandibular right quadrant. (a and b) Parallax radiographs reveal a slightly more diffuse trabecular bone pattern (yellow arrow in a) in the periapical region of the distal root of the mandibular right first molar tooth, however the lamina dura is intact (yellow arrow in b). (c) Reconstructed sagittal CBCT images again show an intact lamina dura and diffuse bone pattern around the distal root. (d) Signs of condensing osteitis (red arrow) associated with the mesial root. (e) Inverting the reconstructed image is sometimes helpful to assess the bony pattern. A diagnosis of chronic AP for the mandibular right first molar tooth was reached.

Fig 7-6 (a and b) Parallax radiographs of a root-treated maxillary left central incisor for which a new crown is planned. The periapical bone adjacent to this tooth reveals a slightly more diffuse trabecular bone pattern, but no obvious periapical radiolucency. (c) Reconstructed sagittal CBCT image reveals well-defined peri-apical radiolucency associated with the maxillary left central incisor tooth.

A further, relatively early radiographic sign of AP is disruption of the lamina dura, the integrity of which may be breached and which may appear to lose density. Any changes will be localised to the affected portal of exit from which the microbes are egressing. However, in isolation, a break in the continuity of the lamina dura should be viewed with caution. Tiny perforations of the lamina dura, although not always seen radiographically, are necessarily present to accommodate vascular and neural supply from the adjacent medullary bone to the teeth. These perforations may manifest on some radiographs and not on others. Furthermore, a certain amount of variation in normal lamina dura radiodensity and thickness can be expected between individuals. These features may also be altered by the angle of the radiographic exposure.

With the development of AP, the mineral content of the cancellous bone trabeculae becomes depleted, and the trabeculae become thinner and less dense, with a resultant increase in the size of the adjacent marrow spaces. The affected area sometimes develops what has been described as a 'shotgun' appearance. This represents an intermediate stage in the progression of the lesion, from the subtle structural changes of the bone described above to the development of a clear periapical radiolucency. However, it is not always identifiable.

When the bone demineralisation has reached a critical threshold, a radiolucency will develop. Diagnosis of

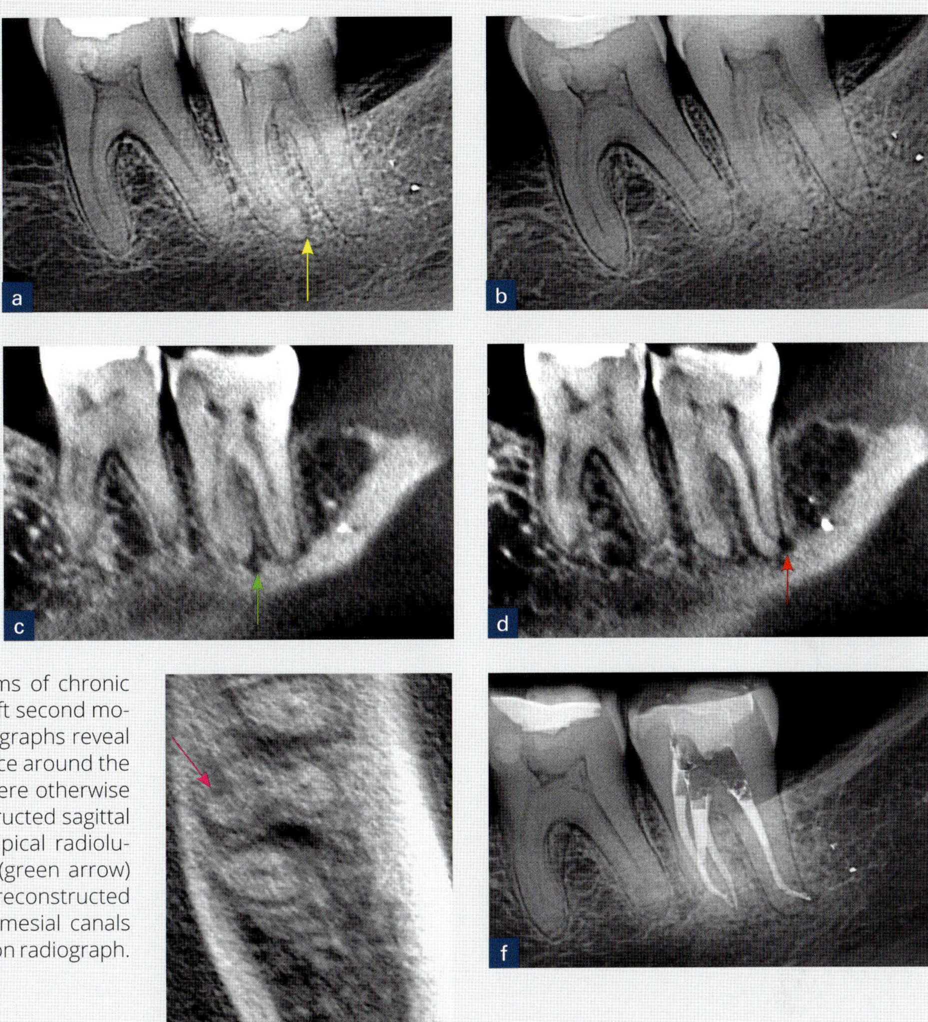

Fig 7-7 A patient with symptoms of chronic AP localised to the mandibular left second molar tooth. (a and b) Parallax radiographs reveal possible widening of the PDL space around the mesial root (yellow arrow), but were otherwise unremarkable. (c and d) Reconstructed sagittal CBCT images clearly show periapical radiolucencies around the mesial root (green arrow) and distal root (red arrow). (e) A reconstructed axial CBCT image reveals three mesial canals (pink arrow). (f) Final post-oburation radiograph.

AP at this stage is less complicated. Nevertheless, depending on the exposure angle of any given radiograph and the site of the subject tooth, adjacent anatomical features may impair interpretation of the radiograph, such that the radiolucency may not be readily identified, or conversely, may look larger. The margins of periapical radiolucencies may be well or poorly defined, and in some instances they will have a corticated appearance.

Another potential precursor of AP is 'condensing osteitis', which is a reactionary production of dense bone in the periapical area of the affected tooth in response to low-grade pulpal irritation. Condensing osteitis manifests radiographically as a localised radiopacity in the area around the apex (or other portal of exit) of the affected root. The nature of the areas of condensing osteitis is variable, and the border of the lesion may be well or poorly defined (Fig 7-8a). In some instances, this reactionary bone can completely obscure the anatomy of the affected root on conventional radiographs.

Historically, it was thought that the histological nature of AP lesions could be determined by radiographic features of the associated periapical radiolucency, such as size and the presence or absence of a radiopaque, corticated rim (Bhaskar, 1966). These associations have since been disproved (Nair, 1998; Nair et al, 1999), and it is believed that the radiographic features of periapical radiolucencies, such as size and the presence of a corticated lamina dura (Ricucci et al, 2006), are in fact poor predictors of the true histological nature of AP lesions.

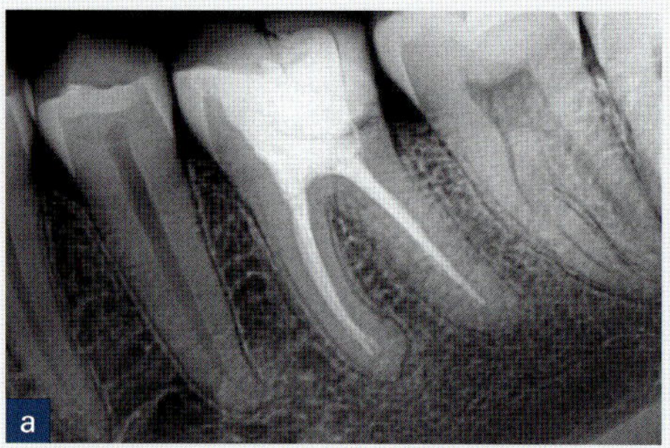
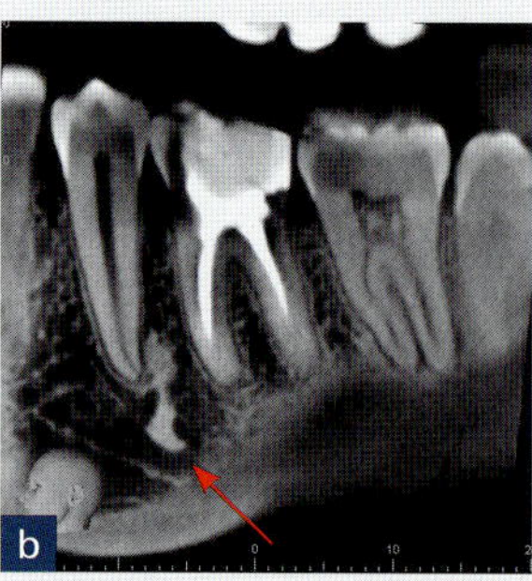

Fig 7-8 (a) Condensing osteitis in the periradicular region of the mandibular left second premolar is not identifiable on the (a) periapical radiograph, but clearly visible on the (b) reconstructed sagittal CBCT images (red arrows). This intact mandibular left premolar tooth has a distal hairline crack running thought it, which is the most likely cause of pulpal irritation.

Due to the difficulties inherent in detecting AP on conventional radiographs, especially at an early stage, a scoring system for the registration of AP, called the 'Periapical Index' (PAI), was developed (Ørstavik et al, 1996). It is a five-point grading system that classifies AP according to some conventional radiographic features (previously described) associated with the development of the disease.

Cone beam computed tomography

The true extent of bone destruction associated with AP is underestimated on conventional radiographs (Paula-Silva et al, 2009c; Abella et al, 2014). Therefore, the absence of (conventional) radiographic signs of AP does not rule out its presence, while the presence of radiographic features of AP are inevitably associated with a true diagnosis of AP (Brynolf et al, 1970a, 1970b; Kanagasingam et al, 2016b). AP presents on a CBCT scan, even in its earliest stages, as a 2-mm, well-defined widening of PDL space, or as a clearly defined periapical radiolucency (Tsai et al, 2013; Abella et al, 2014) (Fig 7-7). These findings may have an impact on the treatment plan of a tooth provisionally diagnosed with reversible pulpitis. An AP lesion may be clearly detected with CBCT, even though conventional radiographs are within normal limits (Hashem et al, 2015), therefore root canal treatment rather than pulp preservation treatment (e.g. pulp capping) would be indicated. With the elimination of anatomical noise comes a more objective appreciation of the presence and extent of bone loss associated with the disease, when compared to conventional radiography (Figs 7-5 and 7-6). Condensing osteitis can also become more evident (Fig 7-8).

As such, AP can be reliably diagnosed, and the nature (i.e. dimensions and extent) of the lesion accurately determined using CBCT. Assessing the true nature of AP and its proximity to important anatomical structures can be especially relevant when considering periapical microsurgery (Bornstein et al, 2011; Patel et al, 2015). Any expansion and perforations of cortical bone can also be accurately identified and related to clinical findings.

The CBCT-PAI has been suggested for use with CBCT (Estrela et al, 2008). This index uses a six-point scale to quantify the maximum diameter of bone loss associated with AP. The scores range from 0 'intact periapical bone structures' to 5 'diameter of periapical radiolucency >8 mm'. The variables +E (expansion of periapical cortical bone) and +D (destruction of periapical cortical bone) may be added to any score if they are detected on the CBCT analysis. Recent reports have suggested that this is a reproducible method of assessing the extent of AP (Esposito et al, 2011).

The improved accuracy of the diagnosis of AP associated with CBCT has potential implications for the assessment of the outcome of endodontic treatment (Patel et al, 2012b; Fernández et al, 2013). Lesions will be identifiable on CBCT for longer periods post-treatment (when compared with conventional radiographs) due to the superior sensitivity of the system (Fig 7-4). It is therefore likely that the way the outcome of endodontic treatment (including prognostic factors) is determined will need to be reassessed in the future (Patel et al, 2011).

Dose reduction protocols should always be considered whenever possible to reduce the effective dose to which a patient is exposed. Recently, Al-Nuaimi et al (2016) demonstrated a good diagnostic accuracy for detecting simulated AP lesions with CBCT when the exposure settings were adjusted away from the manufacturer's default settings. In this study, there was no significant reduction in diagnostic yield when the radiation was reduced by up to 74%.

Conclusion

The current evidence suggests that CBCT is more sensitive and accurate compared with periapical radiography in detecting AP.

CBCT must not be used as a default imaging system to detect AP (Patel et al, 2015). Instead, it should be used in those instances where clinical and conventional radiographic assessment is equivocal for the diagnosis of odontogenic and/or non-odontogenic disease (European Society of Endodontolgy CBCT position statement, 2014).

References

Abella F, Patel S, Durán-Sindreu F, Mercadé M, Bueno R, Roig M. Evaluating the periapical status of teeth with irreversible pulpitis by using cone-beam computed tomography scanning and periapical radiographs. J Endod 2012;38:1588–1591.

Abella F, Patel S, Durán-Sindreu F, M. Mercadé M, Bueno R, Roig M. An evaluation of the periapical status of teeth with necrotic pulps using periapical radiography and cone-beam computed tomography. Int Endod J 2014;47:387–396.

Al-Nuaimi N, Patel S, Foschi F, Mannocci F. The detection of simulated periapical lesions with CBCT—a dose reduction study. Int Endod J 2016 (accepted for publication).

Barbat J, Messer HH. Detectability of artificial periapical lesions using direct digital and conventional radiography. J Endod 1998;24:837–342.

Bender IB, Seltzer S. Roentgenographic and direct observation of experimental lesions in bone: I. J Am Dent Assoc 1961a;62:152–160.

Bender IB, Seltzer S. Roentgenographic and direct observation of experimental lesions in bone: II. J Am Dent Assoc 1961b;62:708–716.

Bhaskar SN. Periapical lesion—types, incidence and clinical features. Oral Surg Oral Med Oral Pathol 1966;21:657–671.

Bornstein MM, Lauber R, Sendi P, von Arx T. Comparison of periapical and limited cone-beam computed tomography in mandibular molars for analysis of anatomical landmarks before apical surgery. J Endod 2011;37:151–157.

Brynolf I. A histological and roentenological study of the periapical region of human upper incisors. Odonto Revy 1967;18, Supplement 11.

Brynolf I. Roentgenolgic periapical diagnosis. IV. When is one roentgenogram not sufficient? Sven Tandlak Tidskr 1970a;63:415–423.

Brynolf I. Roentgenolgic periapical diagnosis III. The more roentgenograms – the better information? Sven Tandlak Tidskr 1970b;63:409–413.

Davies A, Mannocci F, Mitchell P, Andiappan M, Patel S. The detection of periapical pathoses in root filled teeth using single and parallax periapical radiographs versus cone beam computed tomography—a clinical study. Int Endod J 2015a;48: 582–592.

Davies A, Patel S, Foschi, F, Andiappan M, Mitchell PJ, Mannocci F. The detection of periapical pathoses using digital periapical radiography and cone beam computed tomography in endodontically retreated teeth – part 2: a 1 year post-treatment follow-up. Int Endod J 2015b; in press.

Esposito S, Cardaropoli M, Cotti E. A suggested technique for the application of the cone beam computed tomography periapical index. Dentomaxillofac Radiol 2011;40:506–512.

Estrela C, Bueno MR, Azevedo BC, Azevedo JR, Pécora DJ. A new periapical index based on cone beam computed tomography. J Endod 2008;34:1325–1331.

European Society of Endodontology position statement: The use of CBCT in Endodontics. Int Endod J 2014;47:502–504.

European Society of Endodontology. Quality guidelines for endodontic treatment: consensus report of the European Society of Endodontology. Int Endod J 2006;39:921–930.

Fernández R, Cadavid D, Zapata SM, Alvarez LG, Restrepo FA. Impact of three radiographic methods in the outcome of nonsurgical endodontic treatment: a five-year follow-up. J Endod 2013;39:1097–1103.

Gröndahl HG, Huumonen S. Radiographic manifestations of periapical inflammatory lesions. Endod Topics 2004;8:55–67.

Hashem D, Mannocci F, Patel S, et al. Clinical and radiographic assessment of the efficacy of calcium silicate indirect pulp capping: a randomized controlled clinical trial. J Dent Res 2015;94:562–268.

Huumonen S, Ørstavik D. Radiological aspects of apical periodontitis. Endod Topics 2002;1:3–25.

Kabak Y, Abbott PV. Prevalence of apical periodontitis and the quality of endodontic treatment in an adult Belarusian population. Int Endod J 2005;38:238–245.

Kanagasingam S, Lim CX, Yong CP, Patel S. Accuracy of single versus multiple images of conventional and digital periapical radiography in diagnosing periapical periodontitis using histopathological findings as a reference standard. Int Endod J 2016a (submitted for publication).

Kanagasingam S, Mannocci F, Lim CX, Yong CP, Patel S. Diagnostic accuracy of cone beam computed tomography scans and periapical radiography in detecting apical periodontitis using histopathological findings as a gold standard. Int Endod J 2016b (submitted for publication).

Kullendorf B, Nilsson M, Rohlin M. Diagnostic accuracy of direct digital dental radiography for the detection of periapical bone lesions: overall comparison between conventional and direct digital radiography. Oral Surg Oral Med Oral Pathol Oral Radiol Endod 1996;82:344–350.

Kullendorf B, Nilsson M. Diagnostic accuracy of direct digital dental radiography for the detection of periapical bone lesions. II. Effects on diagnostic accuracy after application of image processing. Oral Surg Oral Med Oral Pathol Oral Radiol Endod 1996;82:585–589.

Liang YH, Li G, Wesselink PR, Wu MK. Endodontic outcome predictors identified with periapical radiographs and cone-beam computed tomography scans. J Endod 2011;37: 326–331.

Lofthag-Hansen S, Huumonen S, Gröndahl K, Gröndahl HG. Limited cone-beam CT and intraoral radiography for the diagnosis of periapical pathology. Oral Surg Oral Med Oral Pathol Oral Radiol Endod 2007;103:114–119.

Low KM, Dula K, Bürgin W, von Arx T. Comparison of periapical radiography and limited cone-beam tomography in posterior maxillary teeth referred for apical surgery. J Endod 2008;34:557–562.

Nair PNR. New perspectives on radicular cysts: do they heal? Int Endod J 1998;31:155–160.

Nair PN, Sjögren U, Figdor D, Sundqvist G. Persistent periapical radiolucencies of root filled human teeth, failed endodontic treatments and periapical scars. Oral Surg Oral Med Oral Pathol Oral Radiol Endod 1999;87:617–627.

Ørstavik D. Time-course and risk analyses of the development and healing of chronic apical periodontitis in man. Int Endod J 1996;29:150–155.

Özen T, Kamburoğlu K, Cebeci AR, Yüksel SP, Paksoy CS. Interpretation of chemically created periapical lesions using 2 different dental cone-beam computerized tomography units, an intraoral digital sensor, and conventional film. Oral Surg Oral Med Oral Pathol Oral Radiol Endod 2009;107:426–432.

Patel S, Dawood A, Mannocci F, Wilson R, Pitt Ford T. Detection of periapical bone defects in human jaws using cone beam computed tomography and intraoral radiography. Int Endod J 2009;42:507–515.

Patel S, Durack C, Abella F, Roig M, Shemesh H, Lambrechts P, Lemberg K. European Society of Endodontology position statement: The use of CBCT in Endodontics. Int Endod J 2014:47:502–504.

Patel S, Mannocci F, Shemesh H, Wu MK, Wesselink P, Lambrechts P. Radiographs and CBCT – time for a reassessment? Int Endod J 2011;44:887–888.

Patel S, Wilson R, Dawood A, Mannocci F. The detection of periapical pathosis using periapical radiography and cone beam computed tomography – Part 1: pre-operative status. Int Endod J 2012a;45:702–710.

Patel S, Wilson R, Dawood A, Foschi, Mannocci F. The detection of periapical pathosis using digital periapical radiography and cone beam computed tomography – Part 2: a 1-year post-treatment follow-up. Int Endod J 2012b;45:711–723.

Patel S, Durack C, Abella F, Shemesh H, Roig M, Lemberg M. Cone beam computed tomography in Endodontics—a review. Int Endod J 2015;48:3–15.

Paula-Silva FW, Wu MK, Leonardo MR, da Silva LA, Wesselink PR. Accuracy of periapical radiography and cone-beam computed tomography scans in diagnosing apical periodontitis using histo-pathological findings as a gold standard. J Endod 2009a;35:1009–1012.

Paula-Silva FW, Hassan B, da Silva LA, Leonardo MR, Wu MK. Outcome of root canal treatment in dogs determined by periapical radiography and cone-beam computed tomography scans. J Endod 2009b;35:723–726.

Paula-Silva FW, Santamaria M Jr, Leonardo MR, Consolaro A, da Silva LA. Cone-beam computerized tomographic, radiographic, and histological evaluation of periapical repair in dogs post-endodontic treatment. Oral Surg Oral Med Oral Pathol Oral Radiol Endod 2009c;108:796–805.

Pauls V, Trott JR. A radiological study of experimentally produced lesions in bone. Dent Pract Dent Rec 1966;16:254–258.

Pope O, Sathorn C, Parashos P. A comparative investigation of cone-beam computed tomography and periapical radiography in the diagnosis of a healthy periapex. J Endod 2014;40:360–540.

Ricucci D, Mannocci F, Ford TR. A study of periapical lesions correlating the presence of a radiopaque lamina with histological findings. Oral Surg Oral Med Oral Pathol Oral Radiol Endod 2006;101:389–394.

Schwartz SF, Foster JK Jr. Roentgenographic interpretation of experimentally produced bony lesions. I. Oral Surg Oral Med Oral Pathol 1971;32:606–612.

Shoha RR, Dowson J, Richards AG. Radiographic interpretation of experimentally produced bony lesions. Oral Surg Oral Med Oral Pathol 1974;38:294–303.

Soğur E, Gröndahl HG, Baksı BG, Mert A. Does a combination of two radiographs increase accuracy in detecting acid-induced periapical lesions and does it approach the accuracy of cone-beam computed tomography scanning? J Endod 2012;38:131–136.

Stavropoulos A, Wenzel A. Accuracy of cone beam dental CT, intraoral digital and conventional film radiography for the detection of periapical lesions: an ex vivo study in pig jaws. Clin Oral Investig 2007;11:101–106.

Tsai P, Torabinejad M, Rice D, Azevedo B. Accuracy of cone-beam computed tomography and periapical radiography in detecting small periapical lesions. J Endod 2013;38:965–970.

Vertucci FJ, Haddix JE. Tooth morphology and access cavity preparation. In: Hargreaves KM, Cohen S (eds). Pathways of the Pulp, ed 10. Missouri, MO: Mosby, 2010: 236–222.

Chapter 8

Non-surgical and Surgical Re-treatment

Shanon Patel, Hagay Shemesh, Navid Saberi

Introduction

Endodontic treatment has a high success rate (Ng et al, 2011); however, on occasion treatment may fail. Several factors have been reported to contribute to the failure of endodontically treated teeth (Siqueira, 2001; Ng et al, 2007; Azim et al, 2015).

The management of failed root canal treatment is dependant on the mode of failure, which may be multi-factorial (Fig 8-1). Treatment options commonly include non-surgical endodontic re-treatment, surgical re-treatment, extraction, and no treatment. Other less-frequent treatment options include root amputation and intentional implantation.

An effective treatment plan can only be devised when firstly, the diagnosis, and secondly the reason behind treatment failure have been determined. This chapter will explore how the data obtained by cone beam computed tomography (CBCT) may influence clinical decision making and the overall treatment planning in managing failed endodontically treated teeth (Fig 8-1).

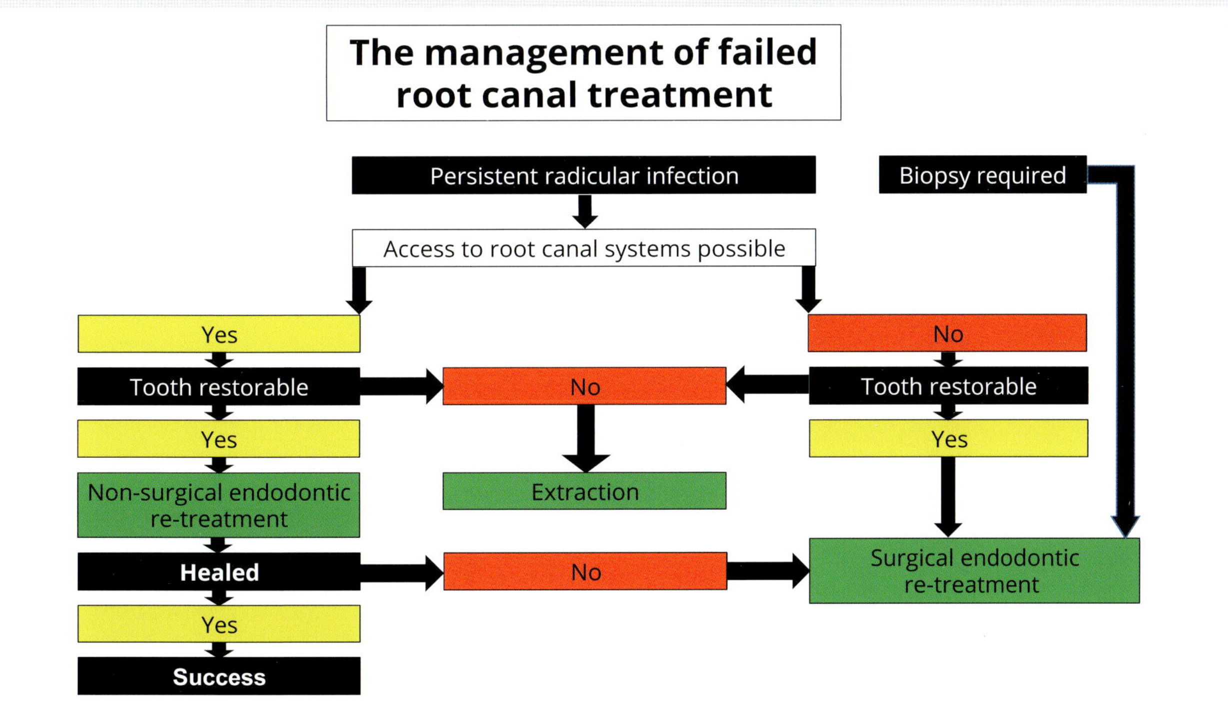

Fig 8-1 Factors involved in clinical decision making in relation to the management of failed root canal treatment. Green boxes indicate the treatment plan. Note that the ability of the clinician to gain access to the root canal systems is at the heart of the decision tree and non-surgical endodontic re-treatment should be attempted first where possible. Occasionally, however, surgical endodontic re-treatment may be indicated as the first line of therapy if a periapical biopsy is required, or in cases where retrieval of extruded endodontic material is necessary.

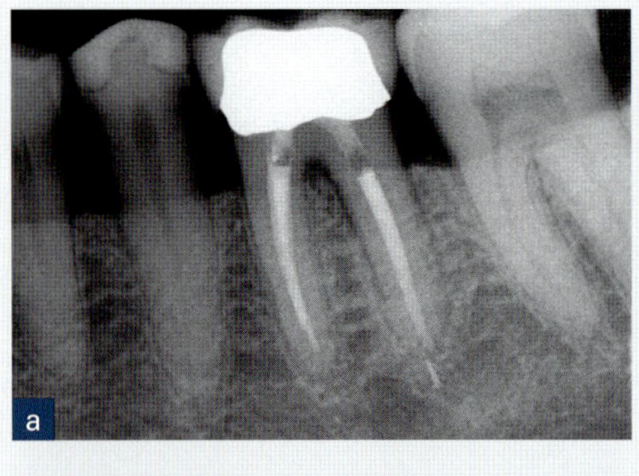
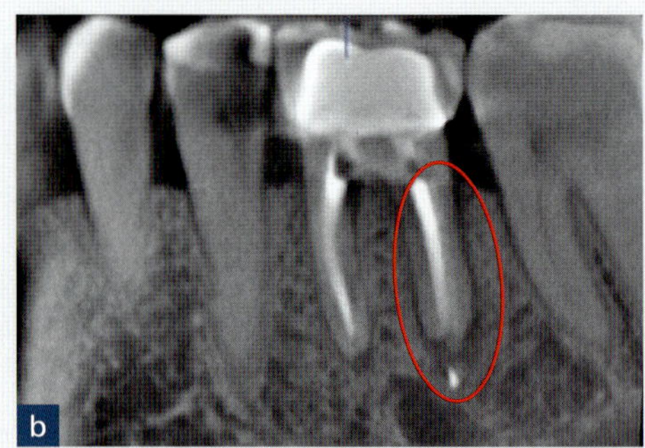
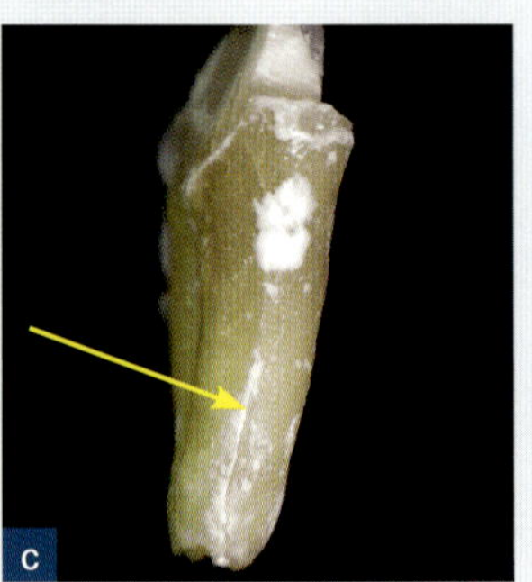
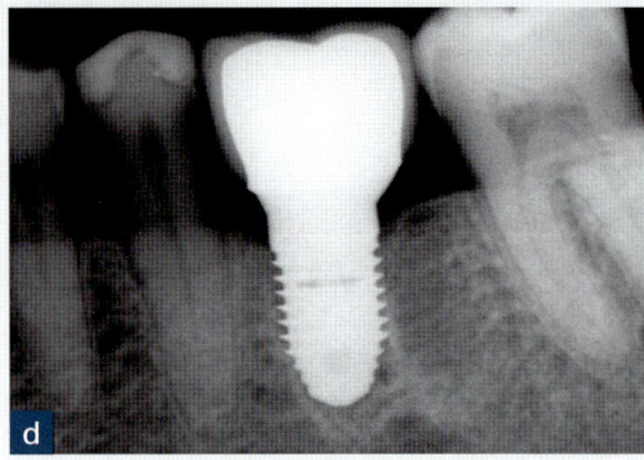

Fig 8-2 (a) A periapical radiograph of a root-treated symptomatic mandibular left first molar showing no sign of periapical or periradicular radiolucency. (b) The sagittal CBCT slice reveals subtle bone loss along the distal aspect of the distal root extending towards the root apex (red outline), indicating a vertical root fracture. (c) The extracted mandibular left first molar confirming the vertical fracture line (yellow arrow). (d) The extracted tooth was replaced with a dental implant (implant placement by Dr Andrew Dawood).

Non-surgical endodontic re-treatment

CBCT has been shown to be useful in the management of failed root canal treatments (Davies et al, 2015b) and may provide information regarding the presence, exact location (root) and nature of periapical lesions that may not be readily detected on conventional radiographs (Simon et al, 2006; Patel et al, 2012; Cheung et al, 2013).

Furthermore, additional root canals (Blattner et al, 2010; Neelakantan et al, 2010) and complications, such as vertical root fractures (Fig 8-2), perforations (Figs 8-3 and 8-4), and the nature and position of resorption

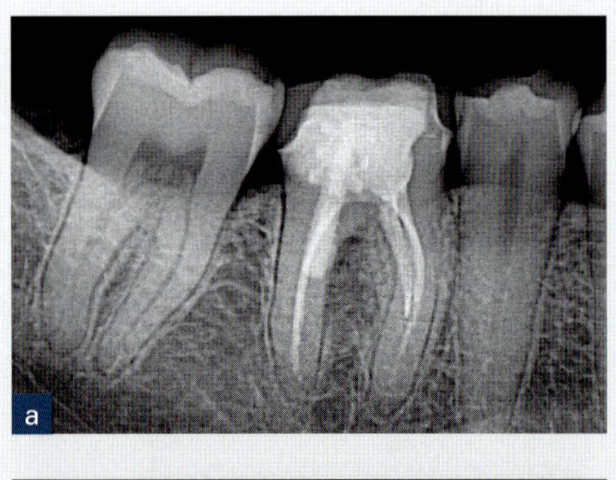
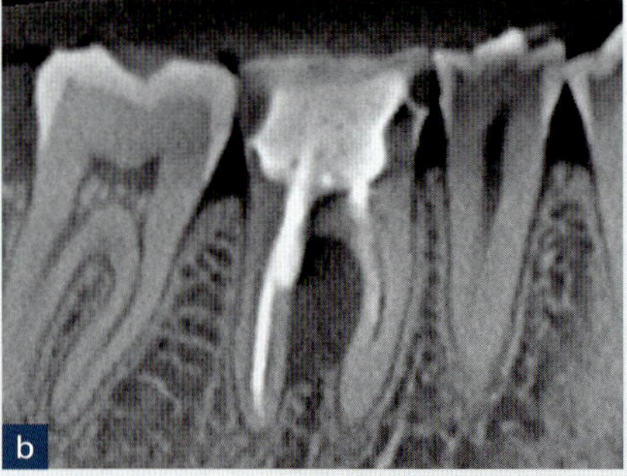
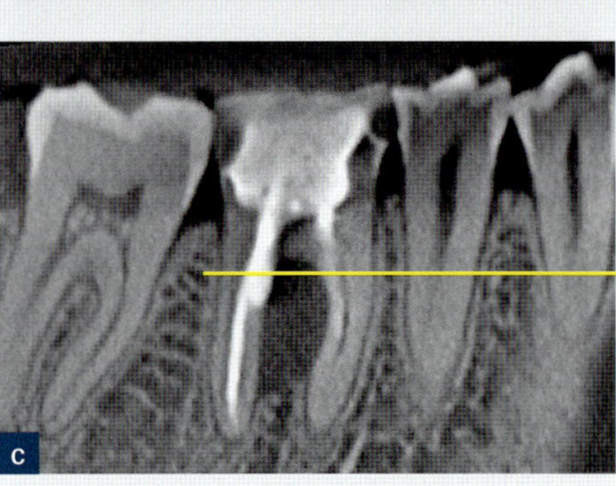
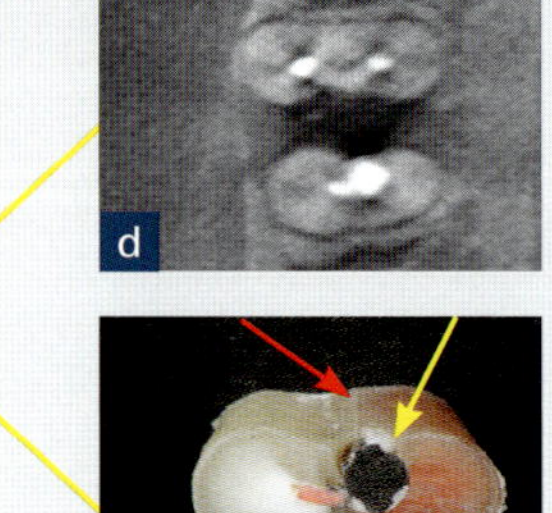

Fig 8-3 (a) A periapical radiograph of a symptomatic root-treated mandibular first molar with slight tenderness to percussion but no other obvious signs of endodontic or periodontal disease and no sign of periapical or periradicular radiolucency. The treatment plan included non-surgical endodontic re-treatment. The post space may have perforatedthe mesial aspect of the distal root. However, this radiographic appearance could also be due to the relationship of the X-ray beam to the digital sensor. (b and c) The CBCT scan changed the treatment plan; the sagittal CBCT slice revealed a large inter-radicular radiolucency, suggesting a perforation. (d) Axial CBCT slice revealing the extent of the perforation and inter-radicular bone loss. (e) The unsalvageable tooth was extracted, confirming the presence not only of the perforation (yellow arrow) but also of a vertical root fracture (red arrow).

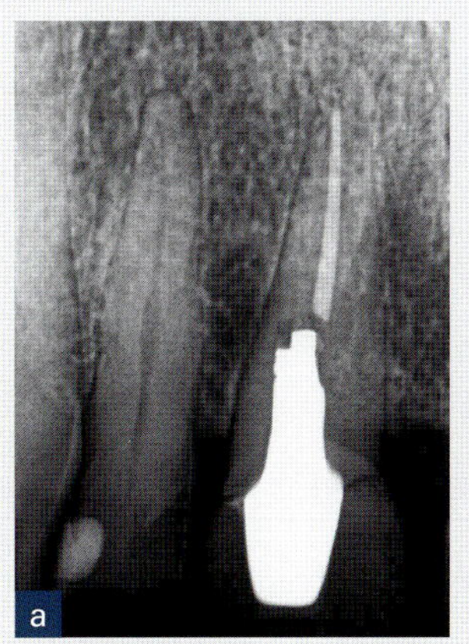

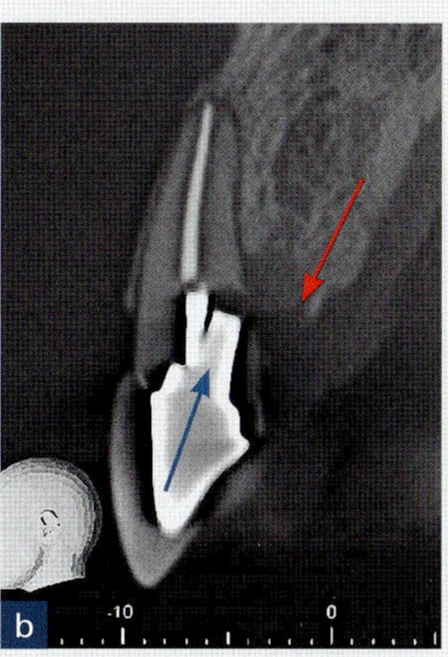

Fig 8-4 (a) A periapical radiograph of a root-treated maxillary right central incisor restored with a post-retained crown. Clinical examination revealed a 4 mm periodontal probing depth palatally, but the examination was otherwise unremarkable. On the periapical radiograph, the post appears to have deviated distally but the lamina dura is intact and there is no sign of widening of the periodontal ligament space or of an obvious periapical or periradicular radiolucency. In addition, the root filling looks acceptable in terms of length and density. (b) Sagittal CBCT slice revealed the palatal angulation of the post preparation (blue arrow) and a coronal third root perforation. The associated palatal bone loss is clearly evident (red arrow).

defects (Figs 8-5 and 8-6) may be readily identified with CBCT (D'Addazio et al, 2011; Shemesh et al, 2011).

Presence of a periapical lesion

It is well established that conventional radiographs may not detect periapical lesions, especially on molar teeth (Cheung et al, 2013; Liang et al, 2014; Venskutonis et al, 2014a). The presence of a periapical radiolucency, not detected on a conventional radiograph, may have an effect on whether an existing root canal treatment should be left alone or re-treated prior to providing a new coronal restoration (Figs 8-2 and 8-3). Davies et

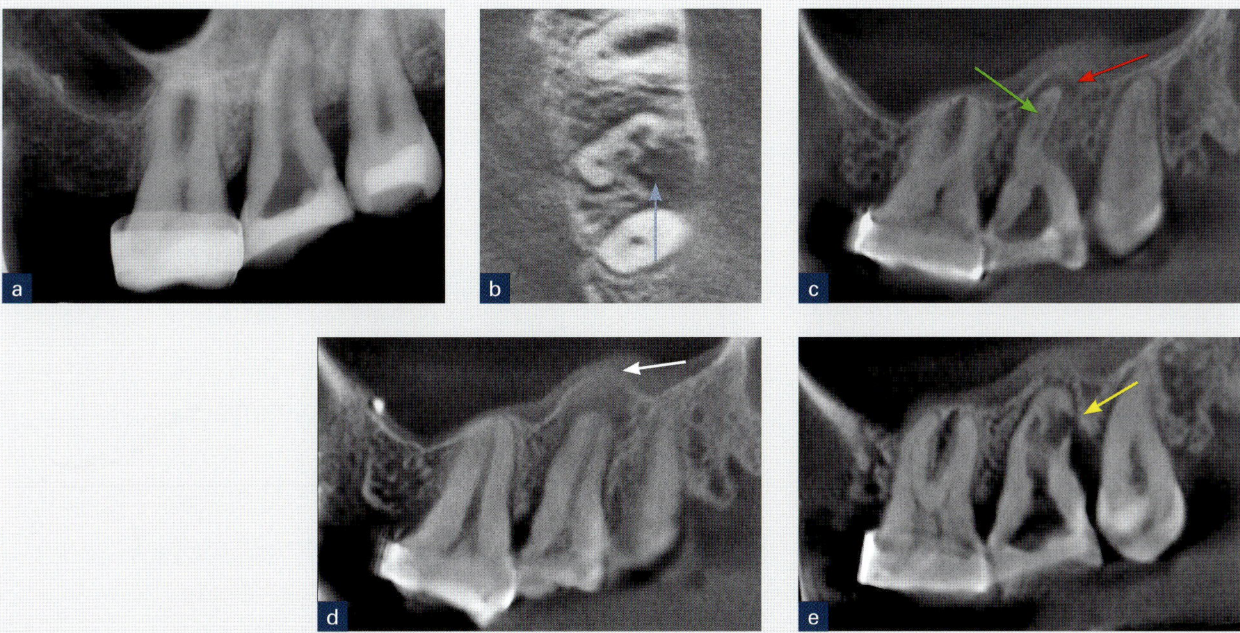

Fig 8-5 (a) A periapical radiograph of a maxillary left second molar, in which endodontic treatment was aborted due to failed anaesthesia. The patient was referred to a specialist endodontist. (b) The axial CBCT slice revealed the presence of internal root resorption, which had perforated the distobuccal, mesiobuccal and palatal root canal walls (blue arrow). (c to e) Sagittal CBCT reconstructed images: (c) the mesiobuccal root; (d) the palatal root; and (e) the distobuccal root. The CBCT images reveal the true size and nature of the resorptive lesion in the mesiobuccal and palatal roots (c and d), which are associated with periapical radiolucencies (red and white arrows); there are also signs of internal resorption associated with the mesiobuccal canal (green arrow) and the distobuccal root (e), which is associated with a very large perforating internal root resorption lesion (yellow arrow). Note the amount of root surface loss due to resorption in (e) and the associated distal bone loss. Without prior knowledge about the presence and nature of the resorptive lesion, there would be a very high risk of causing a hypochlorite accident during chemomechanical root canal treatment. This unsalvageable tooth was extracted.

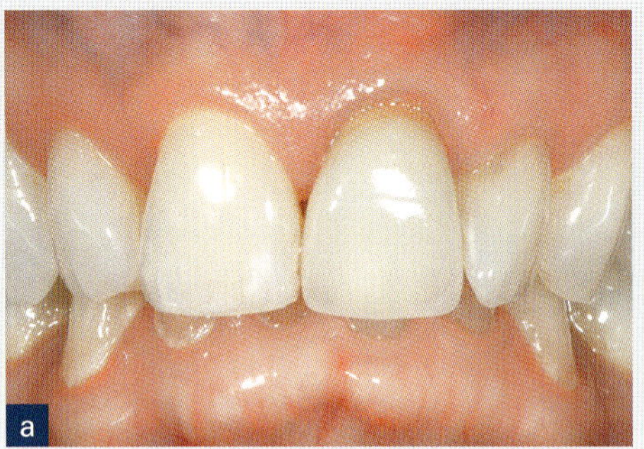

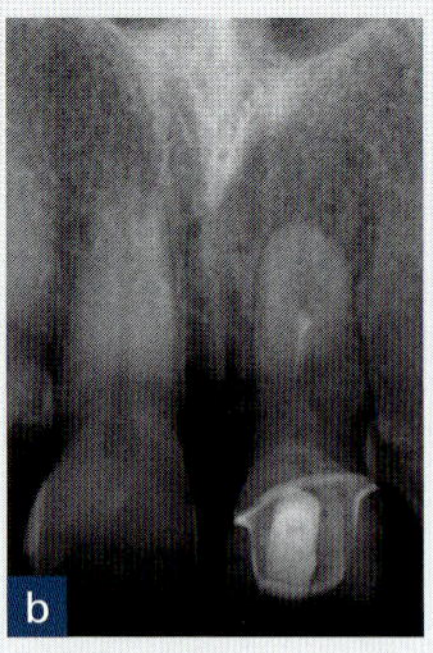

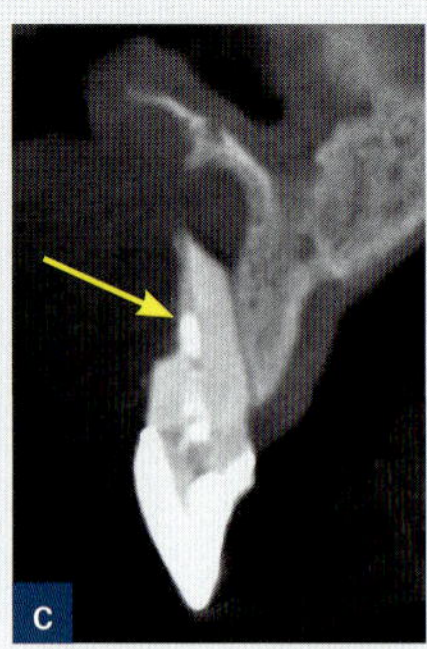

Fig 8-6 (a) A photograph and (b) periapical radiograph of the maxillary left central incisor tooth. The symptomatic tooth has been root-treated and there is an associated persistent round and well-circumscribed periapical radiolucency. The root filling lacks adequate length and density. During non-surgical endodontic re-treatment, the apex locator reading was erratic and the zero reading and working length could not be reliably established. (c) Sagittal CBCT reconstructed image through the same tooth revealed significant loss of labial root structure from the coronal third to the apex (yellow arrow) and associated periapical bone loss. Root canal re-treatment was not possible and the tooth was extracted.

al (2015b) assessed the outcome of non-surgical root canal re-treatment radiographically and found a lower number of favourable outcomes with CBCT compared to periapical radiographs. The assessment with CBCT affected the management of the reviewed cases. The ability of CBCT to diagnose periapical disease is further discussed in Chapter 7.

The differential diagnosis of a cyst from a periapical granuloma using CBCT has also been investigated (Simon et al, 2006; Rosenberg et al, 2010; Guo et al, 2013). In a clinical study, Bornstein et al (2015) concluded that CBCT could not reliably differentiate between a granuloma and a cyst. At present, the only reliable diagnosis can be made by in-toto excision and subsequent serial sectioning of the lesion (Nair et al, 1996).

CBCT has been shown to be beneficial in the diagnosis of vertical root fractures (VRFs). Subtle periradicular signs of bone loss indicating a VRF associated with a root-treated tooth (Fig 8-2), which may be challenging to diagnose by other means, may be evident on CBCT examination (Bernades et al, 2009; Wang et al, 2011; Kajan and Taromsari, 2012). The presence or absence of a VRF will have an impact on treatment planning and is described in more detail in Chapter 11.

Quality of existing root canal treatment

Clinical and population studies have shown a strong correlation between the quality of root canal fillings and the outcome of treatment (Liang et al, 2012a; Kirkevang et al, 2014). The quality of the root canal filling is usually assessed by periapical radiographs and is focused on the length and density of the filling (Fig 8-7). A root canal filling that terminates 0 to 2 mm from the radiographic apex has been shown to be more likely to result in a favourable outcome, compared to long or short fillings (European Society of Endodontology, quality guidelines , 2006; Liang et al, 2012a). A void-free root canal filling also results in a higher success rate (Sjögren et al, 1990; Song et al, 2011; Ng et al, 2011).

Liang et al (2012a) demonstrated an overestimation of root canal filling quality by radiographs compared to CBCT. On conventional radiographs when the root filling was flush at the radiographic apex, it was actually long on CBCT. Furthermore, CBCT was also found to be superior to conventional radiography in detecting root filling voids, especially in the buccolingual plane of the root filling (Liang et al, 2012a).

The additional information from a CBCT scan may influence whether the clinician decides to carry out non-surgical or surgical endodontic re-treatment in refractory cases. In some instances, extraction may be the only viable treatment option (D'Addazio et al, 2011; Shemesh et al, 2011; Eskandarloo et al, 2012).

Missed root canals and anatomical features

Inadequate disinfection of the root canal system may lead to failure of root canal treatment. (Ng et al, 2008). One of the reasons for persistent intra-radicular in-

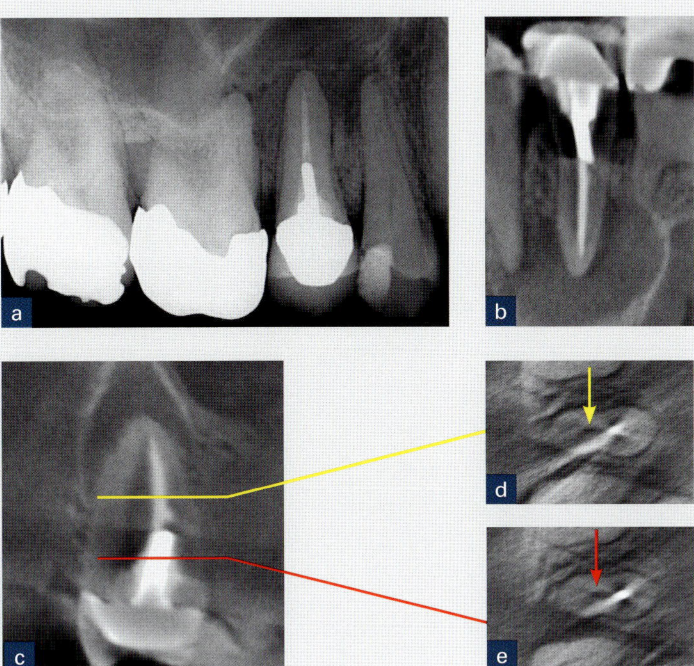

Fig 8-7 (a) A periapical radiograph of a root-treated maxillary right second premolar revealing a large, well-circumscribed periapical radiolucency associated with this tooth. The density and length of the root filling appear to be satisfactory. (b) Sagittal CBCT slice confirms the findings on the periapical radiograph. However, (c) a coronal CBCT slice through the same tooth shows that the palatal canal has not been identified, and around 75% of the canal system has not been obturated. Axial CBCT slices through the middle (d) and coronal (e) thirds of the same tooth also reveal the untreated palatal canal (arrows). The diagnosis of apical periodontitis was confirmed with the aid of a periapical radiograph. However, the presence of the palatal canal could not be confirmed from the periapical radiograph. This knowledge is essential to allow for thorough and predictable instrumentation.

fection is failure to identify and treat all canals during treatment. The ability of CBCT to detect supplemental canals (Figs 8-8 and 8-9) and anatomic aberrations is well established (Tu et al, 2007, 2009; Abella et al, 2012; Davies et al, 2015a). Nevertheless, incorrect interpretations of images resulting in false positive diagnoses of supplemental canals may occur from scatter caused by filling materials in an adjacent root filled canal (Krithikadatta et al, 2010).

Root canal location(s) can be readily identified from CBCT scans before commencing treatment, thus allowing the clinician to plan the access cavity design

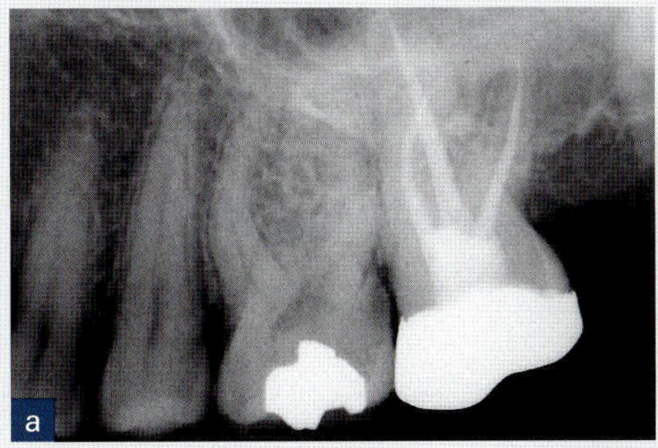

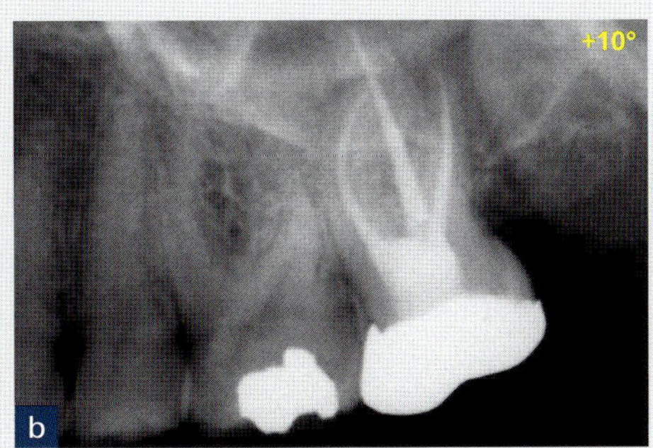

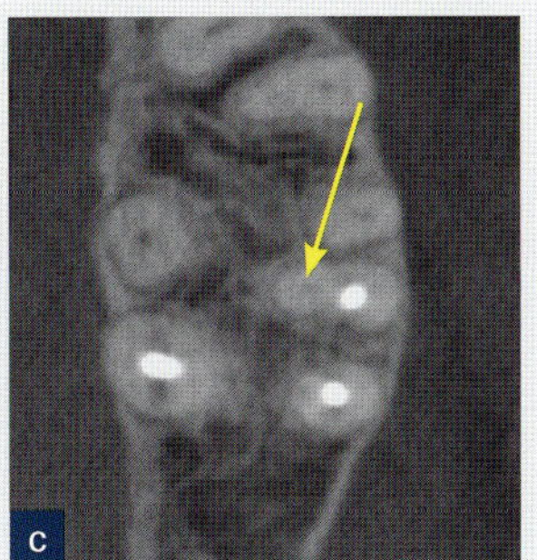

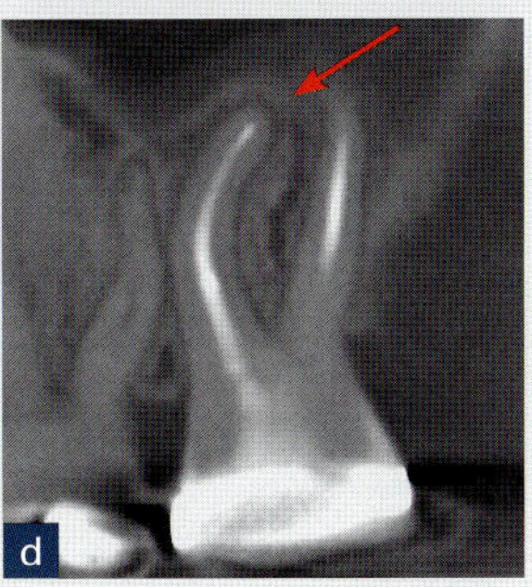

Fig 8-8 (a and b) Parallax periapical radiographs of a symptomatic root-treated maxillary left second molar revealing an acceptable root filling in terms of length and density. The periapical radiographs did not show the presence of any periapical radiolucency. (c) Axial CBCT reconstructed image revealed an unfilled second mesiobuccal canal (yellow arrow), and (d) sagittal CBCT reconstructed image revealed a periapical radiolucency (red arrow) associated with the mesiobuccal root. The existing root canal treatment was carried out by an experienced endodontist, and there was doubt whether it could be improved upon. It was also unclear whether the patient's symptoms were due to an endodontic infection or a vertical root fracture. The CBCT scan confirmed that the patient's symptoms were endodontic in nature, and that non-surgical root canal treatment was the ideal treatment option.

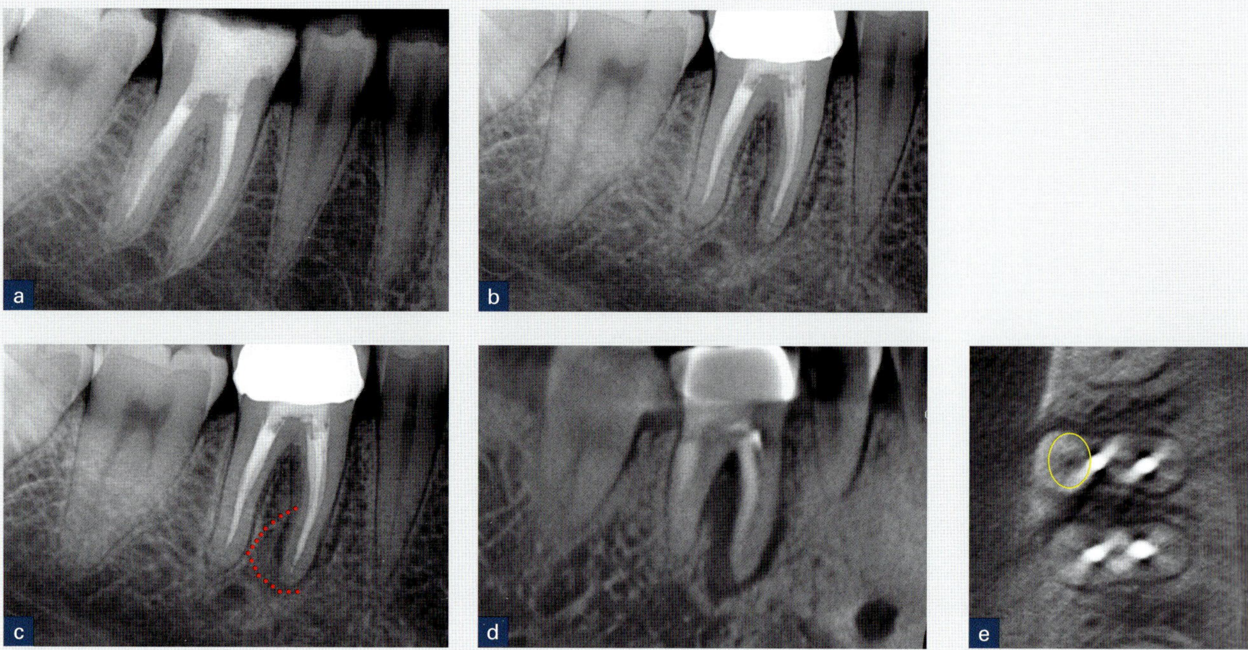

Fig 8-9 (a) A periapical radiograph of the mandibular right first molar showing a well-executed root canal filling in terms of length and density. (b) A 5-year review reveals a periradicular radiolucency along the distal aspect of the mesial root (J-shaped radiolucency), potentially indicating bone loss associated with a vertical root fracture. (c) A 10-degree distal X-ray tube shift confirmed the presence of the radiolucency (red dotted line). (d) Sagittal CBCT reconstructed image revealed the full extent of bone loss, suggesting the possibility of a vertical root fracture. (e) However, the axial CBCT reconstructed image revealed an unfilled (missed) third mesial canal (yellow circle). After various treatment options were discussed, the patient decided to have the tooth extracted.

accurately and minimise removal of sound dentine (Tu et al, 2009; Patel, 2010). The presence of isthmuses and fins that may not have been debrided in the root canal systems may also be assessed and subsequently managed (Liang et al, 2012b) (Fig 8-10). In addition, a high prevalence of C-shaped molar root canal anatomy has also been confirmed using CBCT (Kim et al, 2015)

An appreciation of the divergence or convergence of root canals using CBCT scanning may also influence how the root canal system is prepared and/or subsequently obturated. For example, what appears to be a well executed, but failed endodontic treatment in a maxillary molar tooth with only one identified mesiobuccal canal may suggest failure due to an unidentified second mesiobuccal canal. Therefore, non-surgical re-treatment would be indicated, with the principal aim being to locate, disinfect and seal the unidentified root canal system. However, a CBCT scan may confirm the absence of a second mesiobuccal canal, indicating that a surgical approach would be more appropriate.

Surgical endodontic re-treatment

Surgical endodontic re-treatment is indicated when persistent periapical periodontitis does not heal after root canal treatment and non-surgical endodontic re-treatment is either not possible due to the presence of irretrievable or impassable fractured instruments, ledges or blockages, or has already been attempted but failed as a result of an extra-radicular infection (Wang et al, 2004; Nair, 2004). Furthermore, the need to obtain a biopsy or perform exploratory surgery are the other factors that necessitate surgical management (Siqueira, 2001; Kim and Kratchman, 2006).

CBCT has been recommended for the planning of surgical endodontic re-treatment (Tsurumachi and Honda, 2007). Rigolone et al (2003) concluded that CBCT might play an important role in planning for surgical endodontic re-treatment on the palatal roots of maxillary first molars. The distance between the cortical plate and the palatal root apex could be measured, and the presence or absence of the maxillary sinus between the roots could be assessed (Fig 8-11).

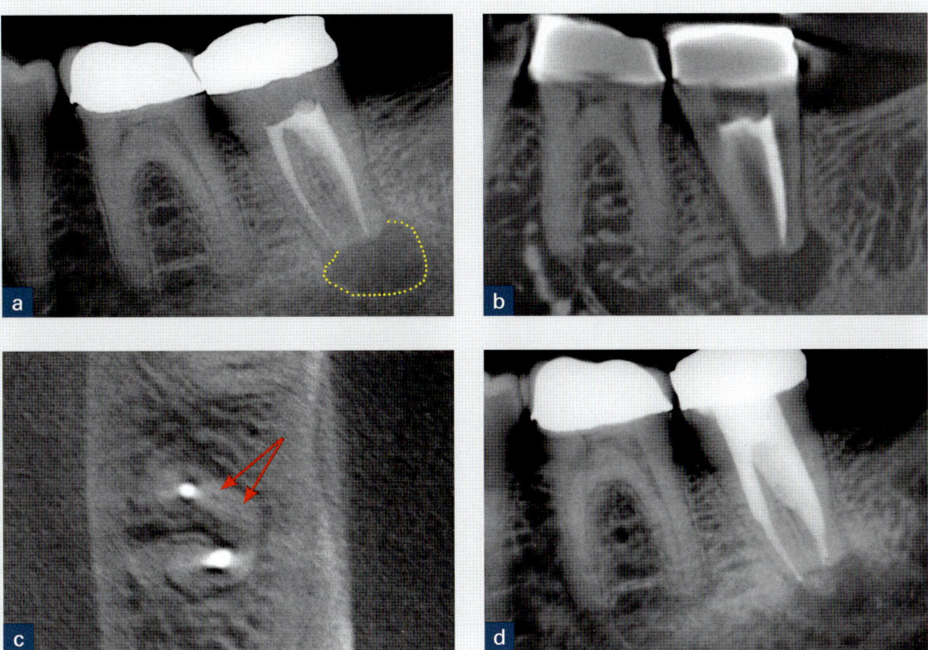

Fig 8-10 (a) Periapical radiograph of a mandibular left second molar with refractory apical periodontitis. The root filling seems satisfactory in terms of length and density. (b) Sagittal CBCT slice through the same tooth showing the true size and outline of the lesion. (c) Axial CBCT slice through the same tooth revealing a C-shape root morphology and the missed root canal anatomy (red arrows). (d) At the 1-year review following endodontic re-treatment, the periapical radiolucency has reduced in size; note the the difference in the shape of the filled root canal system after a well-executed chemomechanical preparation and obturation when compared with (a).

CBCT allows the anatomical relationship of the root apices to important neighbouring anatomical structures, such as the inferior dental canal, mental foramen, and maxillary sinus, to be clearly identified in any plane the clinician wishes to view (Patel et al, 2007; Lofthag-Hansen et al, 2007; Bornstein et al, 2011). The information from a CBCT scan may result in deciding against surgical endodontic re-treatment of maxillary molar teeth where the sinus floor has been perforated by a larger-than-estimated periapical lesion, which may not have been readily detected on periapical radiographs (Maillet et al, 2011).

By selecting relevant CBCT slices, the thickness of the cortical plate, the cancellous bone pattern, the presence and position of fenestrations (Fig 8-12), and the inclination of the roots of teeth planned for surgical endodontic re-treatment can be accurately determined preoperatively (Nakata et al, 2006; Lofthag-Hansen et al, 2007; Low et al, 2008). Root morphology and bony topography can be visualised in three dimensions, as can the number of root canals and whether they converge or diverge from each other; this information is essential to improve the outcome of treatment. Unidentified (and untreated) root canals may be identified using axial slices (Lofthag-Hansen et al, 2007; Low et al, 2008). The true size, location and extent of the periapical lesion can also be appreciated, while the actual root with which the lesion is associated may be confirmed (Patel et al, 2012). This information may have a bearing on non-surgical and surgical endodontic re-treatment.

Low et al (2008) compared the findings of periapical radiographs with those of CBCT in root-treated maxillary posterior teeth, that were being assessed for periapical surgery. In this study, 34% of periapical lesions detected by CBCT were not detected with periapical radiographs. The likelihood of detecting periapical lesions with periapical radiographs was reduced when the root apices were in close proximity to the floor of the maxillary sinus and when there was less than 1 mm of bone between the periapical lesion and the sinus floor. Therefore, periapical radiographs were less sensitive for detecting periapical lesions associated with maxillary molar teeth.

Bornstein et al (2011) carried out a similar study on root-treated mandibular posterior teeth and had similar results—26% of periapical lesions were missed by periapical radiographs.

Kurt et al (2014) performed surgical endodontic re-treatment on 40 maxillary first molars. Two groups of patients were included; one had a preoperative CBCT scan and the other was evaluated only with periapical radiographs. The CBCT group had fewer sinus perforations during surgery and the procedure was more efficient to carry out.

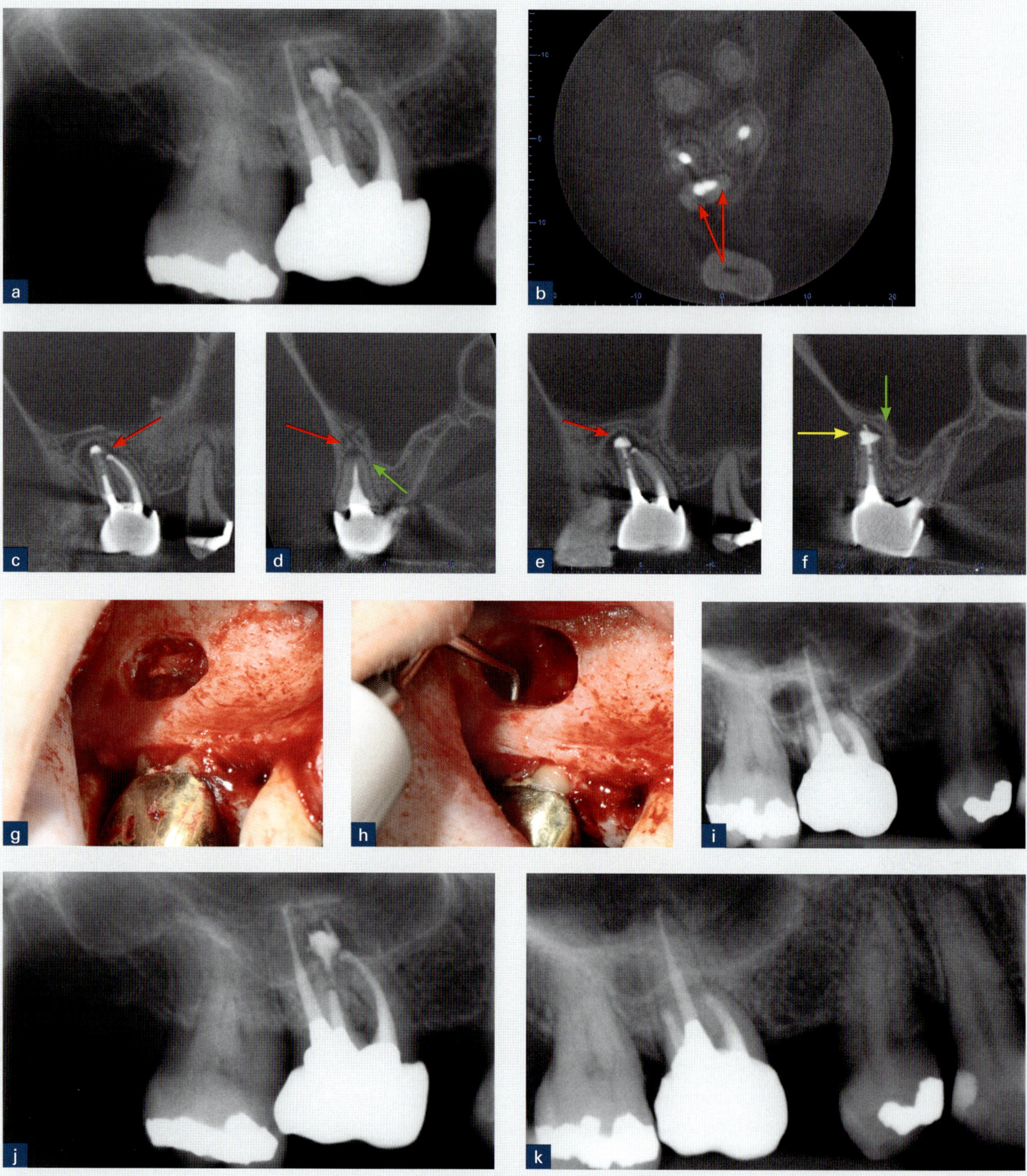

Fig 8-11 (a) Periapical radiograph of a failed root treatment and periapical extrusion of the root filling material in the maxillary right first molar, with periapical radiolucencies around the mesiobuccal and distobuccal root apices. (b) Axial CBCT slice of the middle third of the tooth reveals that both mesiobuccal canals have been identified and their isthmus has been shaped, cleaned and filled (red arrows). Sagittal and coronal CBCT reconstructed images, respectively, of (c) and (d) mesiobuccal, and (e) and (f) distobuccal roots reveal the location and extent of apical radiolucencies (red arrows) and the position of the extruded root filling. Note the close proximity of the roots to the maxillary sinus (green arrows) and the existing buccal alveolar bone perforation (yellow arrow). The sinus floor is, however, intact (c, d, e, f). The coronal CBCT slices also aid in examining the presence or absence of the maxillary sinus between the roots before surgical endodontic re-treatment (e and f). In this case, the inter-radicular extension of the sinus in between the buccal and palatal roots is evident (d and f). (g and h) Intra-operative photographs showing the osteotomy site and ultrasonic retro preparation of the resected buccal roots. (i) Immediate postoperative situation showing a well-executed surgical endodontic re-treatment of the mesiobuccal and distobuccal roots. (j) Preoperative and (k) 1-year postoperative radiograph of the same tooth showing healing.

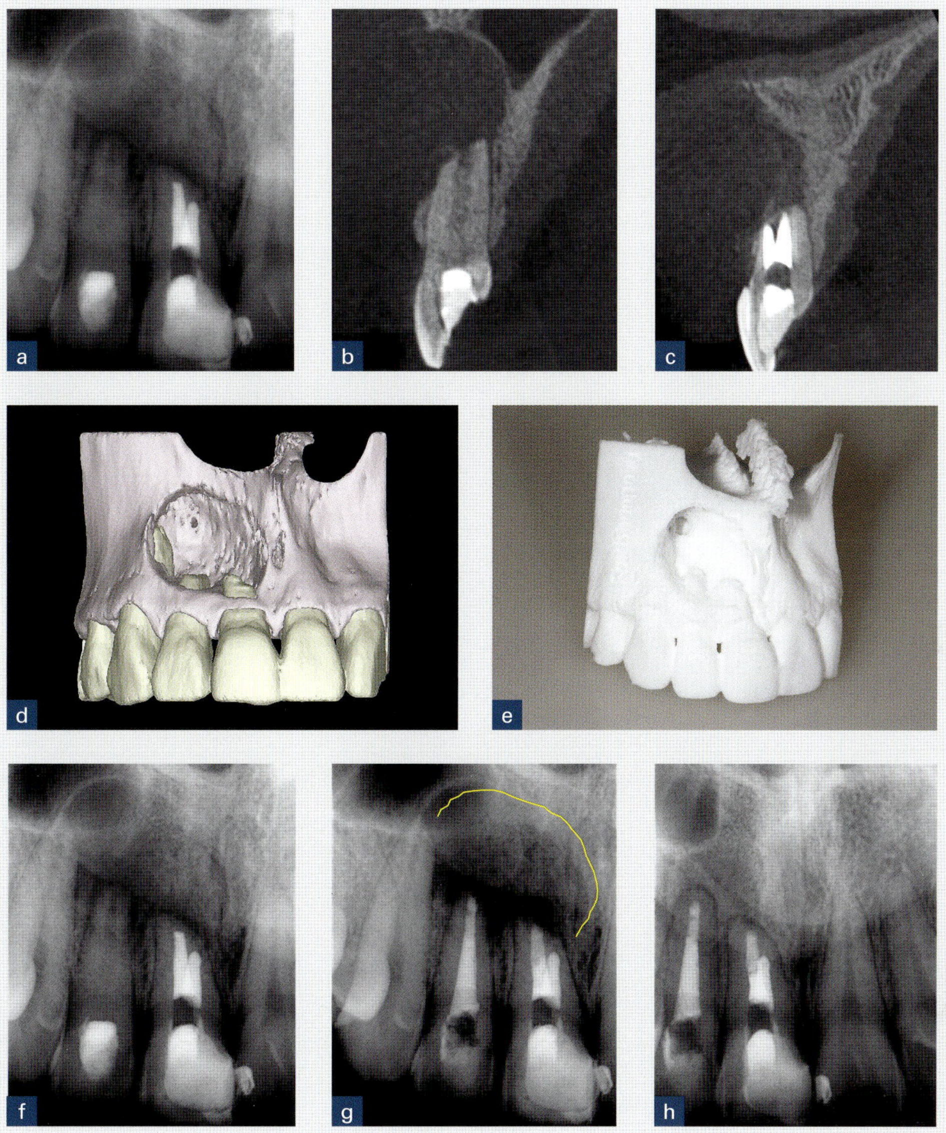

Fig 8-12 (a) Periapical radiograph of the maxillary right central and lateral incisors associated with a large periapical radiolucency. The central incisor has been root-treated to an acceptable standard in terms of density and length of the root filling. (b) Sagittal CBCT slice through the maxillary right lateral incisor showing apical root resorption and a very large and well-circumscribed radiolucency associated with this tooth. Note the loss of labial alveolar bone. (c) Sagittal CBCT slice through the maxillary right central incisor revealing the involvement of this tooth and associated periapical bone loss. (d) To aid management, dental implant planning software can be used to create a three-dimensionally rendered image of the entire lesion and the surrounding anatomy. (e) The DICOM data set may be used to fabricate a nylon model of the scanned anatomy for better visualisation and surgical treatment planning (Cavendish Imaging, London, UK). (f and g) The lesion was managed by surgical endodontic re-treatment of the right central incisor and a combined endodontic treatment and root-end resection of the right lateral incisor. (h) 1-year periapical radiograph of the same teeth, showing significant bony infill and a healed outcome.

Conclusion

A pre-treatment CBCT scan can supplement existing modalities and provide valuable additional information on failed root canal treatments (Venskutonis et al, 2014b). The information obtained from a CBCT scan in complex endodontic cases may influence treatment planning strategies (Ee et al, 2014; Mota de Almeida et al, 2015) and ultimately the treatment outcome.

Identification of the presence and location of previously undetected periapical lesions, complex tooth anatomy, adjacent anatomical structures, and complications such as procedural errors (e.g. perforations) may improve the management of non-surgical and surgical endodontic treatment.

A CBCT scan should only be considered when conventional radiographic techniques do not provide adequate information for the diagnosis and/or management of endodontic problems (Patel et al, 2015). The relative benefits of the CBCT scan should outweigh the risk to the patient. Each scan must be justified, and the patient radiation dose must be optimised (European Society of Endodontolgy CBCT position statement, 2014).

References

Abella F, Patel S, Durán-Sindreu F, Mercadé M, Roig M. Mandibular first molars with disto-lingual roots: review and clinical management. Int Endod J 2012;45:963–978.

Azim AA, Griggs JA, Huang GT. The Tennessee study: factors affecting treatment outcome and healing time following non-surgical root canal treatment. Int Endod J 2015; doi: 10.1111/iej.12429 [Epub ahead of print].

Bernardes RA, de Moraes IG, Húngaro Duarte MA, Azevedo BC, de Azevedo JR, Bramante CM. Use of cone-beam volumetric tomography in the diagnosis of root fractures. Oral Surg Oral Med Oral Pathol Oral Radiol Endod 2009;108:270–277.

Blattner TC, Goerge N, Lee CC, Kumar V, Yelton CD. Efficacy of cone-beam computed tomography as a modality to accurately identify the presence of second mesiobuccal canals in maxillary first and second molars: a pilot study. J Endod 2010;36:867–870.

Bornstein MM, Bingisser AC, Reichart PA, Sendi P, Bosshardt DD, von Arx T. Comparison between radiographic (2-dimensional and 3-dimensional) and histologic findings of periapical lesions treated with apical surgery. J Endod 2015;41:804–811.

Bornstein MM, Lauber R, Sendi P, von Arx T. Comparison of periapical and limited cone-beam computed tomography in mandibular molars for analysis of anatomical landmarks before apical surgery. J Endod 2011;37:151–157.

Cheung GSP, Wei WL, McGrath C. Agreement between periapical radiographs and cone-beam computed tomography for assessment of periapical status of root filled molar teeth. Int Endod J 2013;46:889–895.

D'Addazio PS, Campos CN, Özcan M, Teixeira HGC, Passoni RM, Carvalho ACP. A comparative study between cone-beam computed tomography and periapical radiographs in the diagnosis of simulated endodontic complications. Int Endod J 2011;44:218–224.

Davies A, Mannocci F, Mitchell P, Andiappan M, Patel S. The detection of periapical pathoses in root filled teeth using single and parallax periapical radiographs versus cone beam computed tomography – a clinical study. Int Endod J 2015a;48:582–592.

Davies A, Patel S, Fosci F, Andiappan M, Mitchell PJ, Mannocci F. The detection of periapical pathosis using digital periapical radiography and cone beam computed tomography in endodontically retreated teeth-part 2: a 1 year post-treatment follow-up. Int Endod J 2015b (in press).

Ee J, Fayad MI, Johnson BR. Comparison of endodontic diagnosis and treatment planning decisions using cone-beam volumetric tomography versus periapical radiography. J Endod 2014;40:910–916.

Eskandarloo A, Mirshekari A, Poorolajal J, Mohammadi Z, Shokri A. Comparison of cone-beam computed tomography with intraoral photostimulable phosphor imaging plate for diagnosis of endodontic complications: a simulation study. Oral Surg Oral Med Oral Pathol Oral Radiol 2012;114:e54–61.

European Society of Endodontology position statement: The use of CBCT in Endodontics. Int Endod J 2014;47:502–504.

European Society of Endodontology. Quality guidelines for endodontic treatment: consensus report of the European Society of Endodontology. Int Endod J 2006;39:921–930.

Guo J, Simon JH, Sedghizadeh P, Soliman ON, Chapman T, Enciso R. Evaluation of the reliability and accuracy of using cone-beam computed tomography for diagnosing periapical cysts from granulomas. J Endod 2013;9:1485–1490.

Kajan ZD, Taromsari M. Value of cone beam CT in detection of dental root fractures. Dentomaxillofac Radiol 2012;41:3–10.

Kim SY, Kim BS, Kim Y. Mandibular second molar root canal morphology and variants in a Korean subpopulation. Int Endod J 2015; doi: 10.1111/iej.12437 [Epub ahead of print].

Kim S, Kratchman S. Modern endodontic surgery concepts and practice: a review. J Endod 2006;32:601–623.

Kirkevang LL, Vaeth M, Wenzel A. Ten-year follow-up of root filled teeth: a radiographic study of a Danish population. Int Endod J 2014;47:980–988.

Krithikadatta J, Kottoor J, Karumaran CS, Rajan G. Mandibular first molar having an unusual mesial root canal morphology with contradictory cone-beam computed tomography findings: a case report. J Endod 2010;36:1712–1716.

Kurt SN, Üstun Y, Erdogan Ö, Evlice B, Yoldas O, Öztunc H. Outcomes of periradicular surgery of maxillary first molars using a vestibular approach: a prospective, clinical study with one year of follow-up. J Oral Maxillofac Surg 2014;72:1049–1061.

Liang YH, Jiang L, Gao XJ, Shemesh H, Wesselink PR, Wu MK. Detection and measurement of artificial periapical lesions by cone-beam computed tomography. Int Endod J 2014;47:332–338.

Liang YH, Li G, Shemesh H, Wesselink PR, Wu MK. The association between complete absence of post-treatment periapical lesion and quality of root canal filling. Clin Oral Investig 2012a;16:1619–1626.

Liang YH, Yuan M, Li G, Shemesh H, Wesselink PR, Wu MK. The ability of cone-beam computed tomography to detect simulated buccal and lingual recesses in root canals. Int Endod J 2012b;45:724–729.

Lofthag-Hansen S, Huumonen S, Gröndahl K, Gröndahl HG. Limited cone-beam CT and intraoral radiography for the diagnosis of periapical pathology. Oral Surg Oral Med Oral Pathol Oral Radiol Endod 2007;103:114–119.

Low KM, Dula K, Bürgin W, von Arx T. Comparison of periapical radiography and limited cone-beam tomography in posterior maxillary teeth referred for apical surgery. J Endod 2008;34:557–562.

Maillet M, Bowles WR, McClanahan SL, John MT, Ahmad M. Cone-beam computed tomography evaluation of maxillary sinusitis. J Endod 2011;37:753–757.

Mota de Almeida JF, Knutsson K, Flygare L. The impact of cone beam computed tomography on the choice of endodontic diagnosis. Int Endod J 2015:48:564–572.

Nair PNR, Pajarola G, Schroeder HE. Types and incidence of human periapical lesions obtained with extracted teeth. Oral Surg Oral Med Oral Pathol Oral Radiol Endod 1996;81:93–102.

Nair PN. Pathogenesis of apical periodontitis and the causes of endodontic failures. Crit Rev Oral Biol Med 2004;15:348–381.

Nakata K, Naitoh M, Izumi M, Inamoto K, Ariji E, Nakamura H. Effectiveness of dental computed tomography in diagnostic imaging of periradicular lesion of each root of a multirooted tooth: a case report. J Endod 2006;32:583–587.

Neelakantan P, Subbarao C, Subbarao C V. Comparative evaluation of modified canal staining and clearing technique, cone-beam computed tomography, peripheral quantitative computed tomography, spiral computed tomography, and plain and contrast medium-enhanced digital radiography in studying root canal morphology. J Endod 2010;36:1547–1551.

Ng YL, Mann V, Gulabivala K. A prospective study of the factors affecting outcomes of nonsurgical root canal treatment: part 1: periapical health. Int Endod J 2011;44:583–609.

Ng YL, Mann V, Rahbaran S, Lewsey J, Gulabivala K. Outcome of primary root canal treatment: systematic review of the literature—part 1. Effects of study characteristics on probability of success. Int Endod J 2007;40:921–939.

Ng YL, Mann V, Rahbaran S, Lewsey J, Gulabivala K. Outcome of primary root canal treatment: systematic review of the literature—part 2. Influence of clinical factors. Int Endod J 2008;41:6–31.

Patel S, Dawood A, Whaites E, Pitt Ford T. The potential applications of cone beam computed tomography in the management of endodontic problems. Int Endod J 2007;40:818–830.

Patel S. The use of cone beam computed tomography in the conservative management of dens invaginatus: a case report. Int Endod J 2010;43:707–713.

Patel S, Wilson R, Dawood A, Mannocci F. The detection of periapical pathosis using periapical radiography and cone beam computed tomography—part 1: pre-operative status. Int Endod J 2012;45:702–710.

Patel S, Durack C, Abella F, Shemesh H, Roig M, Lemberg K. Cone beam computed tomography in endodontics—a review. Int Endod J 2015;48:3–15.

Rigolone M, Pasqualini D, Bianchi L, Berutti E, Bianchi SD. Vestibular surgical access to the palatine root of the superior first molar: "low-dose cone-beam" CT analysis of the pathway and its anatomic variations. J Endod 2003;29:773–775.

Rosenberg PA, Frisbie J, Lee J, et al. Evaluation of pathologists (histopathology) and radiologists (cone beam computed tomography) differentiating radicular cysts from granulomas. J Endod 2010;36:423–428.

Shemesh H, Cristescu RC, Wesselink PR, Wu MK. The use of cone-beam computed tomography and digital periapical radiographs to diagnose root perforations. J Endod 2011;37:513–516.

Simon JH, Enciso R, Malfaz JM, Roges R, Bailey-Perry M, Patel A. Differential diagnosis of large periapical lesions using cone-beam computed tomography measurements and biopsy. J Endod 2006;32:833–837.

Siqueira Jr JF. Aetiology of root canal treatment failure: why well-treated teeth can fail. Int Endod J 2001;34:1–10.

Sjögren U, Hägglund B, Sundqvist G, Wing K. Factors affecting the long-term results of endodontic treatment. J Endod 1990;16:498–504.

Song M, Jung IY, Lee SJ, Lee CY, Kim E. Prognostic factors for clinical outcomes in endodontic microsurgery: a retrospective study. J Endod 2011;37:927–933.

Tsurumachi T, Honda K. A new cone beam computerized tomography system for use in endodontic surgery. Int Endod J 2007;40:224–232.

Tu MG, Tsai CC, Jou MJ, et al. Prevalence of three-rooted mandibular first molars among Taiwanese individuals. J Endod 2007;33:1163–1166.

Tu MG, Huang HL, Hsue SS, et al. Detection of permanent three-rooted mandibular first molars by cone-beam computed tomography imaging in Taiwanese individuals. J Endod 2009;35:503–507.

Venskutonis T, Daugela P, Strazdas M, Juodzbalys G. Accuracy of digital radiography and cone beam computed tomography on periapical radiolucency detection in endodontically treated teeth. J Oral Maxillofac Res 2014a;1;5:e1.

Venskutonis T, Plotino G, Juodzbalys G, Mickevičienė L. The importance of cone-beam computed tomography in the management of endodontic problems: a review of the literature. J Endod 2014b;40:1895–1901.

Wang N, Knight K, Dao T, Friedman S. Treatment outcome in endodontics-The Toronto Study. Phases I and II: apical surgery. J Endod 2004;30:751–761.

Wang P, Yan XB, Lui DG, Zhang WL, Zhang Y, Ma XC. Detection of dental root fractures by using cone-beam computed tomography. Dentomaxillofac Radiol 2011;40:290–298.

Chapter 9

Traumatic Dental Injuries

Mitsuhiro Tsukiboshi, Conor Durack

Introduction

The World Health Organisation (WHO) created a classification system for the varying types of traumatic dental injuries (TDIs) in 1992 (WHO, 1992). Two years later, this classification was modified by Andreasen and Andreasen (1994) in order to define and categorise trauma entities not presented in the original WHO classification (Tables 9-1 to 9-4).

Reports on the prevalence of TDI vary considerably due to the lack of homogeneity between studies examining this epidemiological measure. A national survey carried out in the USA, with a cohort of 154 million people between the ages of 6 and 50, revealed that almost one in three 6 to 20-year-olds and one in four 20 to 50-year-olds had suffered TDI (Kaste et al, 1996).

The accurate diagnosis of TDI is reliant on the acquisition of a thorough history, coupled with a systematic examination of the patient. This examination includes special clinical diagnostic tests and an appropriate radiographic assessment of the injured area(s) of the dentition, supporting tissues and, when indicated, adjacent soft tissues. The radiographic assessment is, and can only be, an adjunct to, and a component part of, the diagnostic process.

TDIs are often associated with the development of post-injury complications, such as pulp canal obliteration (Andreasen et al, 1987), pulp necrosis (Andreasen and Pedersen, 1985), the development of apical periodontitis (AP), root resorption (Andreasen and Pedersen, 1985), and marginal periodontal breakdown (Andreasen and Pedersen, 1985; Oikarinen et al, 1987). Any of these undesirable sequelae may occur in isolation or in combination with one or more of the others, and may result in tooth loss. As such, it is important that traumatically injured teeth are followed up clinically and radiographically in a systematic manner and according to the International Association of Dental Traumatology (IADT) guidelines, to ensure the earliest possible detection and management of these complications (IADT, 2012a). In many cases, radiographic signs of pulpal and/or periapical pathosis may be the first indication of the development of these types of complications.

Radiographic assessment of TDI

Background

Contemporary guidelines for the radiographic assessment and follow-up of traumatically injured permanent teeth advise that two periapical radiographs and an anterior occlusal radiograph be taken to assess the injured tooth (Flores et al, 2007a, b; IADT, 2012a, b). Further radiographs are specifically indicated to identify debris or tooth segments that have become embedded in soft tissues. The periapical radiographs should be taken with a beam aiming device, with the central X-ray beam centred on the tooth in question. The X-ray beam in the second periapical (parallax) radiograph should be laterally orientated to the tooth being imaged (Flores et al, 2007a, b; IADT, 2012a). However, due to the limitations of conventional radiography, the true nature of certain TDIs are extremely difficult to visualise using conventional radiographic examinations, and this is reflected in the number of radiographs recommended by the guidelines to assess the affected teeth.

Injuries occurring in the plane of the radiographic exposure (e.g. palatal luxation injuries, and fractures and comminution injuries to the labial cortical plate) and those obscured by overlying and adjacent anatomy (e.g. horizontal root fractures in which the X-ray beam is not orientated along the fracture line) may be very difficult to diagnose using conventional radio-

Table 9-1 Classification of injuries to the hard dental tissues and the pulp (Andreasen and Andreasen, 1994).

Type of injury	Description
Enamel infraction	An incomplete fracture (crack) of the enamel without loss of tooth substance
Enamel fracture	A fracture with loss of tooth substance confined to enamel
Enamel–dentine fracture (uncomplicated crown fracture)	A fracture with loss of tooth substance confined to enamel and dentine, but not involving the pulp
Complicated crown fracture	A fracture involving enamel and dentine, exposing the pulp
Uncomplicated crown–root fracture	A fracture involving enamel, dentine and cementum, but not exposing the pulp
Complicated crown–root fracture	A fracture involving enamel, dentine and cementum, and exposing the pulp
Root fracture	A fracture involving dentine, cementum and the pulp. Root fractures can be further classified according to displacement of the coronal fragment

graphy (Andreasen, 1970; Bender and Freedland, 1983; Andreasen and Andreasen, 1985; Andreasen and Andreasen, 1988; Andreasen, 2007).

Though not yet considered routine in the assessment of TDI, cone beam computed tomography (CBCT) has been shown to improve the visualisation and nature of dentoalveolar injuries (IADT, 2012a), and is indicated in situations where conventional radiographs yield limited information (Patel and Saunders, 2013; European Society of Endodontology CBCT position statement, 2014).

CBCT is indicated in current IADT guidelines as a tool that improves the monitoring of healing and assessment of complications following TDI (IADT, 2012a). Systematic conventional radiographic follow-up of traumatically injured teeth is advised and may be necessary for up to 5 years, depending on the nature of the injury (IADT, 2012a, b).

Radiographic assessment of specific TDI

a. Injuries to the hard tissues and dental pulp

Conventional radiography

Crown fracture. The extent and nature of crown fractures (enamel infraction, uncomplicated crown fracture, and complicated crown fracture; see Table 9-1) are generally diagnosed from the history provided and the clinical examination carried out. Radiographic assessment of crown fractures is nonetheless necessary in order to rule out more serious concomitant TDI not necessarily evident clinically. Furthermore, radiographs taken at the time of the injury provide information about the size of the pulp and the stage of root development of the affected tooth/teeth (Fig 9-1). These radiographs are a baseline record with which subsequent follow-up radiographs can be compared in order to assess the pulpal and periapical status of the tooth and the development of complications over time.

In the case of complicated crown fractures that have been treated using vital pulp therapy techniques, the baseline radiographs can also be used to evaluate the development of a hard tissue barrier over the pulpal exposure with time. Uncomplicated and complicated crown fractures should be assessed according to the IADT guidelines (IADT, 2012a).

Enamel infractions should be assessed with a single periapical radiograph only, unless signs or symptoms indicative of other problems are present. In the event of a crown fracture (of any type) occurring in isolation, the radiographic appearance of the affected tooth (apart from the loss of coronal tooth tissue) should appear normal. The tooth will have normal periapical architecture and the root form should be appropriate for the stage of development of the tooth.

Crown–root fracture. Crown–root fractures (Table 9-1) are most often clinically diagnosed based on the history provided, the symptoms the patient is experiencing, and visualisation of the fracture. Crown–root fractures in anterior teeth commonly have an oblique orientation and may be minimally displaced (Figs 9-2 and 9-3), as the fractured portion is retained in position by the fibres of the periodontal ligament (PDL). As such, they can be missed clinically, especially when occurring in posterior teeth, where the fracture orientation will be similar to that in anterior teeth but may involve the occlusal surface instead of extending onto the labial aspect of the tooth crown.

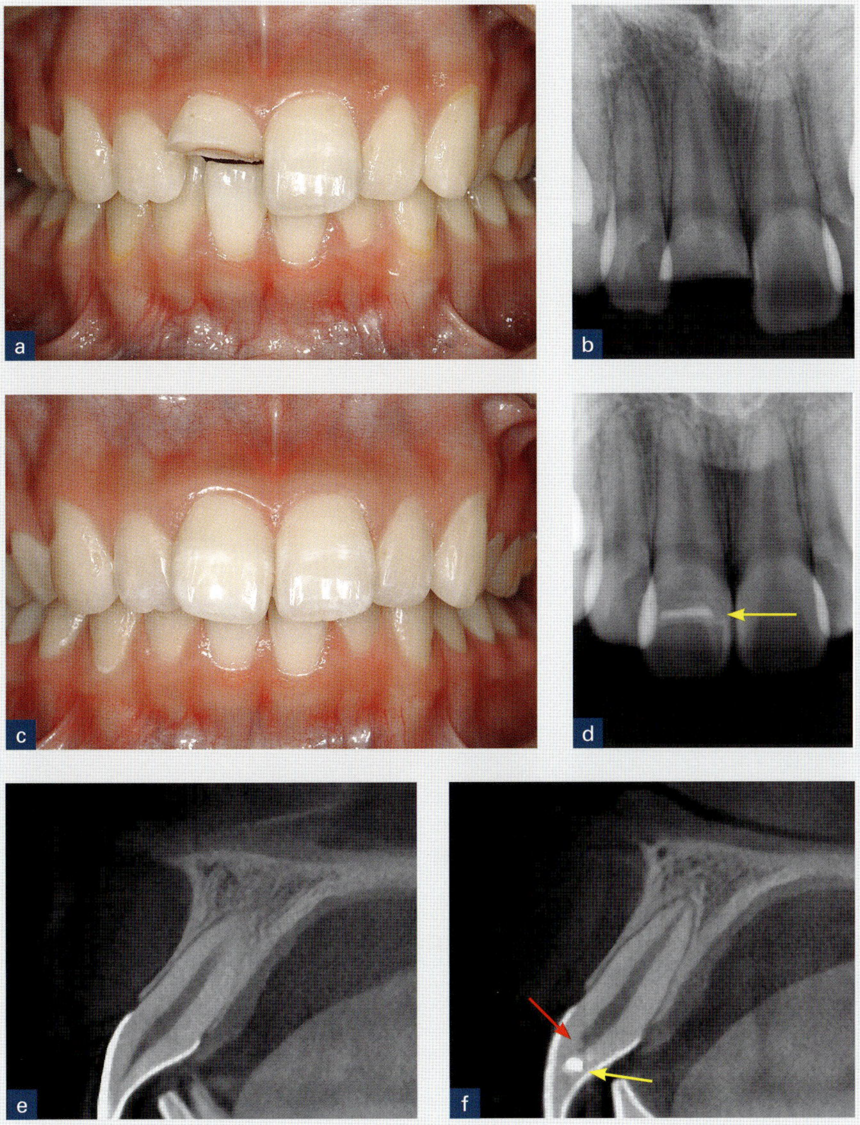

Fig 9-1 Crown fracture. (a) Clinical examination revealed a complicated crown fracture of the maxillary right central incisor (tooth 11). (b) A periapical radiograph showed that the periapical tissues appear normal. (c) Clinical view 1 year after treatment of the injury, which involved a coronal pulpotomy, a direct pulp capping procedure with CaOH and rebonding of the fractured coronal portion of the crown. (d) The 1-year review radiograph is unremarkable. The pulpal dressing is evident radiographically (yellow arrow), but there is no radiographic evidence of dentine bridge formation. (e) Sagittal CBCT view of tooth 21, which was uninjured, 1 year after the injury. The dental hard tissues and supporting periodontal tissues appear healthy. (f) Sagittal CBCT view of tooth 11, 1 year after the injury. The dental hard tissues and the periodontal tissues appear healthy. Of significance is the evidence of the formation of a hard tissue barrier (red arrow) just apical to the pulp dressing (yellow arrow).

Crown–root fractures should be assessed according to the IADT guidelines (IADT, 2012a). However, the apical extent of crown–root fractures with the common oblique orientation is very often difficult to visualise using conventional radiographic examinations, regardless of the number of parallax exposures. This is because the oblique fracture will tend to run almost perpendicular to the X-ray beam in each of the examinations, and the fractured subgingival fragment is generally well adapted to the root of the tooth. The limitations of conventional radiographic examination (see Chapter 1) means it tends not to add to the information obtained from the clinical examination (Andreasen et al, 2007b).

Crown–root fractures with a buccolingual orientation will be more readily evident on conventional radiographs, as the X-ray beam will pass through the fracture line. Crown–root fractures with a mesiodistal orientation will be more difficult to detect with conventional radiographic views, as the fracture orientation will be perpendicular to the plane of the X-ray source. The periapical anatomy of the injured tooth will appear normal on conventional radiographs immediately after the injury, as long as there is not a concomitant luxation injury.

Horizontal root fracture. The diagnosis of horizontal root fractures (HRFs) is reliant on the radiographic

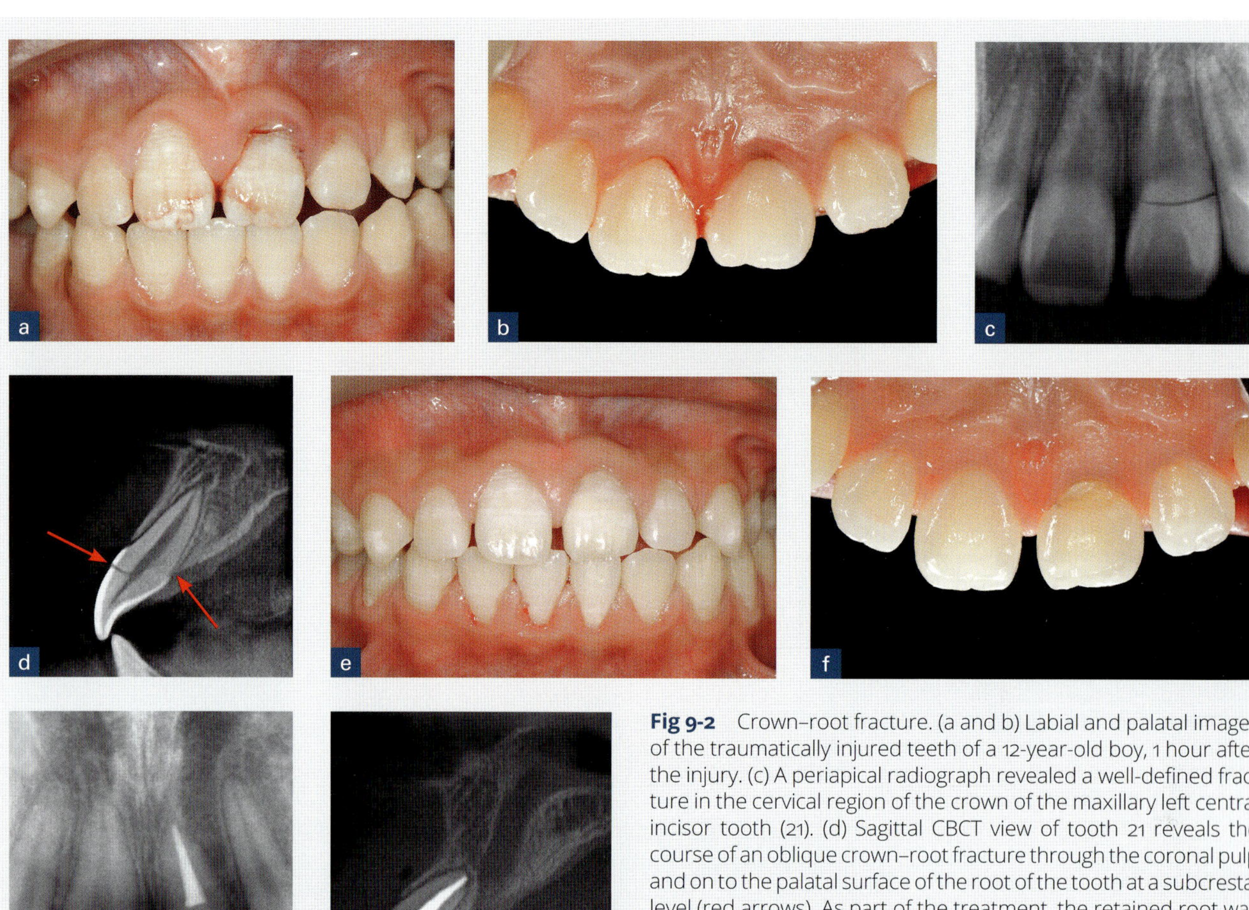

Fig 9-2 Crown–root fracture. (a and b) Labial and palatal images of the traumatically injured teeth of a 12-year-old boy, 1 hour after the injury. (c) A periapical radiograph revealed a well-defined fracture in the cervical region of the crown of the maxillary left central incisor tooth (21). (d) Sagittal CBCT view of tooth 21 reveals the course of an oblique crown–root fracture through the coronal pulp and on to the palatal surface of the root of the tooth at a subcrestal level (red arrows). As part of the treatment, the retained root was extracted, rotated 180 degrees and replanted, such that the fracture line was situated supragingivally on the labial and palatal surfaces of the tooth. The crown of the tooth was rebonded with composite 3 weeks after the surgery. (e and f) Clinical appearance at the 3-year review. (g and h) The periapical radiograph and sagittal CBCT image of tooth 21, 3 years after the injury, are unremarkable.

demonstration of the injury (Andreasen et al, 2007a). However, HRFs are generally only visible on conventional intraoral radiographs when the central X-ray beam is orientated either directly through the fracture line, or within a maximum range of 15- to 20-degrees of the orientation of the fracture line (Bender and Freedland, 1983; Andreasen and Andreasen, 1988). When the X-ray beam passes directly through the fracture line, it will be represented radiographically as a single transverse radiolucency across the root. As the X-ray beam deviates from the plane of the fracture line (within the 15 to 20 degree range), the fracture will take on a more ellipsoid appearance on the radiograph (Figs 9-4 and 9-5). With greater deviations of the X-ray beam from the fracture plane, the fracture line becomes undetectable (Andreasen and Hjørting-Hansen, 1967). These are the findings in the presence of a single transverse fracture line. Multiple root fractures will have an irregular appearance radiographically (Andreasen and Hjørting-Hansen, 1967).

The course of HRFs can vary considerably, but is generally obliquely (more common in apical or mid-root fractures) or horizontally (more common in cervical third fractures) orientated. As such, periapical radiographs with a 90-degree horizontal angulation relative to the tooth under examination will be more useful at detecting horizontally orientated fractures, while occlusal views will be more useful at detecting oblique fractures. Multiple radiographic exposures are therefore necessary to assess teeth for HRFs (May et al, 2013; IADT, 2012a). However, even in situations where multiple exposures are utilised, HRFs may not always be detected in the immediate aftermath of the injury, especially if the fractured portions are still

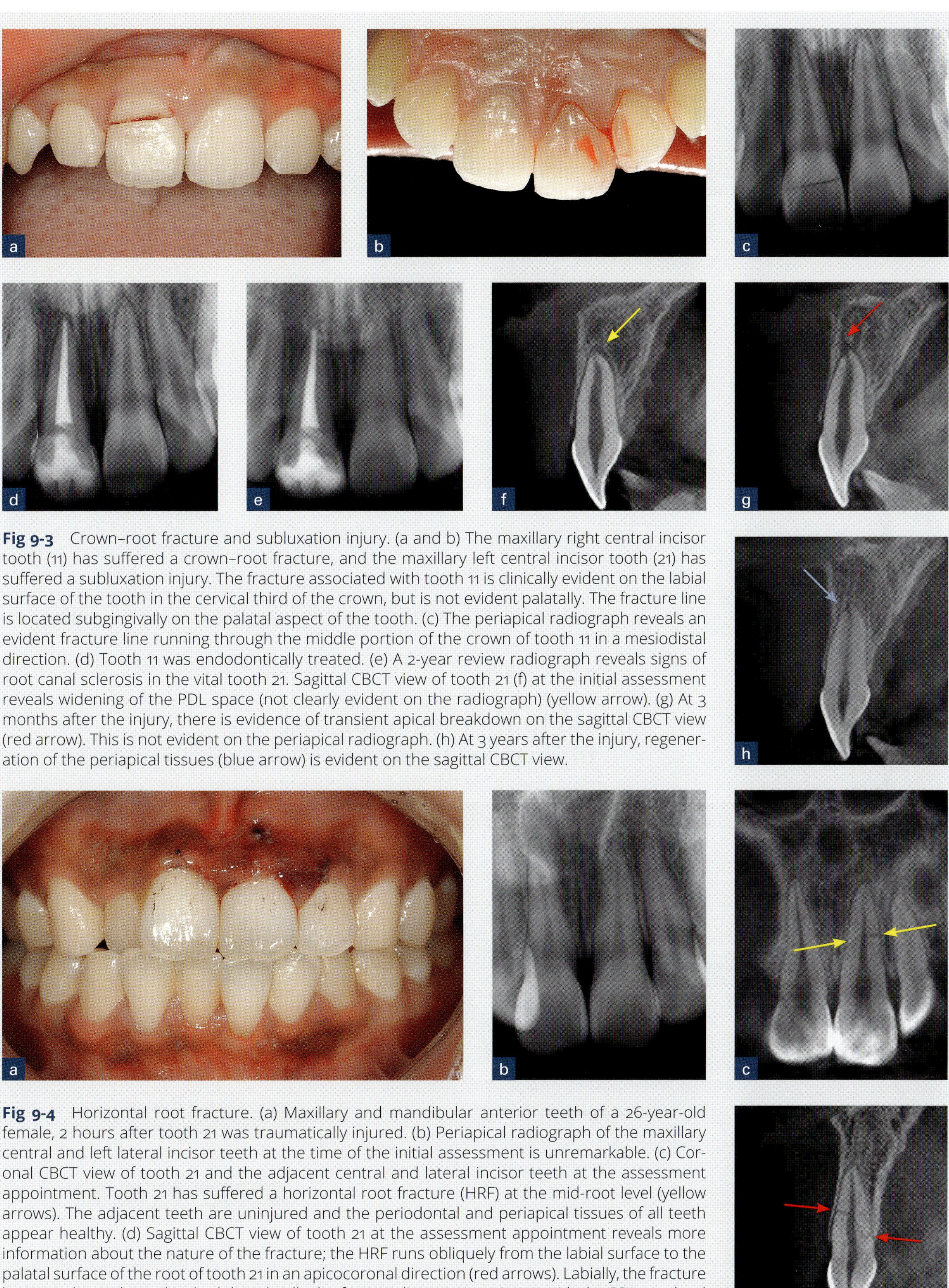

Fig 9-3 Crown–root fracture and subluxation injury. (a and b) The maxillary right central incisor tooth (11) has suffered a crown–root fracture, and the maxillary left central incisor tooth (21) has suffered a subluxation injury. The fracture associated with tooth 11 is clinically evident on the labial surface of the tooth in the cervical third of the crown, but is not evident palatally. The fracture line is located subgingivally on the palatal aspect of the tooth. (c) The periapical radiograph reveals an evident fracture line running through the middle portion of the crown of tooth 11 in a mesiodistal direction. (d) Tooth 11 was endodontically treated. (e) A 2-year review radiograph reveals signs of root canal sclerosis in the vital tooth 21. Sagittal CBCT view of tooth 21 (f) at the initial assessment reveals widening of the PDL space (not clearly evident on the radiograph) (yellow arrow). (g) At 3 months after the injury, there is evidence of transient apical breakdown on the sagittal CBCT view (red arrow). This is not evident on the periapical radiograph. (h) At 3 years after the injury, regeneration of the periapical tissues (blue arrow) is evident on the sagittal CBCT view.

Fig 9-4 Horizontal root fracture. (a) Maxillary and mandibular anterior teeth of a 26-year-old female, 2 hours after tooth 21 was traumatically injured. (b) Periapical radiograph of the maxillary central and left lateral incisor teeth at the time of the initial assessment is unremarkable. (c) Coronal CBCT view of tooth 21 and the adjacent central and lateral incisor teeth at the assessment appointment. Tooth 21 has suffered a horizontal root fracture (HRF) at the mid-root level (yellow arrows). The adjacent teeth are uninjured and the periodontal and periapical tissues of all teeth appear healthy. (d) Sagittal CBCT view of tooth 21 at the assessment appointment reveals more information about the nature of the fracture; the HRF runs obliquely from the labial surface to the palatal surface of the root of tooth 21 in an apicocoronal direction (red arrows). Labially, the fracture line is at the mid-root level, while palatally the fracture line communicates with the PDL at a level just apical to the crestal bone.

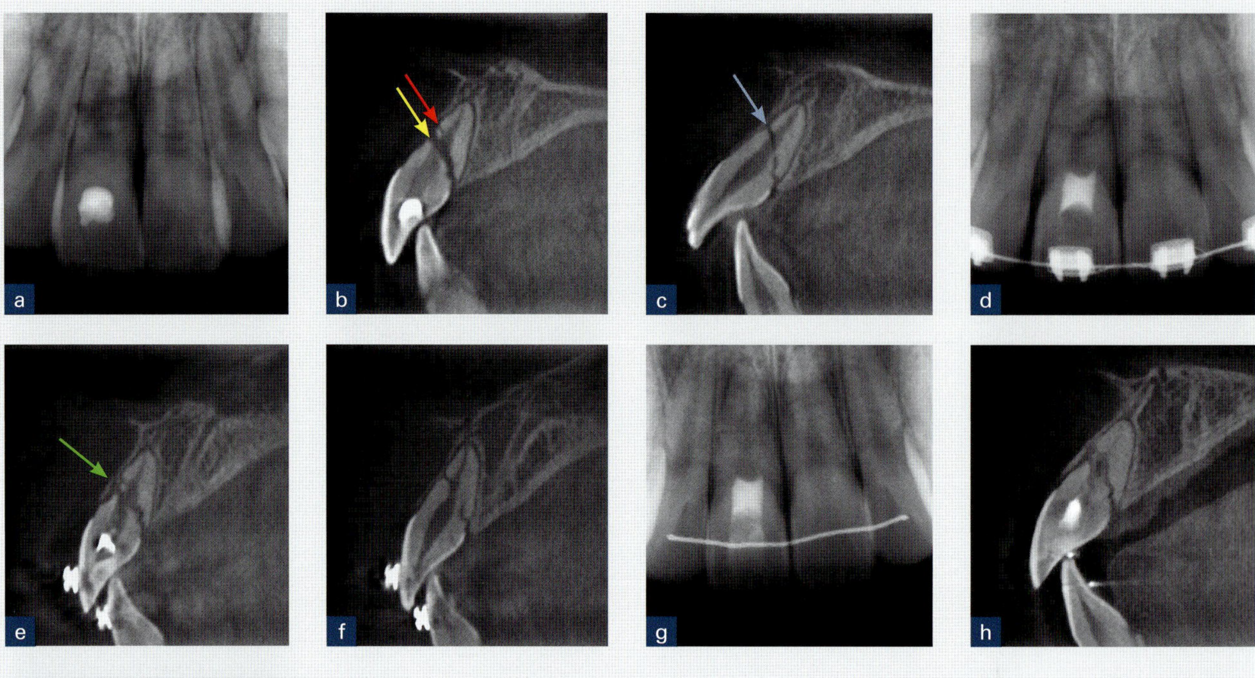

Fig 9-5 Horizontal root fracture. (a) Periapical radiograph of the maxillary central incisor teeth of a 13-year-old boy reveals HRFs associated with both central incisor teeth following a TDI 3 months earlier. It is unclear whether there are multiple fractures associated with the teeth, or whether the radiographic projection is producing an ellipsoid appearance of the fracture lines on the radiograph in one or both teeth. Endodontic treatment of the coronal portion of the root canal of the maxillary right central incisor tooth (11) was initiated 1 month earlier by the patient's clinician following the development of a gingival abscess. (b) Sagittal CBCT of tooth 11 reveals a primary fracture running obliquely, in an apicocoronal direction, from the mid-root level of the labial root surface to the palatal surface of the root at the level of the crestal bone. The coronal fragment is significantly displaced in a coronal direction. A smaller fracture (red arrow) is evident on the labial aspect of the root, immediately apical to, and communicating with, the primary fracture. The labial alveolar bone overlying the fracture has resorbed. (c) Sagittal CBCT view of the maxillary left central incisor tooth (21) taken at the initial appointment. The root has suffered a single fracture (blue arrow). There is only minor separation of the fractured root segments. (d to f) At the 3-year review: (d) the periapical radiograph of the maxillary incisor teeth does not reveal the exact nature and degree of healing, while (e) the sagittal CBCT view of tooth 11 reveals that the labial cortical plate has regenerated and remodelled (green arrow). The apical root canal has sclerosed and there is deposition of mineralised tissue in the root canal coronal to the fracture line. The fracture line has further reduced and repaired with hard tissue deposition. The fracture has most likely repaired with connective tissue. (f) Sagittal CBCT view of tooth 21, 13 months after the injury. The fracture shows signs of repair, with interposition of some dental hard tissue in the fracture line on the palatal aspect of the root. (g) Periapical radiograph of the maxillary incisor teeth, 3 years after the injury. There appears to be continued healing of the fracture, but the exact nature and degree of healing is difficult to assess from the periapical radiograph. (h) Sagittal CBCT view of tooth 11 reveals that the labial cortical plate has healed further so that the integrity of the plate is intact. The apical root canal has sclerosed further and there is more deposition of mineralised tissue in the root canal coronal to the fracture line. The fracture line has further reduced and repaired with hard tissue deposition. (i) Sagittal CBCT view of tooth 21 reveals that the fracture has repaired completely with hard tissue, labially. There is continued repair of the palatal fracture with hard tissue. The fracture line at its junction with the PDL space, palatally, has not healed completely with hard tissue.

closely juxtaposed. Subsequent radiographs may then reveal a fracture. This may be due to separation of the fractured segments following subsequent haemorrhage, or granulation tissue build-up at the site of the fracture, or in the adjacent alveolar bone (Andreasen and Andreasen, 1988).

CBCT

Crown fracture. In cases of crown fracture, a CBCT examination might be prescribed to assess the affected tooth, or teeth, for more serious concomitant injuries. In the event that the injury is an isolated crown fracture, the CBCT data will provide a more

Table 9-2 Classification of injuries to the periodontal tissues (Andreasen and Andreasen, 1994).

Type of injury	Description
Concussion	An injury to the tooth-supporting structures without abnormal loosening or displacement, but with marked reaction to percussion
Subluxation	An injury to the tooth-supporting structures with abnormal loosening, but without clinically or radiographically demonstrable displacement of the tooth
Extrusive luxation	Partial displacement of the tooth out of its socket
Lateral luxation	Displacement of the tooth in a direction other than axially. This is accompanied by comminution or fracture of the alveolar socket
Intrusive luxation	Displacement of the tooth into the alveolar bone. This injury is accompanied by comminution or fracture of the alveolar socket
Avulsion	Complete displacement of the tooth out of its socket

diagnostically accurate and reliable assessment of the health of the periodontal tissues and the root of the affected tooth than that which can be provided by conventional intraoral radiography (Patel et al, 2009a; Durack et al, 2011) (Fig 9-1). In uncomplicated crown fractures, the thickness of the dentine wall at the base of the fracture and overlying the coronal pulp can be measured and compared with future scans to obtain a reliable qualitative and quantitative assessment of the degree of tertiary dentine formation following the injury. This provides some adjunctive information about the health of the pulp. In the same manner, in complicated crown fractures, review CBCT scans can be compared to the assessment scan taken at the time of the injury to objectively assess the presence and thickness (using measuring tools) of any dentine bridge formation over the exposed pulp. Conventional intraoral radiography can only offer a subjective assessment of dentinal bridge and tertiary dentine formation following crown fractures (Fig 9-1).

Crown–root fracture. We have already outlined the difficulties associated with assessing the course and apical extent of crown–root fractures using conventional intraoral radiography. When assessing these injuries using CBCT, adjacent and overlying anatomy masking the view of the oblique fracture line can be eliminated, permitting the entire course of the fracture to be traced with certainty (Fig 9-2). An appreciation of the relationship of the fracture line to the pulp as well as the crestal bone and periodontium can therefore be elucidated before removal of the fractured segment, facilitating treatment planning.

Horizontal root fracture. CBCT enables removal of anatomical noise that obscures the area of interest and allows assessment of the root in all planes (Figs 9-4 and 9-5). The detection of HRFs using CBCT is not impaired by the often oblique nature of the fracture. The presence and nature of HRFs can be identified more reliably using this imaging modality when compared with conventional intraoral radiography (Bernardes et al, 2009; Bornstein et al, 2009; Kamburoğlu et al, 2009).

While CBCT may be associated with an increased effective radiation dose to the patient, a recent study found that altering the exposure parameters to reduce the radiation dose does not impair the diagnostic yield of CBCT scans in the detection of simulated HRFs when using an *ex vivo* model (Jones et al, 2015). In this study, a dose reduction of up to 80% had little impact on the diagnostic ability of CBCT to detect simulated HRFs.

b. Injuries to the periodontal tissues

Conventional radiography

Concussion and subluxation. The nature of concussion and subluxation injuries is such that there is typically no conventional radiographic evidence of displacement of the affected teeth (Table 9-2). As such, in the immediate aftermath of the injury, the root of the affected tooth, the PDL space and the periapical anatomy should maintain a normal radiographic appearance (Fig 9-3). The diagnosis of these injuries is based on a combination of the history, clinical signs (marked tenderness to percussion in concussion injuries and abnormal loosening without displacement in subluxation injuries), and the absence of conventional radiographic evidence of tooth displacement. The only exception may be in cases of severe subluxation injuries with associated grade III mobility, where minimal widening of the PDL space may be evident radiographically (Andreasen and Andreasen, 2007). However, this will only be evident on the proximal aspects of the tooth. Any potential widening of the buccal and/or palatal PDL spaces will not be detected due to the two-dimensional nature of conventional radiography.

Concussion and subluxation injuries should be assessed radiographically according to the IADT guidelines, even in the absence of clinical evidence of tooth displacement (IADT, 2012a). This is because the clinical appearance of some milder luxation injuries may not disclose the true extent of the injury, potentially resulting in the injury having a similar clinical appearance to a subluxation injury. As such, a full radiographic assessment is indicated to reduce the risk of missing a luxation injury (or other more serious injury) in these cases.

Extrusive luxation (extrusion). Conventional radiographic examination of extrusive luxation injuries should reveal an increase in the width of the PDL space. The extent of the widening of the PDL space should reflect the degree of extrusion for the tooth out of its socket. The crown of the tooth should also have a more coronal position relative to the adjacent teeth. This feature would also be clinically evident, but relies on accurate knowledge of the tooth position before the injury.

Lateral luxation. Lateral luxation injuries usually result in fractures of the alveolar socket wall, which may even be comminuted. Lateral luxation injuries (especially ones associated with mild or moderate displacement) are difficult to visualise using conventional radiographic imaging (Fig 9-6). Depending on the direction of the tooth displacement and the orientation of the central X-ray beam in relation to the injured tooth, widening of the PDL space may be evident radiographically. Widening of the PDL space will mainly occur on that aspect of the root from which the tooth was displaced. This makes buccal and palatal luxation injuries more difficult to diagnose radiographically (even with maxillary occlusal radiographs), as the tooth displacement predominantly occurs in the plane of the X-ray beam. However, in some instances of palatal luxation, widening of the PDL space may be evident (Fig 9-6). Fractures of the alveolar socket wall associated with lateral luxation injuries are typically not evident on conventional intraoral radiographic examination, except in cases where the alveolar process is also fractured (Andreasen, 2007) (Figs 9-6 and 9-7).

Intrusive luxation (intrusion). Intrusive luxation injuries result in fracture of the alveolar socket wall. Conventional radiographic examination should reveal that the tooth occupies a more apical position relative to the adjacent teeth (Figs 9-7 and 9-8). The PDL space may be reduced in width or diminished as a result of the injury. The injury to the alveolar socket wall is typically not visible radiographically.

CBCT

Concussion and subluxation. Given that concussion and subluxation injuries are not associated with displacement of the affected tooth, a normal radiographic appearance on CBCT examination should be expected following these types of injury. However, it may be the case that in severe subluxation injuries associated with significant mobility, widening of the PDL space may be evident using CBCT without any evidence of this on conventional radiographs (Fig 9-3). This follows the principle that CBCT is significantly more sensitive than periapical radiographs at detecting PDL widening and small lesions of AP (Cheung et al, 2013; Tsai et al, 2013; Al-Nuaimi et al, 2015), even in vital, pulpitic cases (Abella et al, 2012). Speculatively, it may be the case that some suspected subluxation injuries may actually prove to be luxation injuries when assessed using CBCT.

Lateral luxation. CBCT reveals more information about the nature and extent of lateral luxation injuries than do conventional radiographs (Cohenca et al, 2007; Patel et al, 2015) (Figs 9-6 and 9-7). The nature of the majority of these injuries is such that the crown of the affected tooth will be displaced in the direction of the force to which it was subjected, with the root of the tooth being displaced in the opposite direction. Effectively, the injuring force is directed through the tooth's crown and the tooth rotates around a fulcrum in the region of the crestal bone. The apical portion of the tooth's root will displace into or through the adjacent socket wall, resulting in a fracture and potential displacement of that wall. This will be evident on CBCT examination; the region from which the root moved will be evident as a radiolucent, partially vacated socket space (Figs 9-6 and 9-7). The crown of the tooth will

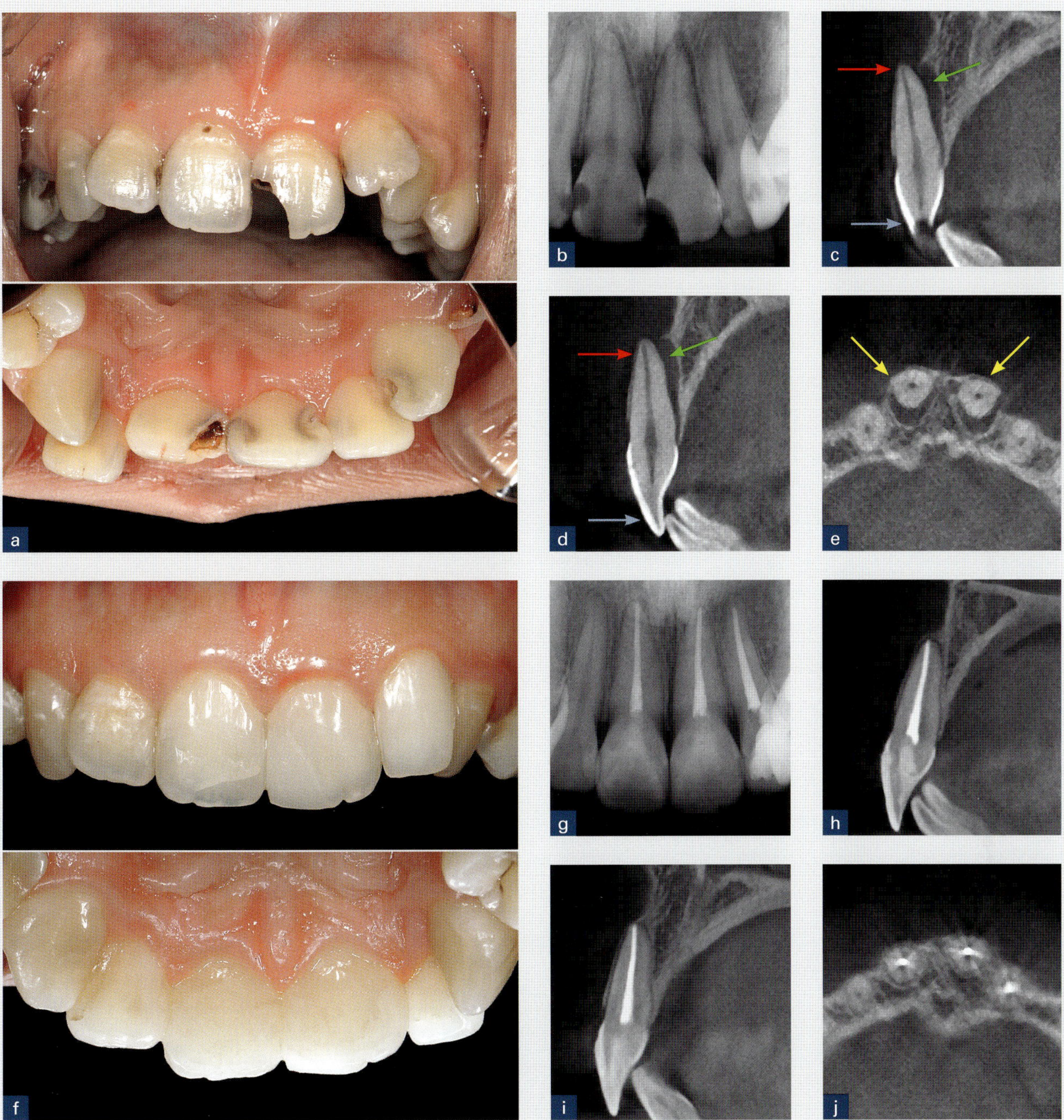

Fig 9-6 Palatal luxation (a to e = TDI assessment; f to j = 15-month review). (a) The grossly carious maxillary right central (11) and maxillary left central (21) incisor teeth have been palatally luxated, but the nature of the injury is not evident clinically. (b) Periapical radiograph of the maxillary central incisors reveals widening of the PDL space associated with both root apices, indicative of a luxation injury. There is no evidence of any other dental hard tissue injury. (c) Sagittal CBCT view of tooth 11 reveals a palatal luxation injury. The crown of the tooth has been displaced palatally (blue arrow) and the root (red arrow) of the tooth has been displaced through the labial wall of the alveolar socket, fracturing the socket wall. The degree of displacement can be quantified by assessing the amount of vacated socket space (green arrow). (d) Sagittal CBCT view of tooth 21 reveals a similar palatal luxation injury to tooth 11 (blue, red and green arrows). (e) Axial CBCT view demonstrates that the teeth have been displaced in a buccolingual direction only. There is no mesiodistal displacement of the teeth. Fractures of the labial alveolar socket wall are evident (yellow arrows). (f) At the 15-month review, after the teeth have been successfully repositioned and the carious cavities treated. (g) Periapical radiograph of the now root-treated maxillary incisor teeth confirms a healthy appearance of the periapical tissues. (h, i and j) The CBCT views confirm that the teeth have been repositioned to their original position and that the periapical tissues appear healthy.

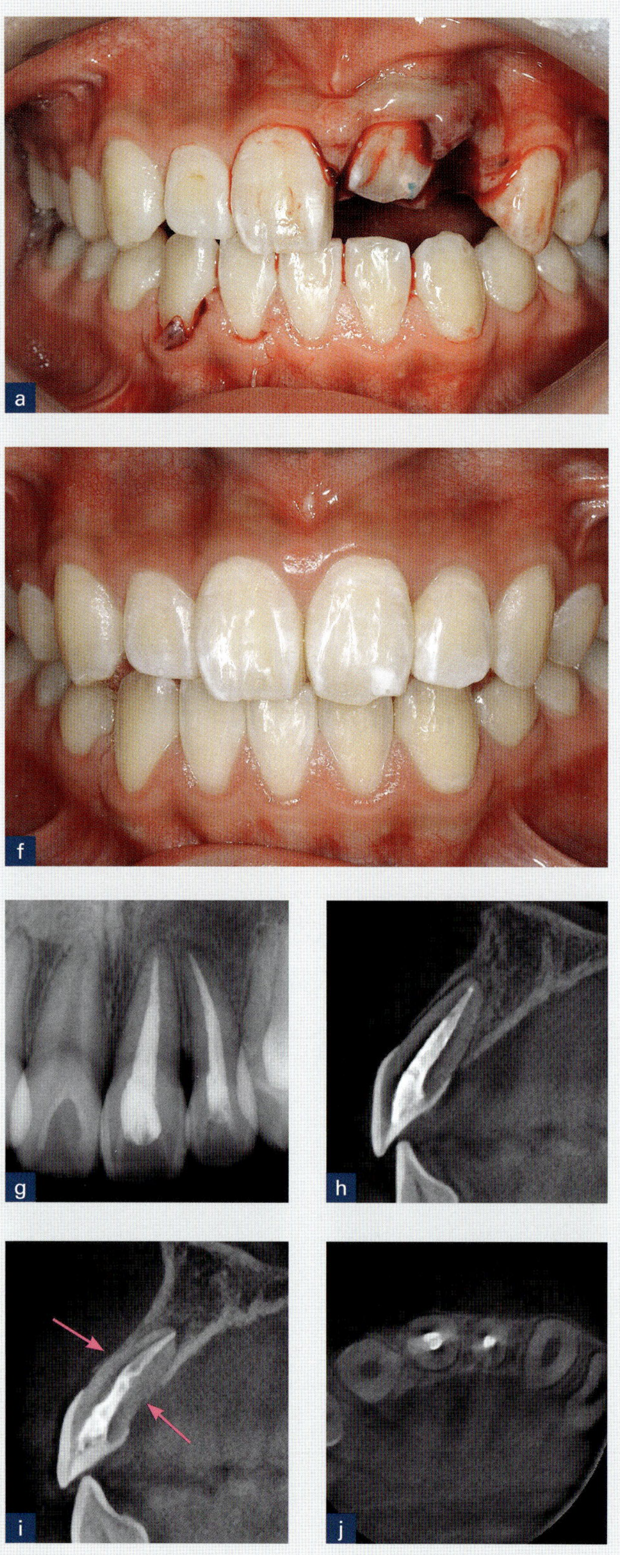

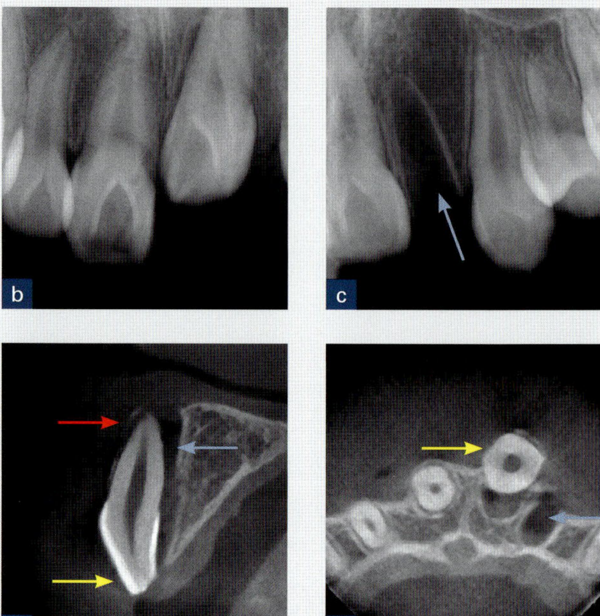

Fig 9-7 Intrusion/lateral luxation. (a) TDI of the maxillary anterior teeth of a 14-year-old boy 45 minutes after the injury. Clinical examination revealed an apparent intruded maxillary left central incisor (21) and an avulsed maxillary left lateral incisor (22). (b and c) The conventional radiographic examination appears to have confirmed the clinical diagnosis. The socket of the avulsed tooth 22 is evident (blue arrow) radiographically, and tooth 21 is occupying a more apical position relative to the adjacent teeth, indicating an intrusion injury. (d) Sagittal CBCT view reveals that, in addition to suffering an intrusion injury, tooth 21 was also luxated palatally (yellow arrow) with concomitant fracture and displacement of the labial alveolar socket wall (red arrow). The degree of displacement of the tooth in an axial direction due to the intrusion injury can be assessed by relating the position of the cementoenamel junction (CEJ) to the crest of the palatal alveolar bone. As in Figure 9-6, information about the degree of labial displacement of the tooth can be obtained by assessing the amount of vacated alveolar socket space (blue arrow). (e) Axial CBCT view confirming the labial displacement of the root of tooth 21 (yellow arrow) and confirming the avulsion of tooth 22 (blue arrow). The degree of labial displacement can be assessed accurately from this view. (f to j) At 6-month review after TDI and tooth repositioning. (f) The teeth are well aligned and there were no visual signs of ongoing problems. (g) Periapical radiograph does not reveal any post-TDI complications (e.g. root resorption, apical periodontitis (AP), canal obliteration); note that tooth 21 and tooth 22 were root-treated. (h and i) Sagittal CBCT views of teeth 21 and 22, respectively; note the periodontal tissues have healed well. Replacement resorption (pink arrows) is evident labially and palatally at the mid-root level of tooth 22, with diminution of the PDL space in these areas as the resorbed root is replaced with alveolar bone. There is also a periapical radiolucency associated with tooth 22. Neither the periapical radiolucency nor the replacement resorption were evident on the periapical radiograph. (j) Axial CBCT view of teeth 21 and 22 was unremarkable.

Table 9-3 Classification of injuries to the supporting bone (Andreasen and Andreasen, 1994).

Type of injury	Description
Comminution of the (maxillary and mandibular) alveolar socket	Crushing and compression of the alveolar socket. This condition is found concomitantly with intrusive and lateral luxation injuries
Fracture of the (maxillary and mandibular) alveolar socket wall	A fracture confined to the facial or oral socket wall
Fracture of the (maxillary and mandibular) alveolar process	A fracture of the alveolar process, which may or may not involve the alveolar socket
Fracture of the mandible or maxilla	A fracture involving the base of the maxilla or mandible and often the alveolar process (jaw fracture). The fracture may or may not involve the alveolar socket

displace into the wall of the alveolar socket on the opposite side from the impact. On CBCT examination, the crown of the tooth will appear proclined or retroclined (in relation to adjacent uninjured teeth) in cases of facial and palatal luxation, respectively, and mesially or distally displaced in cases of luxation injuries occurring in these directions (Figs 9-6 and 9-7).

Lateral luxation injuries may also be associated with more bodily displacement (as opposed to rotational movements) of the tooth. In these situations, the orientation of the long axis of the tooth will remain the same, as the tooth will move as a whole. The direction of force necessary to cause bodily movement of the tooth in this manner tends to be directed through, and roughly perpendicular to, the root of the tooth (as opposed to through the crown). On CBCT examination, the tooth will be notably displaced in the direction of the force, with concomitant fractures of the alveolar socket wall on the side to which the tooth is being displaced. The portion of the socket from which the tooth was displaced will be evident as radiolucent vacant space.

Fractures of the socket wall at the site of impact and/or fractures of the alveolar process may also occur, and these will be identifiable from the CBCT assessment (Fig 9-6).

Extrusive luxation (extrusion). CBCT examination of extrusive luxation injuries will show evidence of displacement of the affected tooth out of the socket (IADT, 2012b). The space between the socket wall and the apex of the tooth will have increased significantly. This will be evident as a well-defined radiolucency on coronal and sagittal CBCT slices and will be representative of the degree of the tooth displacement.

Fractures of the alveolar socket wall are not commonplace in these types of injury, but may occur, and if present will be evident on CBCT examination. Coronal slices through the injured tooth will reveal that its crown is more coronally positioned than the adjacent teeth.

Intrusive luxation (intrusion). Intrusive luxation injuries viewed using CBCT will demonstrate the tooth occupying a more apical position in the socket (Fig 9-8), with a largely diminished or undetectable PDL space around the root end. Diminution of the PDL space may not be evident in cases of intrusion in immature permanent teeth due to the dental papilla space (Fig 9-8). The cementoenamel junction (CEJ) of the affected tooth will be positioned subcrestally, a characteristic of the injury that can be identified on coronal or sagittal slices.

Coronal CBCT slices through the injured tooth will also reveal that the crown of the tooth is more apically positioned relative to the adjacent teeth. If the tooth is predominantly contained within the socket during the injury, a minimally displaced fracture of the alveolar wall will often occur. This normally occurs on the facial side of the socket, where the bone is thinner and the fracture can be viewed by selecting appropriate axial and/or sagittal CBCT slices (Fig 9-8). With more severe intrusive luxation injuries, the affected tooth may be displaced through the facial or oral alveolar socket wall, as well as being displaced apically. On CBCT examination, these types of injury will have characteristics of both intrusive (subcrestal CEJ, more apical tooth position) and lateral luxation injuries (displacement of the tooth or root end through the lateral alveolar socket wall, unoccupied socket space), as they are in fact combination injuries (Fig 9-7).

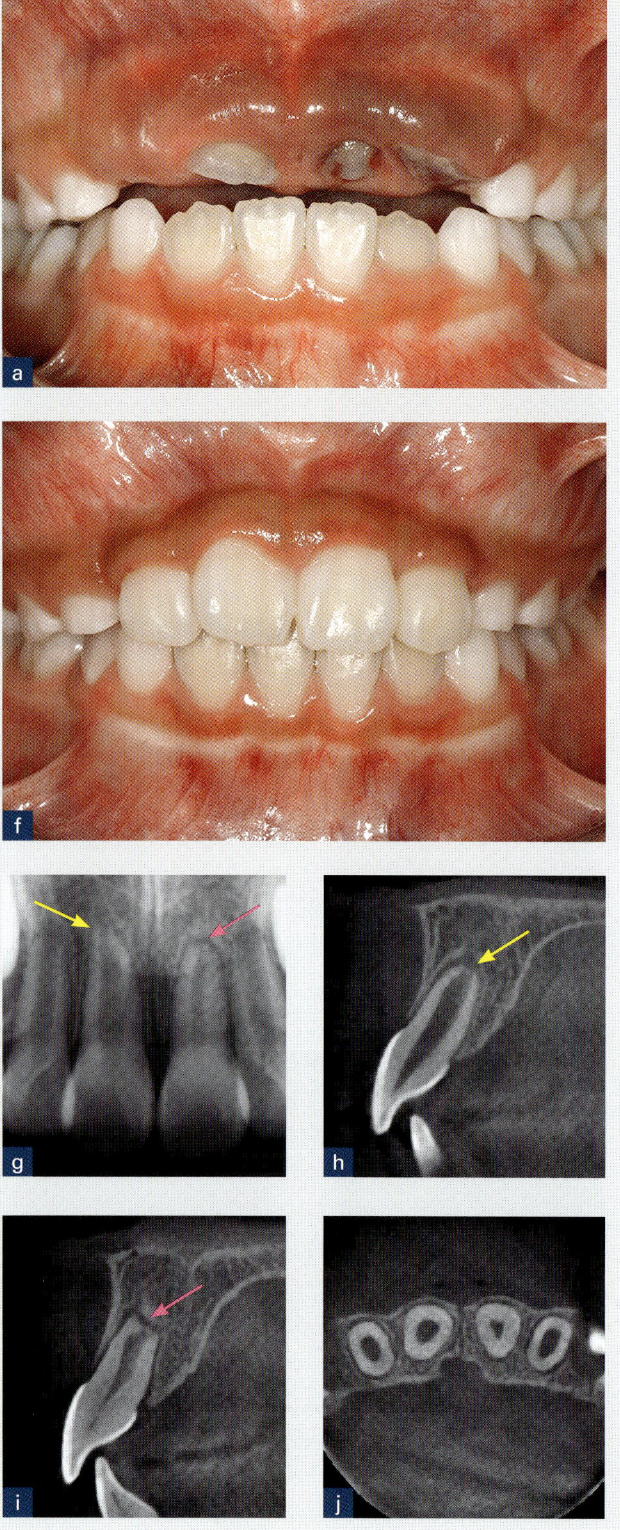

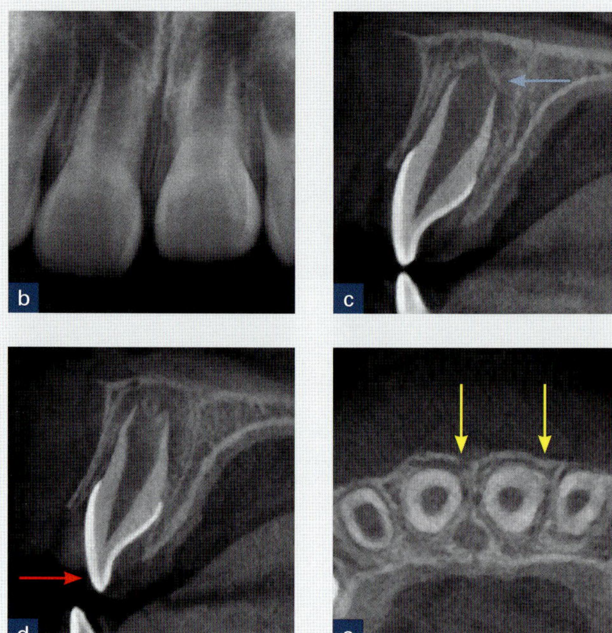

Fig 9-8 Intrusion. (a to e) Presentation 2 days after a TDI to the maxillary anterior teeth of a 7-year-old boy. (a) Clinical photo and (b) periapical radiograph reveal immature roots with open apices. The apicocoronal position of the central incisors appears to be on a level similar to the unerupted lateral incisor teeth, indicating intrusion of the central incisor teeth. (c) Sagittal CBCT view of the maxillary right central incisor tooth (11) reveals axial displacement of the tooth into the socket (blue arrow) to occupy the space of the underlying dental follicle. The CEJ is located subcrestally. Relating the CEJ to the level of the crestal bone allows the degree of intrusion to be quantified. (d) Sagittal CBCT view of tooth 21 showing the degree of intrusion of the tooth and also showing that the crown of the tooth has rotated palatally (red arrow), as indicated by the relationship of the tooth to the opposing dentition. (e) Axial CBCT view reveals fractures of the labial alveolar socket walls due to the force of the injury (yellow arrows). (f to j) At 1-year review. (f) The teeth have spontaneously re-erupted, while (g) a periapical radiograph reveals that the root of tooth 11 has undergone continued development and root formation is almost complete (yellow arrow). Root development of tooth 21 appears to have stopped and the apex is closed (pink arrow). (h and i) Sagittal CBCT views reveal that both teeth have spontaneously re-erupted and that the CEJ is located at the appropriate position. Tooth 11 has undergone continued root development, with the root walls converging apically (yellow arrow). The stage of root development and the root wall thickness are commensurate with that of a child of this age. Root development of tooth 21 has stopped. The root apex has closed, with lateral deposition of dentine to form a flattened root end (pink arrow). However, the tooth has maintained vitality and the root canal space has undergone sclerosis. (j) Axial CBCT view of the maxillary incisor teeth. The alveolar socket fractures have healed and a normal PDL space width has re-established around the root.

c. Injuries to the supporting bone

Conventional radiography

Comminution and fracture of the alveolar socket wall. Fractures and comminutions of the alveolar socket wall (Table 9-3) occur as a matter of course in lateral luxation and intrusive luxation injuries (Fig 9-6 to 9-8). However, the injuries to the alveolar socket wall are rarely, if ever, evident on intraoral radiographic examination. In fractures involving the alveolar process, a distinct fracture line (represented radiographically as a radiolucent line) should be evident on intraoral and extraoral radiographs (e.g. a dental panoramic tomograph) if the fracture separation is significant. However, even in cases where the clinical examination indicates an alveolar fracture, conventional intraoral radiographs may fail to detect it (Andreasen, 2007).

Fractures of the alveolar process. Fractures of the alveolar process may or may not involve the alveolar socket wall of a tooth or teeth. Those involving dental sockets may occur in any area of the socket wall. Fractures involving the alveolar socket walls and/or fractures crossing the interdental septa of the alveolar bone are frequently associated with luxation injuries and/or root fractures of the involved teeth. These concomitant injuries can complicate accurate diagnosis, and their potential occurrence should be borne in mind when assessing alveolar process fractures using conventional intraoral radiography.

An alveolar fracture that traverses the bone on the facial or oral side of an uninjured root may be misinterpreted as a root fracture. A true root fracture associated with a fractured alveolus may be overlooked for similar reasons. In order to minimise these types of diagnostic error, the radiographs should be examined carefully with particular attention being paid to the integrity and continuity of the external root surface and the root canal wall. True root fractures will be associated with steps or breaks in the root wall or root canal wall, while the continuity of intact roots with superimposed alveolar fractures can be traced through the fracture line. Vertical parallax techniques can be utilised to obtain further information. The position of alveolar fracture lines will move in relation to the root surface when the vertical angulation of the X-ray source is altered (Andreasen, 2007).

Fractures of the mandible and maxilla. Fractures of the mandible or maxilla may occur in isolation or in conjunction with injuries to the hard dental tissues and/or the PDL tissues (Table 9-3). Diagnosis and management of these fractures is generally the remit of a dedicated oral and maxillofacial specialist. Displaced fractures may often be diagnosed from clinical signs and symptoms but should always be confirmed radiographically.

The diagnosis of non-displaced fractures is reliant on radiographic assessment. Extraoral radiographs are essential to determine the presence and position of these types of fracture, and the information obtained should be supplemented with intraoral radiographs when there are associated dental injuries. When assessing mandibular fractures, generally a panoramic and a lateral cephalometric radiograph are used to provide two views of the fracture line from opposing perspectives. Posteroanterior and lateral views of the skull, and occasionally a submentovertex, are generally the conventional radiographs used to diagnose maxillary fractures.

CBCT

Comminution and fracture of the alveolar socket wall. In contrast to conventional radiography, CBCT is sufficiently sensitive to detect fractures of the alveolar socket wall in specific cases of TDI where conventional radiographic imaging proves inconclusive (Cohenca et al, 2007) (Figs 9-6 to 9-8). Furthermore, by selecting the appropriate slice to view, any displacement of the socket wall can also be identified (Figs 9-6 and 9-7).

Fractures of the alveolar process. Fractures of the alveolar process and any associated displacement may be diagnosed and qualitatively and quantitively evaluated using CBCT (Patel et al, 2009b). Alveolar process fractures traversing the interdental septa and running through the bone on the facial and/or oral aspects of a tooth can be readily differentiated from root fractures by eliminating the adjacent bony anatomy and assessing the tooth in isolation (Fig 9-9).

Fractures of the mandible and maxilla. In a report on a case of a severe TDI in which a patient suffered multiple mandibular and maxillary bone fractures, combined lateral cephalometric, panoramic and lateral skull radiographs failed to detect fractures of the maxilla and a palatal root fracture of a maxillary tooth, which were subsequently detected using CBCT (Dölekoğlu et al, 2010). Furthermore, in a case series compar-

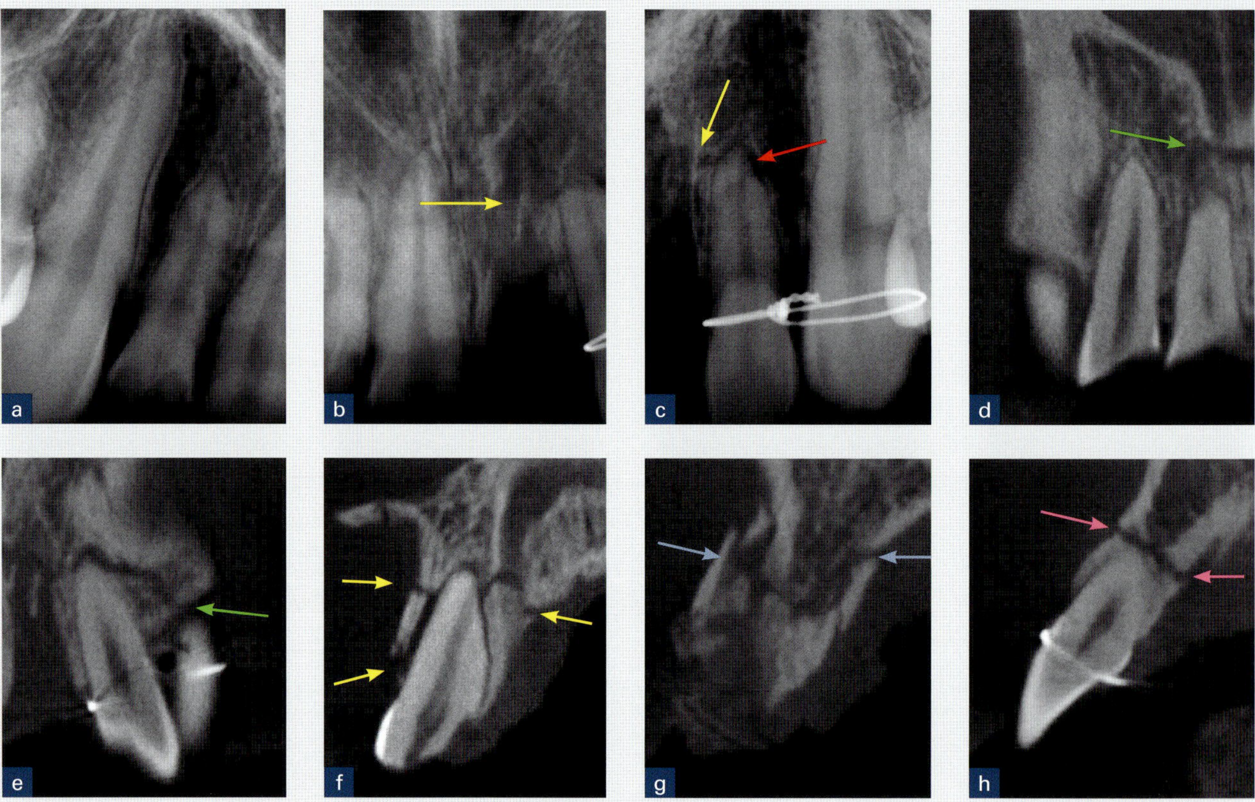

Fig 9-9 Avulsion and fracture of the alveolar process of the maxilla. A 27-year-old male presented 2 days after his maxilla and maxillary anterior teeth were traumatically injured in a bicycle accident. Remedial treatment of the injuries was carried out in a hospital emergency setting. Based on the clinical examination, it was clear that the patient's maxillary right central and lateral incisors suffered crown–root fractures and that the maxillary left central incisor was avulsed. Periapical radiographs (a to c) confirmed these injuries. There was also potential evidence of a fracture line running in close proximity to the apical third of the root of tooth 22 and apparently through the socket of the avulsed tooth (yellow arrows), although the fracture line is not clear cut. It is also unclear whether the root of tooth 22 has suffered a root fracture, is uninjured, or whether a potential fracture of the alveolar process is superimposed on the root of the tooth (red arrow). (d and e) Coronal and sagittal, respectively, CBCT views of the maxillary anterior teeth and the premaxilla reveal a fracture of the alveolar process extending from the right central incisor (d) to the left lateral incisor (e) (green arrow). (f to h) Sagittal CBCT slices through tooth 11 (f), the empty socket of tooth 21 (g) and through tooth 22 (h). The alveolar process fracture involves the cortical plate of tooth 11 (yellow arrows), and tooth 22 (pink arrows), and the socket of tooth 21 (blue arrows). The root of tooth 22 has not suffered a fracture.

ing the efficacy of CBCT and panoramic radiography in the detection of mandibular condylar fractures, it was reported that panoramic radiography failed to detect these fractures in six of eleven cases, while CBCT detected the fractures in all cases (Matsumoto et al, 2013)

d. Injuries to the soft tissues

Conventional radiography

TDIs are frequently associated with concomitant injuries to the oral soft tissues (lip, tongue, gingiva and oral mucosa). Soft tissue injuries of this nature can be classified by type into abrasion, contusion and laceration (Table 9-4), and should be considered for radiographic assessment as part of the overall examination in cases of TDI. Tooth fragments and foreign bodies, such as gravel and glass, may have become embedded in the soft tissue during the injury and may be clinically undetectable.

Radiographs can be utilised to assess the injured soft tissues in these situations. This form of assessment is particularly appropriate when crown fractures have occurred, the broken tooth fragments cannot be located, or there are associated penetrating lip or tongue lacerations. The radiographic technique involves placing an X-ray image receptor on one side of the injured soft tissue and exposing the tissues from the opposite side, utilising an exposure time appropriate for soft tissue evaluation. In the case of tongue

Table 9-4 Classification of soft tissue injuries (Andreasen and Andreasen, 1994).

Type of injury	Description
Laceration of the gingiva or oral mucosa	A shallow or deep wound in the mucosa resulting from a tear, and usually produced by a sharp object
Contusion of the gingiva or oral mucosa	A bruise produced by impact with a blunt object and not accompanied by a break in the mucosa, usually causing a submucosal haemorrhage
Abrasion of gingiva or oral mucosa	A superficial wound produced by rubbing or scraping of the mucosa, leaving a raw, bleeding surface

injuries, the tongue should be protruded such that the injury is in an extraoral position before exposure (Andersson and Andreasen, 2007).

Periapical or occlusal image receptors may be employed, depending on the size of the injury and the anatomical constrictions of the mouth. Occlusal receptors placed extraorally are particularly useful when assessing the lips with a lateral view. The embedded matter will be evident on the radiograph as a radiopaque object(s), the shape and radiodensity of which will reflect the type of material.

A major restriction of using conventional imaging techniques is that multiple radiographs may have to be taken to identify the location of the embedded material, as it may be missed in initial exposures. Even in situations where the material is identified with the first radiograph, the examination represents an increase in the radiation exposure to which the patient is subject above that necessary to diagnose any TDI to the teeth and the PDL tissues. Furthermore, these radiographic examinations are difficult to execute in situations where cooperation is not optimal due to existing patient discomfort and anxiety.

CBCT

As CBCT is an extraoral imaging system, any radiodense matter embedded in the soft tissues captured within the field of view will be identified by the scan. The field of view, even in cases of small volume images, will generally include the relevant region of the lips and the tongue. The location of the tooth fragment or foreign body can be precisely identified and related to reproducible anatomical landmarks, such as adjacent teeth. An accurate assessment of the size and shape of the object can be obtained from the scan, providing information that will help minimise the surgical access required to retrieve it.

Of special significance is the fact that all of this information is obtained as part of the scan taken to assess the area of interest for any TDI to the dental hard tissues, the periodontal tissues and the supporting bone. Supplementary specific soft tissue imaging is not required, minimising the effective radiation dose to the patient.

Radiographic follow-up of TDI

Contemporary guidelines suggest the clinical and conventional radiographic follow-up of traumatically injured permanent teeth for between 1 and 5 years after the injury, depending on the nature of the TDI. The radiographic protocol is the same as that suggested for the initial assessment of the injury, with as many as five radiographic re-assessments suggested in the first 12 months, depending on the nature of the TDI (IADT, 2012 a, b).

The purpose of the follow-up procedure is to diagnose, at the earliest possible stage, the development of unfavourable outcomes such as AP and root resorption following TDI (Figs 9-10 and 9-11), so that treatment of these disease processes can be implemented. It has been established that CBCT has a higher diagnostic accuracy than periapical radiography in the detection of root resorption (Patel et al, 2009b; Durack et al, 2011), HRF (Bernardes et al, 2009; Jones et al, 2015), and AP (Patel et al, 2012; Tsai et al, 2013; Cheung et al, 2013). As such, it could be speculatively argued that strategically prescribed radiographic follow-up of TDI using CBCT might yield as much or more information about the development of these disease processes in fewer and earlier follow-up appointments and with similar or less effective radiation dose to the patient than conventional radiography.

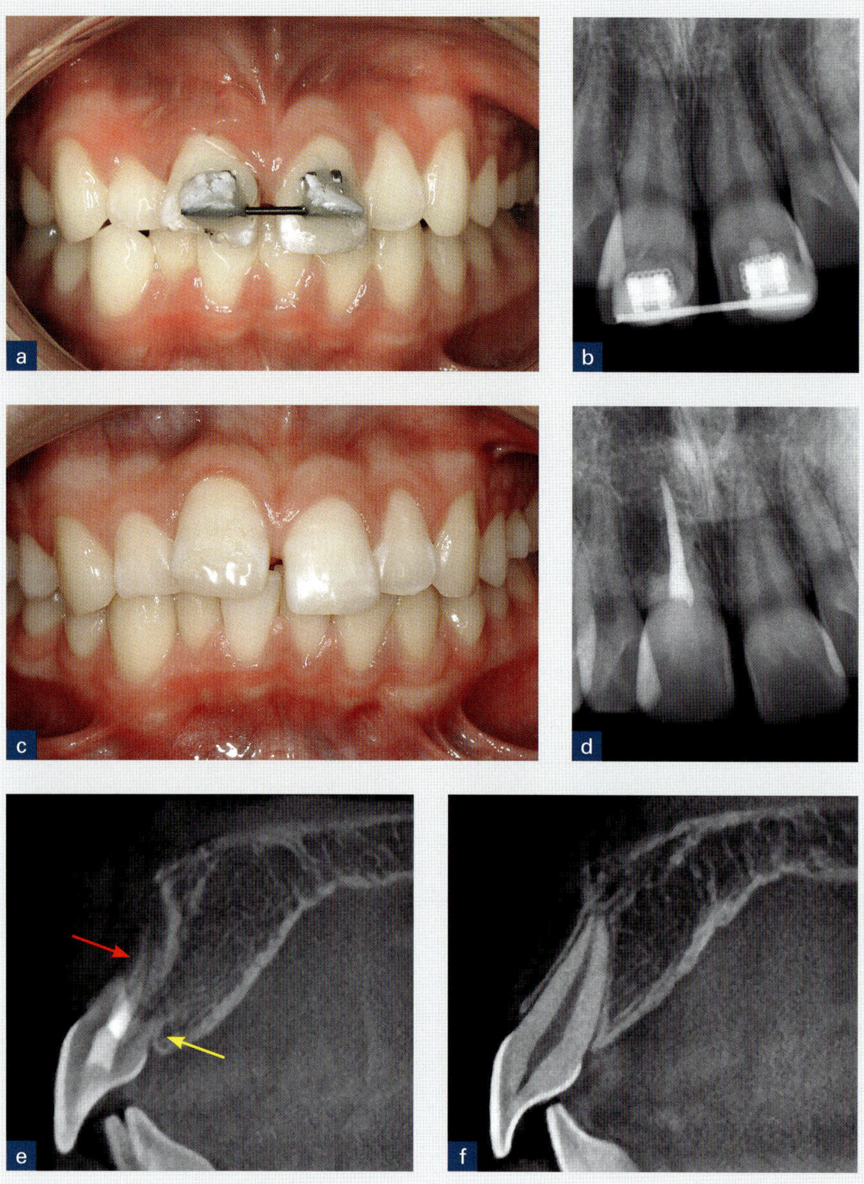

Fig 9-10 Delayed replantation and ankylosis in a mature tooth. (a) A 12-year-old boy, the day after a TDI in which the maxillary right central incisor (11) was avulsed. The tooth was replanted and splinted 30 minutes after the injury and the patient was subsequently referred to one of the authors. (b) Periapical radiograph of tooth 11 and the maxillary left central incisor tooth (21) at the assessment appointment the day after the injury. The avulsed tooth appears to have been appropriately repositioned, and the periapical tissues and the dental hard tissues appear healthy. Root canal treatment was carried out on the tooth 2 weeks after the injury. (c to f) At 42-month review. (c) Tooth 11 is in infraocclusion and the gingival margin of the tooth is at a more apical level, relative to tooth 21. These features are indicative of replacement resorption (ankylosis) of tooth 11. (d) A periapical radiograph reveals that tooth 11 has undergone replacement resorption. (e) Sagittal CBCT view of tooth 11 reveals that the root has been partially resorbed and replaced with alveolar bone (yellow arrow). The buccal cortical plate associated with the ankylosed tooth has completely resorbed such that the tooth has no bone support labially (red arrow). The palatal cortical plate is intact. (f) Sagittal CBCT view of tooth 21 confirms healthy dental and periapical tissues.

Conclusion

CBCT provides more information about the presence and nature of dentoalveolar injuries than conventional radiography (Patel et al, 2015). With improved diagnosis comes better management, and ultimately better outcomes. However, as with all radiographic examinations, the exposure of patients to ionising radiation must be justifiable, and the dose must be as low as reasonably achievable. This is particularly important in the management of TDI in younger patients who are more susceptible to the effects of ionising radiation (Theodorakou et al, 2012).

In cases where the diagnosis of TDI is inconclusive following clinical and conventional radiographic examination, the use of a small field of view CBCT should be considered (European Society of Endodontology, CBCT position statement, 2014). Furthermore, credence should be afforded to strategically prescribed CBCT assessments of traumatically injured teeth in the months following the injury.

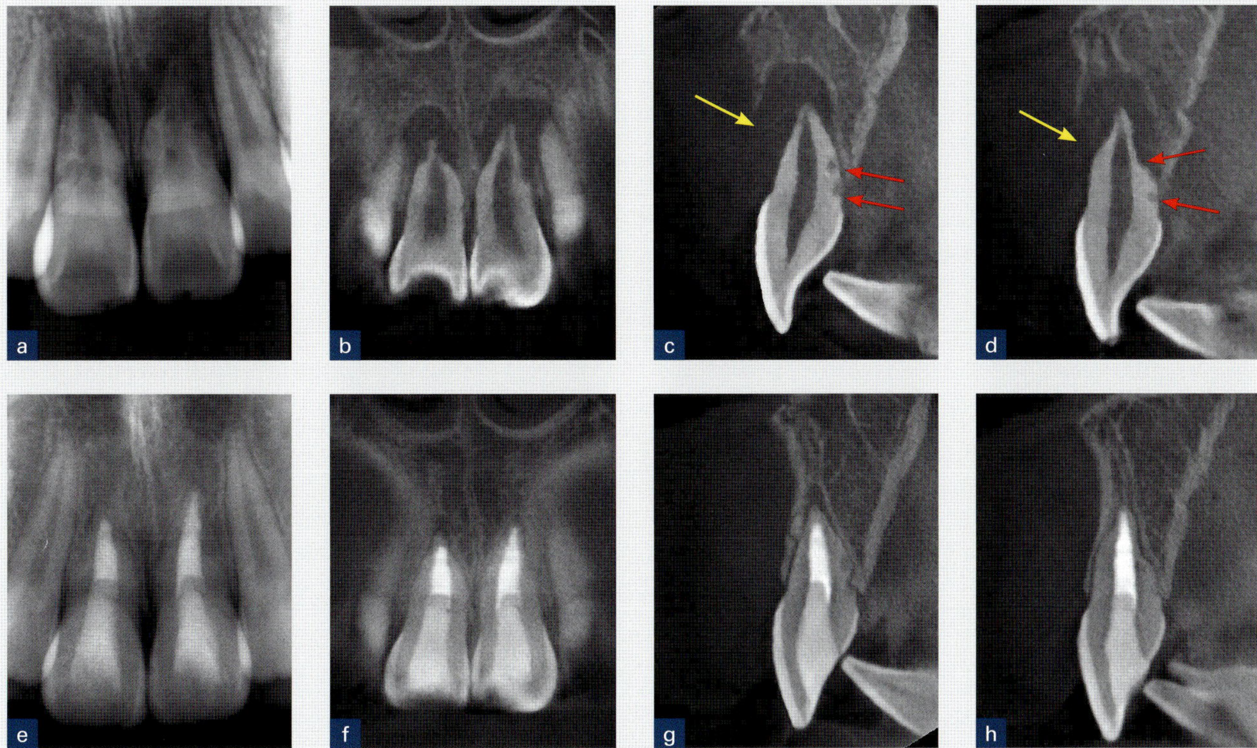

Fig 9-11 Delayed replantation and external inflammatory resorption. An 11-year-old girl presented 3.5 months after a TDI in which the maxillary right central incisor tooth (11) and the maxillary left central incisor tooth (21) were avulsed. Both teeth were replanted after an extra-alveolar period of in excess of 1 hour, and were left untreated thereafter. (a) A periapical radiograph of teeth 11 and 21 at the assessment appointment. Both the maxillary central incisors have undergone external inflammatory resorption. The root ends have been resorbed and shortened, and have adapted a ragged appearance. Saucer-shaped radiolucencies are evident on the root surfaces, and there are periapical radiolucencies associated with both teeth. Coronal (b) and sagittal (c and d) CBCT views of teeth 11 and 21 at the assessment appointment reveal the true nature of the resorptive lesions. It is clear from the sagittal views that the periapical inflammatory process has eroded the labial cortical plate adjacent to both teeth (yellow arrows). Note the saucer-shaped excavations on the palatal surfaces of both roots (red arrows). Although these were evident on the periapical radiograph, their exact location on the root surface could not be identified. The nature and degree of hard tissue loss affecting each root surface can also be appreciated using CBCT. Although the root walls of both teeth have been resorbed significantly in certain areas, the resorptive process has not breached the root canal wall. This information has a bearing on treatment planning. Non-surgical endodontic treatment of teeth 11 and 21 was carried out, based on this information. (e to h) At 2-year review. (e) A periapical radiograph of the maxillary central incisor teeth reveals that resorption has ceased, with apparent repair of the resorption defects. Also, the periapical radiolucencies appear to have completely resolved. (f) Coronal and (g and h) sagittal CBCT views confirm that the periapical radiolucency associated with tooth 21 has completely resolved (h). The periapical radiolucency associated with tooth 11 has significantly reduced in size but has not completely resolved (g). The residual radiolucency is not evident on the periapical radiograph. The labial cortical plates have regenerated and repaired. The resorptive process has ceased with the re-establishment of the PDL space in the area of the defects.

References

Abella F, Patel S, Durán-Sindreu F, Mercadé M, Bueno R, Roig M. Evaluating the periapical status of teeth with irreversible pulpitis by using cone-beam computed tomography scanning and periapical radiographs. J Endod 2012;38:1588–1591.

Al-Nuaimi N, Patel S, Foschi F, Mannocci F. The detection of simulated periapical lesions with CBCT—a dose reduction study. J Endod 2015 doi: 10.1111/iej.12565 [Epub ahead of print].

Andersson L, Andreasen JO. Soft tissue injuries. In: Andreasen JO, Andreasen FM, Andersson L (eds). Textbook and Colour Atlas of Traumatic Injuries to the Teeth, ed 4. Oxford, UK: Blackwell Munksgaard, 2007:577–597.

Andreasen JO. Luxation of permanent teeth due to trauma. A clinical and radiographic follow-up of 189 injured teeth. Scand J Dent Res 1970;78:273–286.

Andreasen JO. Injuries to the supporting bone. In: Andreasen JO, Andreasen FM, Andersson L (eds). Textbook and Colour Atlas of Traumatic Injuries to the Teeth, ed 4. Oxford, UK: Blackwell Munksgaard, 2007:489–515.

Andreasen FM, Andreasen JO. Diagnosis of luxation injuries: the importance of standardized clinical, radiographic and photographic techniques in clinical investigations. Endod Dent Traumatol 1985;1:160–169.

Andreasen FM, Andreasen JO. Resorption and mineralization processes following root fracture of permanent incisors. Endod Dent Traumatol 1988;4:202–214.

Andreasen JO, Andreasen FM. Classification, etiology and epidemiology of traumatic dental injuries. In: Andreasen JO, Andreasen FM (eds). Textbook and Colour Atlas of Traumatic Injuries to the Teeth, ed 3. Copenhagen, Denmark: Munksgaard, 1994:151–177.

Andreasen JO, Andreasen FM. Injuries to the supporting bone. In: Andreasen JO, Andreasen FM, Andersson L (eds). Textbook and Colour Atlas of Traumatic Injuries to the Teeth, ed 4. Oxford, UK: Blackwell Munksgaard, 2007:404–410.

Andreasen JO, Andreasen FM, Cvek M. Root fractures. In: Andreasen JO, Andreasen FM, Andersson L (eds). Textbook and Colour Atlas of Traumatic Injuries to the Teeth, ed 4. Oxford, UK: Blackwell Munksgaard, 2007a:337–371.

Andreasen JO, Andreasen FM, Tsukiboshi M. Crown-root fractues. In: Andreasen JO, Andreasen FM, Andersson L (eds). Textbook and Colour Atlas of Traumatic Injuries to the Teeth, ed 4. Oxford, UK: Blackwell Munksgaard, 2007b:314–336.

Andreasen FM, Pedersen BV. Prognosis of luxated permanent teeth—the development of pulp necrosis. Endod Dent Traumatol 1985;1:207–220.

Andreasen FM, Zhijie Y, Thomsen BL, Andersen PK. Occurrence of pulp canal obliteration after luxation injuries in the permanent dentition. Endod Dent Traumatol 1987;3:103–115.

Andreasen JO, Hjørting-Hansen E. Intraalveolar root fractures: radiographic and histologic study of 50 cases. J Oral Surg 1967;25:414–426.

Bender IB, Freedland JB. Clinical considerations in the diagnosis and treatment of intra-alveolar root fractures. J Am Dent Assoc 1983;107:595–600.

Bernardes RA, de Moraes IG, Duarte MAH, Azevedo BC, de Azevedo JR, Bramante CM. Use of cone-beam volumetric tomography in the diagnosis of root fractures. Oral Surg Oral Med Oral Pathol Oral Radiol Endod 2009;108:270–277.

Bornstein MM, Wölner-Hanssen AB, Sendi P, von Arx T. Comparison of intraoral radiography and limited cone-beam computed tomography in the assessment of root-fractured permanent teeth. Dent Traumatol 2009;25:571–577.

Cheung GS, Wei WL, McGrath C. Agreement between periapical radiographs and cone-beam computed tomography for assessment of periapical status of root filled molar teeth. Int Endod J 2013;46:889–895.

Cohenca N, Simon JH, Roges R, Morag Y, Malfaz JM. Clinical indications for digital imaging in dento-alveolar trauma. Part 1: traumatic injuries. Dent Traumatol 2007a:23:95–104.

Dölekoğlu S, Fişekçioğlu E, Ilgüy D, Ilgüy M, Bayirli G. Diagnosis of jaw and dentoalveolar fractures in a traumatized patient with cone beam computed tomography. Dent Traumatol 2010;26:200–203.

Durack C, Patel S, Davies J, Wilson R, Mannocci F. Diagnostic accuracy of small volume cone beam computed tomography and intraoral periapical radiography for the detection of simulated external inflammatory root resorption. Int Endod J 2011;44:136–147.

European Society of Endodontology, Patel S, Durack C, et al. European Society of Endodontology position statement: the use of CBCT in Endodontics (2014) Int Endod J 2014;47:502–504.

Flores MT, Andersson L, Andreasen JO, et al. Guidelines for the management of traumatic dental injuries. I. Fractures and luxations of permanent teeth. Dent Traumatol 2007a;23:66–71.

Flores MT, Andersson L, Andreasen JO, et al. Guidelines for the management of traumatic dental injuries. II. Avulsion of permanent teeth. Dent Traumatol 2007b;23:130–136.

International Association of Dental Traumatology. International Association of Dental Traumatology guidelines for the management of traumatic dental injuries: 1. Fractures and luxations of permanent teeth. Dent Traumatol 2012a;28:2–12.

International Association of Dental Traumatology. International Association of Dental Traumatology guidelines for the management of traumatic dental injuries: 2. Avulsion of permanent teeth. Dent Traumatol 2012b;28:88–96.

Jones D, Mannocci F, Andiappan M, Brown J, Patel S. The effect of alteration of the exposure parameters of a cone-beam computed tomography scan on the diagnosis of simulated horizontal root fractures. J Endod 2015;41:520–525.

Kamburoğlu K, Cebeci AR, Gröndahl HG. Effectiveness of limited cone-beam computed tomography in the detection of horizontal root fracture. Dent Traumatol 2009;25:256–261.

Kaste LM, Gift HC, Bhat M, Swango PA. Prevalence of incisor trauma in persons 6–50 years of age: United States, 1988–1991. J Dent Res 1996;75:696–705.

Matsumoto K, Sawada K, Kameoka S, Yonehara Y, Honda K. Cone-beam computed tomography for the diagnosis of mandibular condylar fractures: 11 case reports. Oral Radiol 2013;29:80–86.

May JJ, Cohenca N, Peters O. Contemporary management of horizontal root fractures to the permanent dentition: diagnosis—radiologic assessment to include cone-beam computed tomography. Dent Traumatol 2013;39:s20–25.

Oikarinen K, Gundlach KK, Pfeifer G. Late complications of luxation injuries to teeth. Endod Dent Traumatol 1987;3:296–303.

Patel S, Saunders W. Radiographs in Endodontics. Faculty of General Dental Practitioners (UK); Selection Criteria for Dental Radiography, 2013.

Patel S, Dawood A, Mannocci F, Wilson R, Pitt Ford T. Detection of periapical bone defects in human jaws using cone beam computed tomography and intraoral radiography. Int Endod J 2009a;42:507–515.

Patel S, Dawood A, Wilson R, Horner K, Mannocci F. The detection and management of root resorption lesions using intraoral radiography and cone beam computed tomography—an in vivo investigation. Int Endod J 2009b;42:831–838.

Patel S, Wilson R, Dawood A, Mannocci F. The detection of periapical pathosis using periapical radiography and cone beam computed tomography–Part 1: pre-operative status. Int Endod J 2012;45:702–710.

Patel S, Durack C, Abella F, Shemesh H, Roig M, Lemberg M. Cone beam computed tomography in Endodontics– a review. Int Endod J 2015;48:3–15.

Theodorakou C, Walker A, Horner K, et al. Estimation of paediatric organ and effective doses from dental cone beam CT using anthropomorphic phantoms. Br J Radiol 2012;85:153–160.

Tsai P, Torabinejad M, Rice D, Azevedo B. Accuracy of cone-beam computed tomography and periapical radiography in detecting small periapical lesions. J Endod 2013;38:965–970.

World Health Organization. Application of the International Classification of Diseases to Dentistry and Stomatology IDC-DA, ed 3. Geneva: WHO, 1992.

Chapter 10

Root Resorption

Conor Durack, Shanon Patel

Introduction

Root resorption is the destruction of dental hard tissue, namely cementum and dentine, as a result of clastic cell action (Hammarström and Lindskog, 1985; Andreasen, 1988; Patel and Ford, 2007). It can be broadly classified according to the site of its occurrence on the root of the affected tooth; internal resorption affects the root canal wall, while external resorption occurs on the root's outer surface. Both types of resorption are subclassified according to the specific histological nature of the resorptive processes occurring, each of which have specific radiographic features.

External root resorption

- External surface resorption
- External inflammatory resorption
- External replacement resorption
- External cervical resorption

Internal root resorption

- Internal inflammatory resorption
- Internal replacement resorption

A diagnosis of root resorption is reliant on the radiographic demonstration of the process (Andreasen et al, 1987). However, several *ex vivo* and *in vitro* studies have demonstrated that conventional periapical radiography is not a reliable technique for detecting external root resorption, especially when the simulated resorptive defects are small (Andreasen et al, 1987; Chapnick, 1989; Goldberg et al, 1998). In contrast, *ex vivo* studies have confirmed improved accuracy with cone beam computed tomography (CBCT) over conventional periapical radiography in the detection of simulated internal (Kamburoğlu et al, 2011) and external (Bernardes et al, 2012; Ren et al, 2013) root resorption including situations where the external defects are minimal (Durack et al, 2011). Furthermore, some *ex vivo* studies have also demonstrated that, compared to periapical radiography, CBCT is a significantly more effective method of determining the exact site of simulated resorptive cavities on the external surfaces of roots (D'Addazio et al, 2011; Durack et al, 2011). It also proved the more successful method of differentiating between simulated resorption defects on the root canal wall and on the external surface of the root (D'Addazio et al, 2011; Kamburoğlu et al, 2011). One *ex vivo* study reported that CBCT could accurately calculate both the volume of resorptive cavities created on the lateral surfaces of roots and the extent of simulated apical root resorption in a linear plane (Ponder et al, 2013).

Clinical studies comparing the diagnostic accuracy of CBCT and conventional radiography in the detection of root resorption are limited. However, one clinical study demonstrated that CBCT is a significantly better imaging modality at determining the presence and extent of external root resorption when compared to conventional radiography (Estrela et al, 2009). In a further clinical study, the performance of periapical radiography and CBCT as diagnostic and treatment planning tools in the management of external cervical and internal root resorption were compared. CBCT could accurately detect the presence and differentiate between the types of resorption (internal and external) in all of the cases examined, and CBCT also performed significantly better than periapical radiography as a treatment planning tool. The overall sensitivity of intraoral radiographs was significantly lower than CBCT (Patel et al, 2009a).

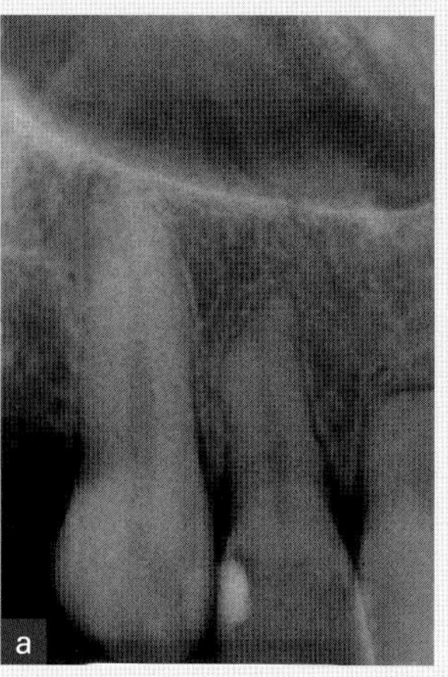

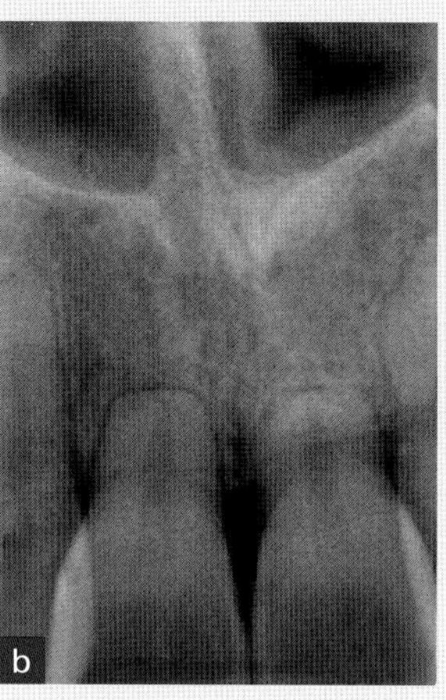

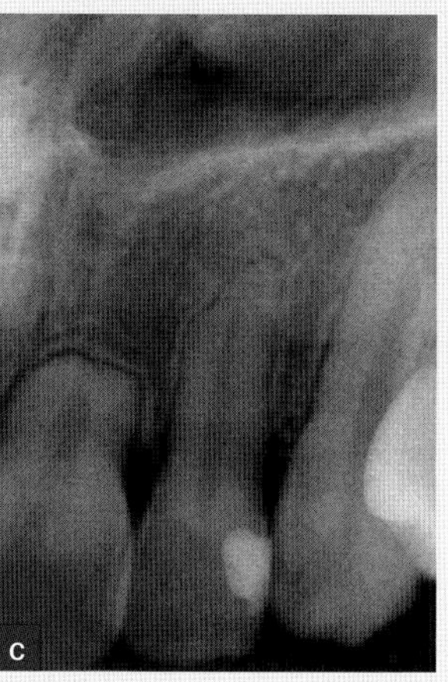

Fig 10-1 External surface resorption. A series of radiographs revealing extensive external surface resorption of the maxillary right first incisor and maxillary left central incisor, and to a lesser extent of the maxillary right second incisor. The patient gave a history of orthodontic treatment and dental trauma.

External root resorption

External surface resorption

Conventional radiography

The conventional radiographic appearance of surface resorption is variable, case-specific, and dependent on the stimulus for resorption. The appearance can vary from small, saucer-shaped, superficial excavations on an otherwise normal root surface outline (as a result of mild traumatic injuries or as a physiological occurrence) to partial or complete destruction of the root (Andreasen and Hjørting-Hansen, 1966a; Andreasen and Pedersen, 1985).

More extensive tissue destruction tends to occur in cases of surface resorption caused by pressure exerted on the roots by orthodontic treatment and/or adjacent impacted masses, such as teeth, cysts, tumours, etc. Teeth with orthodontic-related surface resorption typically present with blunted or uniformly shortened root ends, while the appearance of resorption associated with impacted masses tends to reflect the shape of the offending body (Fig 10-1). Regardless of the aetiology of surface resorption and the extent of the tissue destruction, an intact periodontal ligament (PDL) space/lamina dura typically surrounds the resorbed area of root in cases of surface resorption (Andreasen and Hjørting-Hansen, 1966a).

CBCT

On CBCT scans, external surface resorption has a similar basic radiographic appearance to that seen on conventional radiographs. However, the true nature of the lesion can be more accurately assessed than on conventional (two-dimensional) radiographs. The exact position of any resorptive defect can be pinpointed, and lesions undetectable on conventional radiographs will manifest on CBCT (Fig 10-2). These findings may alter the prognosis of the tooth/teeth under investigation.

External inflammatory resorption

Conventional radiography

External inflammatory resorption associated with dental trauma is characterised radiographically by radiolucent, concave, and sometimes ragged excavations along the root surface, with corresponding and associated radiolucencies in the adjacent alveolar bone (Fig 10-3). There is complete loss of the lamina dura in the area of the resorption (Andreasen and Hjørting-Hansen, 1966b).

External inflammatory resorption is also commonly associated with teeth with infected necrotic root canal systems, and is not always the result of traumatic dental injuries (TDIs) (Laux et al, 2000). In these cases, the resorption site on the affected root will reflect the portal of exit of the bacterial toxins from the root canal. More than one location on the root surface may therefore be affected. However, typically, the apical portion of the root is most commonly affected due to the proximity of the apical foramen (Patel et al, 2016). Conventional radiography may reveal an irregular root at the resorption site. The root may be shortened if the process is occurring apically. The degree of the hard tissue destruction is variable and will reflect the

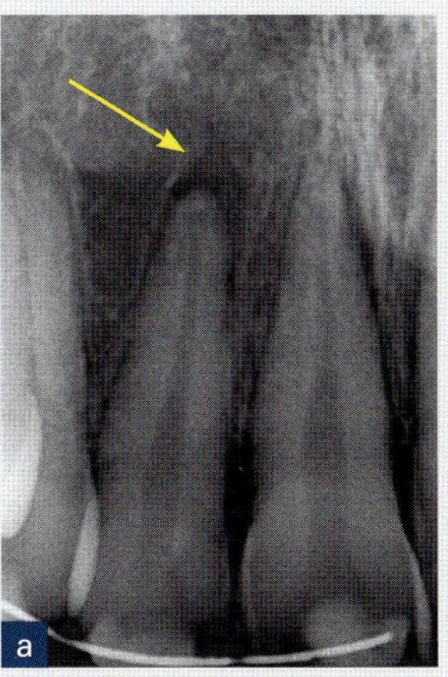

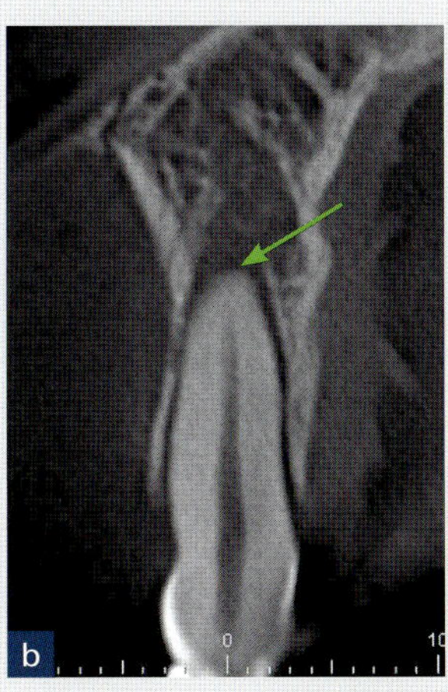

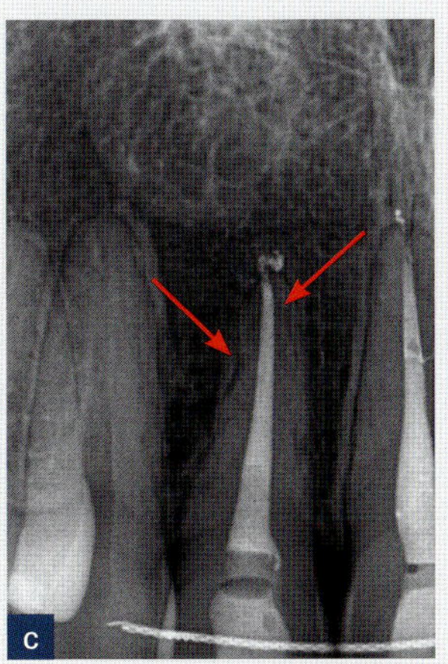

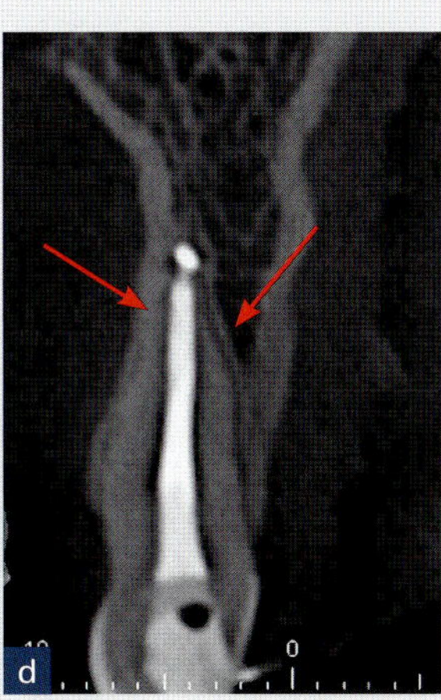

Fig 10-2 External surface resorption. (a) Periapical radiograph of the maxillary right incisor and canine teeth immediately after dental trauma. The maxillary right second incisor had been extruded; the yellow arrow reveals the extent of the extrusion. (b) The sagittal CBCT slice confirms the extent of the extrusion (green arrow). The traumatised non-vital teeth were subsequently endodontically treated and orthodontically repositioned. (c) A 4-year review radiograph reveals signs of external surface resorption (red arrows) on the mesial and distal aspects of the maxillary right incisor. (d) The sagittal CBCT slice confirms surface resorption of the labial and palatal surfaces of the root of the tooth. Note the presence of the intact PDL space and lamina dura around the entire root.

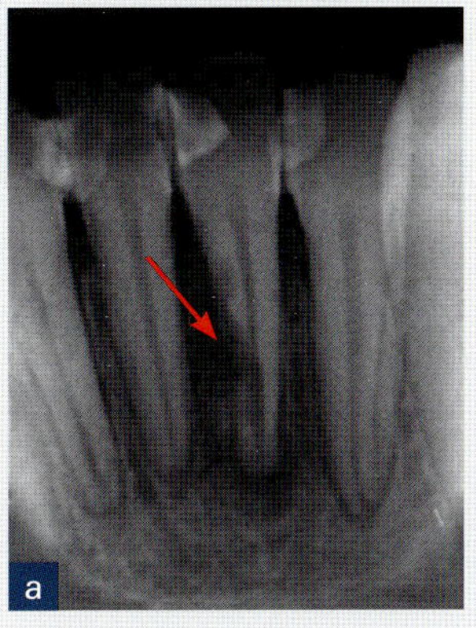

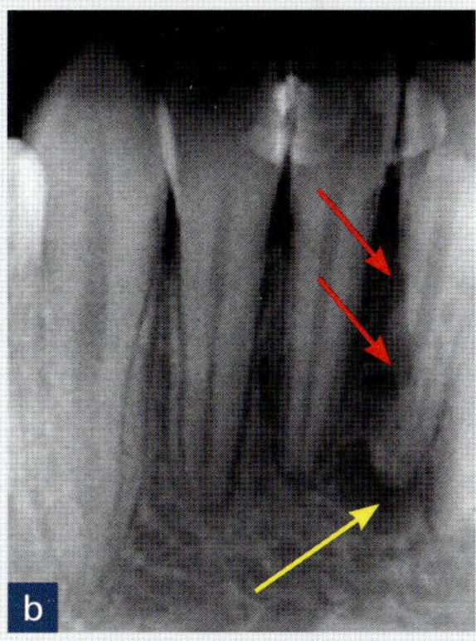

Fig 10-3 External inflammatory resorption. (a and b) Parallax periapical radiographs of the mandibular incisors reveal the classic saucer-shaped excavations on the root surface with associated radiolucencies in the adjacent alveolar bone (red arrows); note there is no intact lamina dura adjacent to the external inflammatory resorption. There is also periapical radiolucency (yellow arrow).

chronicity of the infection. Regardless of the site of the resorption, radiolucency will be present in the adjacent alveolar bone, in addition to the lamina dura, and PDL space will be absent.

CBCT

On CBCT scans, external inflammatory resorption has a similar radiographic appearance to that seen on conventional radiographs. However, the extent of the lesion can be better appreciated, as can the associated periradicular radiolucencies in the adjacent bone (Figs 10-4 and 10-5). Furthermore, the exact position of any resorptive defect can be localised, and lesions undetectable by conventional radiography (buccal/palatal surfaces) can be seen on CBCT (Durack et al, 2011). These incidental findings, however, do not mean that CBCT should be used as a screening tool to routinely assess external inflammatory resorption.

External replacement resorption

Conventional radiography

The distinguishing radiographic features of ankylosis are replacement of the root with adjacent bone and associated disappearance of the normal PDL space (Fig 10-6). There is no radiolucency in the adjoining bone related to the area of resorption (Andreasen and Hjørting-Hansen, 1966a). External replacement resorption (ERR) can affect any portion of the root and may cause varying levels of tissue destruction..

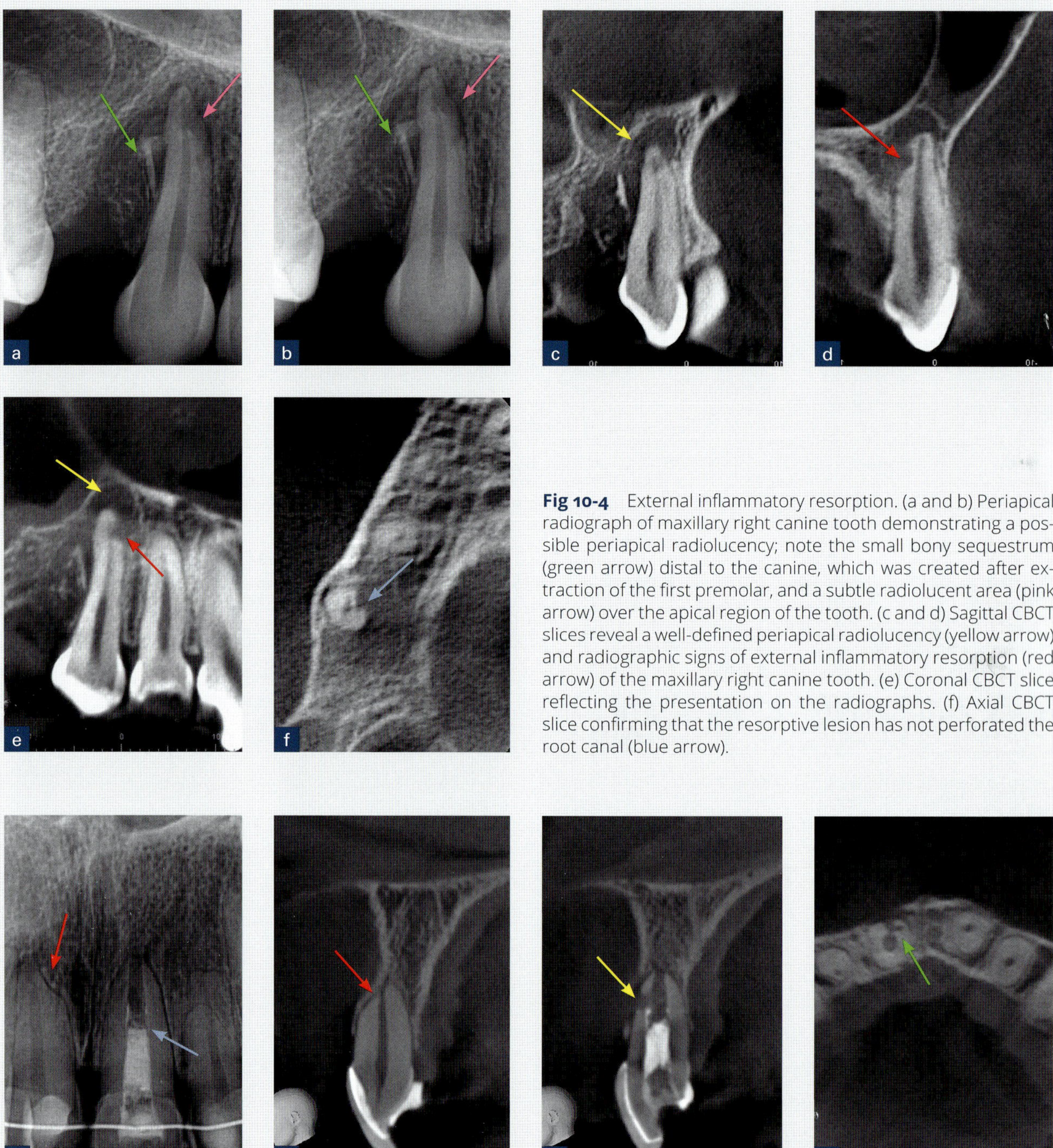

Fig 10-4 External inflammatory resorption. (a and b) Periapical radiograph of maxillary right canine tooth demonstrating a possible periapical radiolucency; note the small bony sequestrum (green arrow) distal to the canine, which was created after extraction of the first premolar, and a subtle radiolucent area (pink arrow) over the apical region of the tooth. (c and d) Sagittal CBCT slices reveal a well-defined periapical radiolucency (yellow arrow) and radiographic signs of external inflammatory resorption (red arrow) of the maxillary right canine tooth. (e) Coronal CBCT slice reflecting the presentation on the radiographs. (f) Axial CBCT slice confirming that the resorptive lesion has not perforated the root canal (blue arrow).

Fig 10-5 External inflammatory resorption. (a) Periapical radiograph of maxillary left central incisor, which has been treated with an intracanal dressing of calcium hydroxide, to a level which is short of the radiographic apex. The apex locator provided a '0' reading at this level and as such the tooth was prepared to this length; note the external surface resorption associated with the mesial root surfaces of the maxillary right central incisor and the maxillary left lateral incisor. This is most likely attributable to a previous TDI suffered by the patient. (b) Sagittal CBCT slice reveals signs of external surface resorption on the mesial aspect of the maxillary left central incisor. (c) Sagittal CBCT slice reveals signs of external inflammatory resorption (yellow arrow) on the mesial aspect of the root of the maxillary left central incisor; note that this may not be seen on the radiograph due to its position on the root surface. (d) Axial CBCT slice reveals signs of external inflammatory resorption on the mesial aspect of the maxillary left central incisor. These CBCT images also confirm that the resorption defect has perforated (green arrow) the root canal system, and will therefore influence the management of this case.

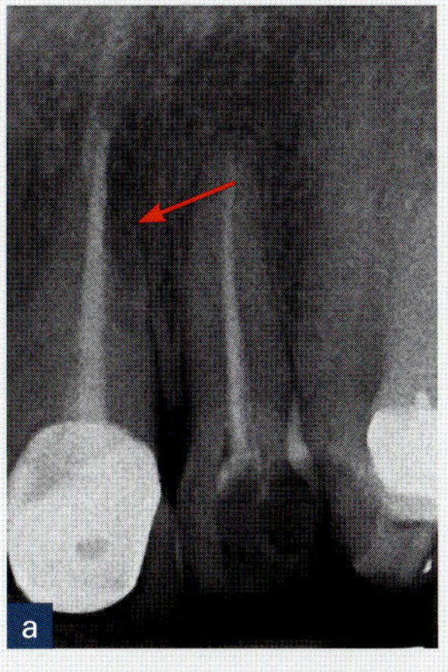

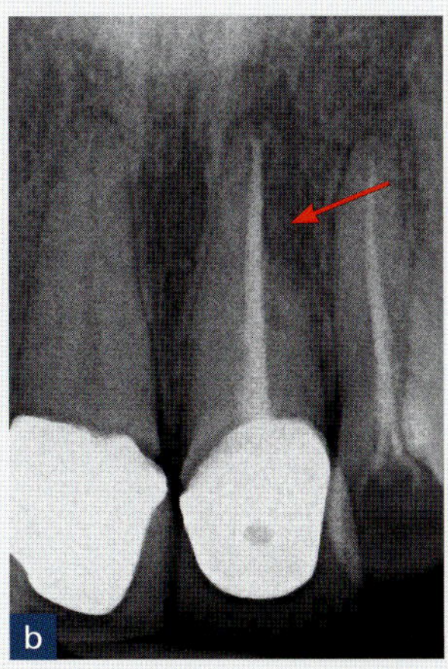

Fig 10-6 External replacement resorption. (a and b) Parallax radiographs of the maxillary left central incisor. Note how bone has directly replaced the root dentine, and how the size of the resorptive defect changes with the second radiograph (red arrow).

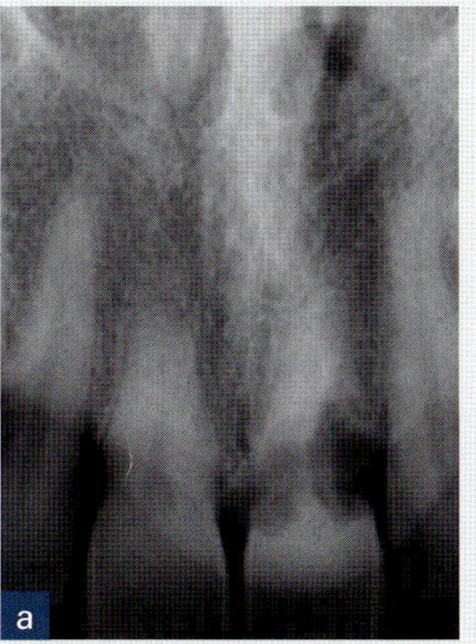

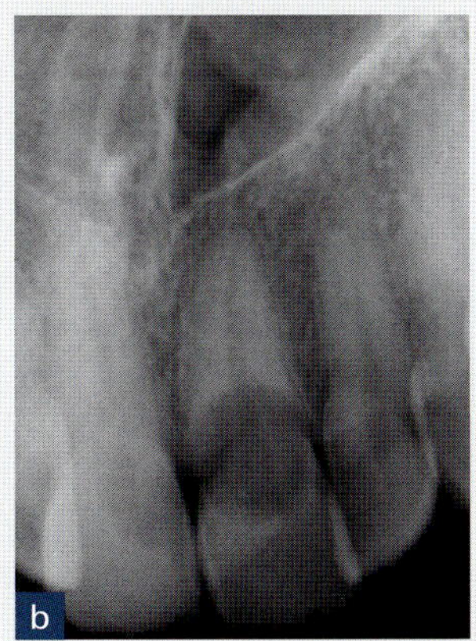

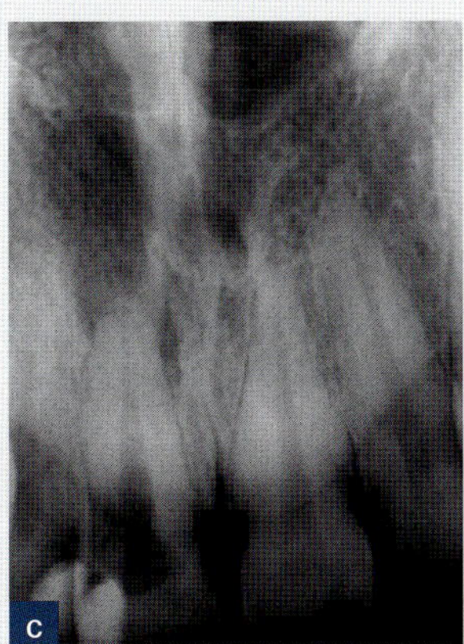

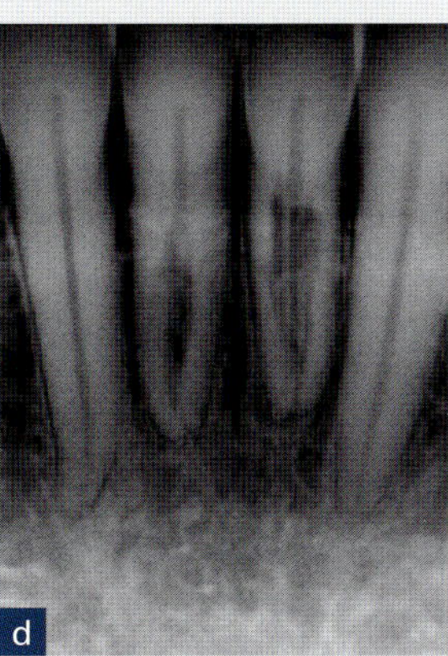

Fig 10-7 External cervical resorption. (a to d) A series of periapical radiographs from different cases demonstrating the variable radiographic presentation of ECR. (a) A 'moth-eaten' radiolucency with irregular margins on the mesial and distal surfaces of the maxillary left central incisor. (b) A well-defined symmetrical radiolucency associated with the cervical region of the maxillary left central incisor. (c) An irregular radiolucency with well-defined borders associated with the cervical region of the maxillary right central incisor. (d) A mottled appearance in the roots of both the mandibular right and left central incisors, indicating bone-like metaplastic changes.

CBCT

The radiographic findings are very similar to conventional radiography. However, small, distinct ERR on the labial and/or palatal aspects of the root can only be reliably detected with CBCT. Conventional radiography is better for detecting proximal defects, which have reached a minimum critical size, but is not able to reliably identify smaller lesions on the labial or palatal root surfaces.

External cervical resorption

Conventional radiography

The conventional radiographic appearance of external cervical resorption (ECR) is highly variable and is influenced by a number of factors, including the site of the defect on the affected tooth, to what extent and in which manner the resorptive process has invaded the root dentine, and the relative proportions of granulomatous and osseous tissue occupying the resorptive defect (Gunst et al, 2011, 2013).

ECR typically affects the cervical region of the affected tooth. However, it may not always appear to involve the tooth's cervical region when assessed on conventional radiographs. ECR may initiate below the cervical region in accordance with the more apical position of the epithelial attachment on the affected tooth. In teeth with a normal periodontal attachment, the lesion may extend some distance apical and/or coronal to the cervical location at which it commenced, reflecting the invasive nature of the process (Heithersay, 1999, 2004).

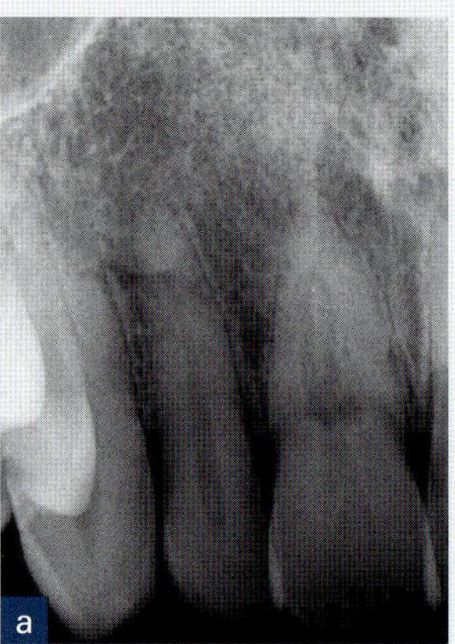
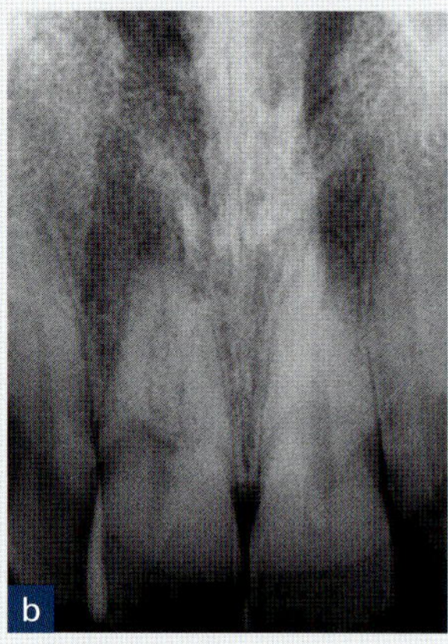
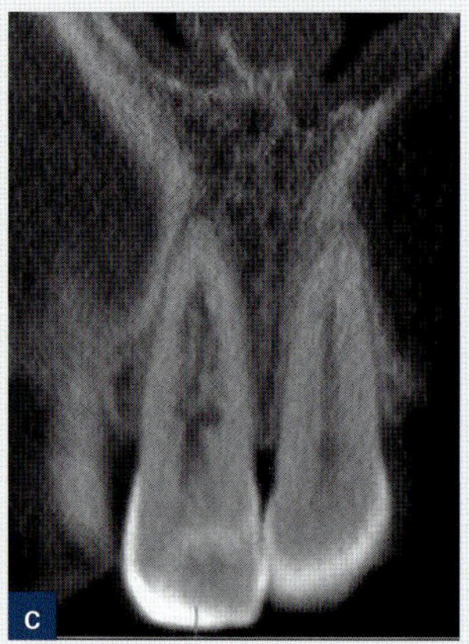
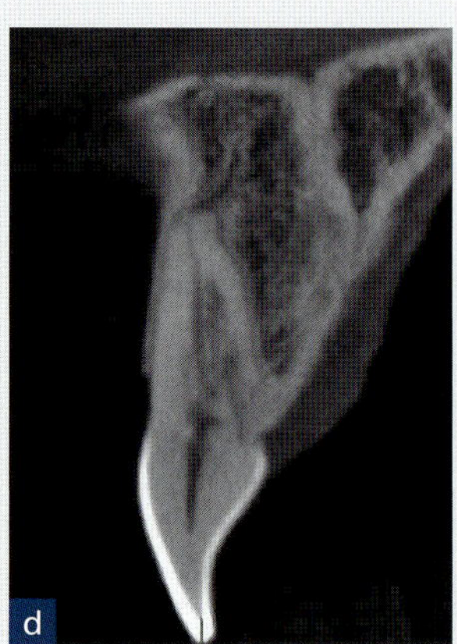
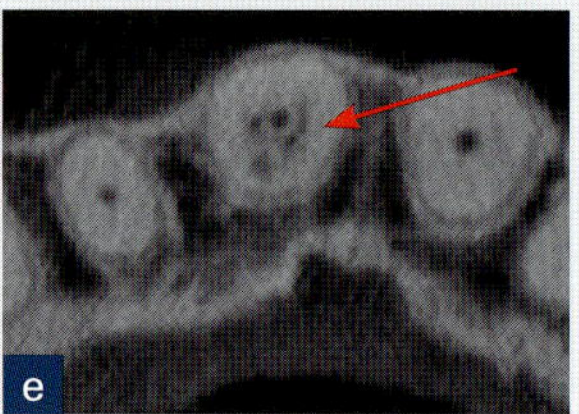

Fig 10-8 External cervical resorption. (a and b) Parallax radiographs of the maxillary right central incisors reveal a 'fuzzy' mottled appearance in the coronal and middle third of the root canal. (c) Reconstructed coronal, (d) sagittal, and (e) axial CBCT slices confirm the presence and true extent of the ECR lesion; note how the ECR is encompassing the root canal (red arrow). There is no significant change in position of the resorptive defect relative to the root canal with the parallax radiographs, possibly indicating an internal resorptive defect; CBCT confirms that defect is ECR (courtesy of Patel S, Dawood A, Wilson R, Horner K, Mannocci F. The detection and management of root resorption lesions using intraoral radiography and cone beam computed tomography - an in vivo investigation. Int Endod J 2009a;42:831–838).

The tissue destruction at the true site of onset may sometimes be minimal and/or obscured by adjacent anatomical noise, and therefore undetectable on conventional radiographs. In such situations, the conventional radiographic appearance may give the impression that the resorptive process has commenced at the site where the bulk of the tissue destruction has occurred. This may be some distance from both the cervical region of the tooth and/or the true site of onset of the resorptive process. This is particularly relevant when conservative management of the lesion is being considered. This is a feature of ECR that has only become appreciated with the advent of CBCT imaging techniques. ECR defects will typically present as radiolucencies of varying radiodensity (Patel et al, 2009b; Gunst et al, 2013).

The ECR lesion will tend to be uniformly radiolucent when the defect is predominantly comprised of fibrovascular, granulomatous tissue. However, except in cases where the lesion is located at supracrestal level, it is relatively uncommon for the resorptive defect to be completely radiolucent. Rather, the lesion will often adopt a partial or completely 'cloudy' appearance, most likely caused by the superimposition of adjacent hard tissue (bone and adjacent root dentine) over the area of interest, and/or a gradual metaplastic change in the tissue occupying the resorptive cavity (Iqbal, 2007; Gunst et al, 2013). It is impossible to make the distinction between the two with conventional radiography (Fig 10-7). The presence of fibro-osseous inclusions in the resorptive defect (i.e. in more long-standing lesions), which have a greater radiodensity than their surrounding granulomatous matrix and may be sparsely or diffusely spread throughout the resorptive cavity, will impart a more 'mottled' appearance to the lesion (Fig 10-8).

When assessed using conventional radiography, the margins of ECR lesions vary from well to poorly defined, depending on the depth of the defect and the proportion and distribution of fibro-osseous inclusions within the lesion. The majority of cases have well-defined margins (Patel et al, 2009b). The parallax technique (see later) may be useful to help identify the nature of the ECR lesion and to differentiate it from internal resorption (Fig 10-9).

Historically, the nature, management, and ultimately, prognosis of ECR have been based on the Heithersay classification (1999). This classification graded ECR according to the extent of ECR invasion within the tooth (I to IV). However, this classification is based on radiographs and therefore can only reliably assess the nature of ECR if it is exclusively confined to the proximal aspects of the tooth (Patel and Dawood, 2007; Gunst et al, 2013).

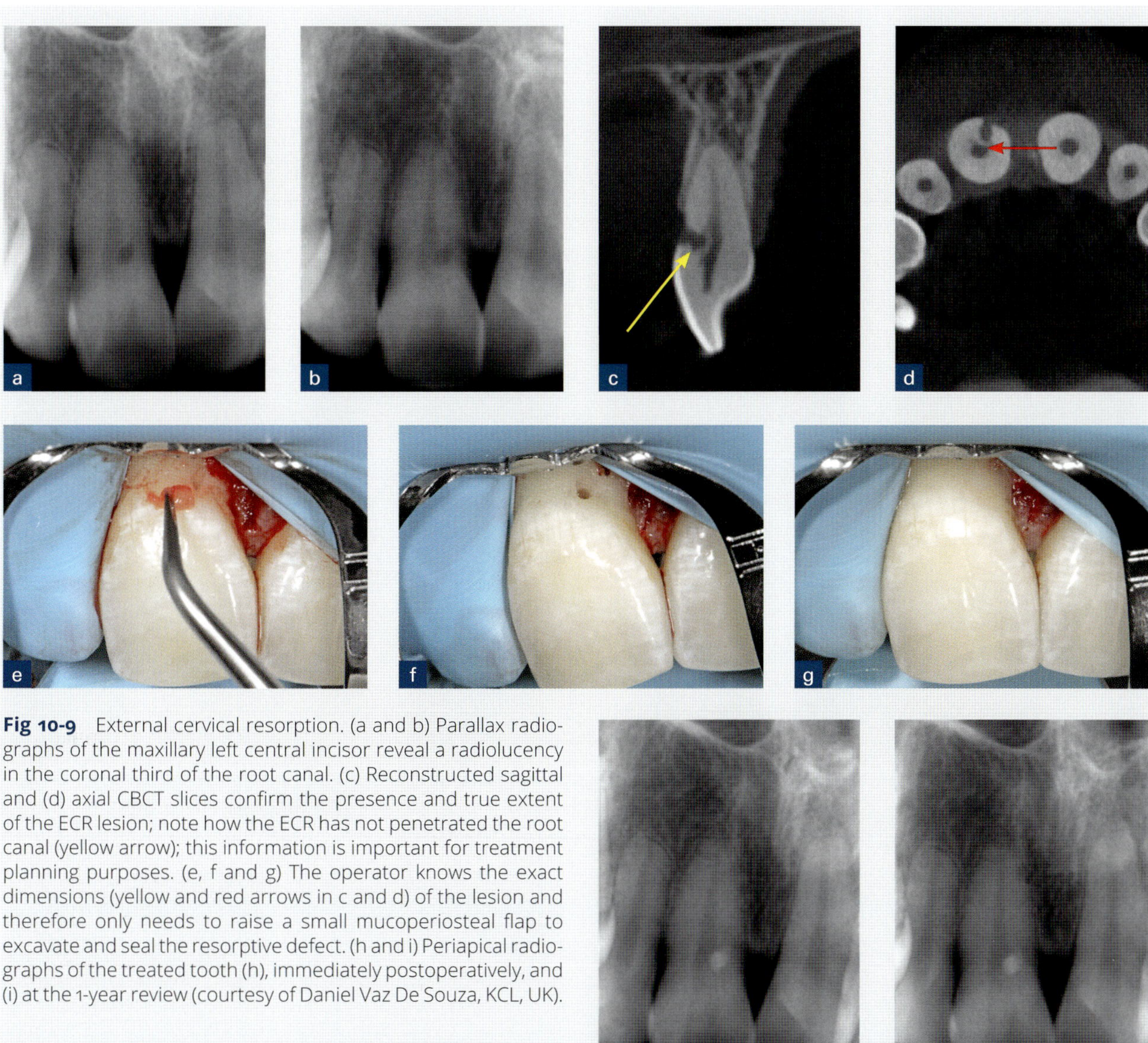

Fig 10-9 External cervical resorption. (a and b) Parallax radiographs of the maxillary left central incisor reveal a radiolucency in the coronal third of the root canal. (c) Reconstructed sagittal and (d) axial CBCT slices confirm the presence and true extent of the ECR lesion; note how the ECR has not penetrated the root canal (yellow arrow); this information is important for treatment planning purposes. (e, f and g) The operator knows the exact dimensions (yellow and red arrows in c and d) of the lesion and therefore only needs to raise a small mucoperiosteal flap to excavate and seal the resorptive defect. (h and i) Periapical radiographs of the treated tooth (h), immediately postoperatively, and (i) at the 1-year review (courtesy of Daniel Vaz De Souza, KCL, UK).

CBCT

With CBCT, all dimensions of an ECR lesion's relationship to the crestal bone can be found, and therefore an estimation of the initiation site(s) of ECR can also be determined. In addition, it can also provide an insight into the nature of the ECR lesion's content (i.e. granulation tissue and/or metaplastic bone-like tissue) (Gunst et al, 2013).

In an *in vivo* study, Patel et al (2009a) found that CBCT was more effective than periapical radiographs for accurately diagnosing external cervical (and internal) resorption. CBCT was also found to increase the likelihood of the correct treatment option being chosen. De Souza et al (2016), in an unpublished study, compared the ability of CBCT and periapical radiographs to assess the nature and location of simulated ECR lesions in dry human mandibles. They found that CBCT was significantly more accurate at determining the exact size and location of these simulated ECR lesions when compared to parallax periapical radiographs. Furthermore, when the simulated lesions were assessed using the Heithersay classification, they found that CBCT was more accurate at correctly classifying the lesions when compared to periapical radiographs.

A main area of tissue destruction, if present, can be easily identified, and is generally represented as radiolucency. As it is possible with CBCT to view the lesion

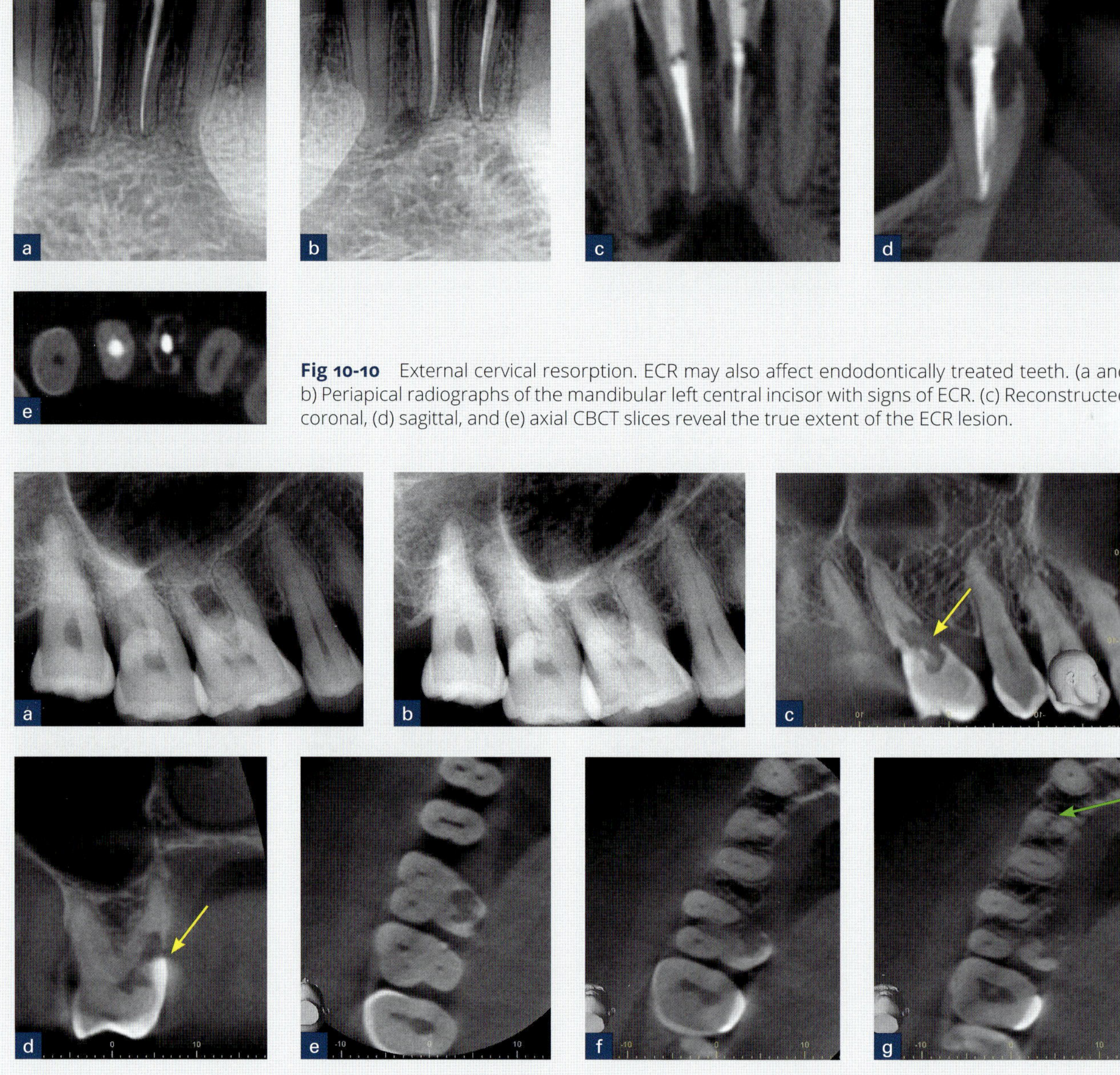

Fig 10-10 External cervical resorption. ECR may also affect endodontically treated teeth. (a and b) Periapical radiographs of the mandibular left central incisor with signs of ECR. (c) Reconstructed coronal, (d) sagittal, and (e) axial CBCT slices reveal the true extent of the ECR lesion.

Fig 10-11 External cervical resorption. (a and b) There are no obvious signs of ECR on these parallax periapical radiographs of the maxillary right first molar. (c) The reconstructed CBCT sagittal, (d) coronal, and (e to g) axial images reveal the true nature of the ECR lesion (yellow arrows). Note that there are signs of ECR on the premolar tooth too (green arrow). (Image courtesy Patel S, Saberi N. External cervical resorption associated with the use of bisphosphonates: a case series. J Endod 2015;41:742-748.)

unobstructed by eliminating anatomical noise and focusing on an area (or areas) of interest, the true radiodensity of the lesions can be established (Figs 10-10 and 10-11). As such, any cloudiness or obvious radiopacity occupying the lesion will represent metaplastic change within the lesion. Specifically, cloudiness within the lesion will represent a transitional stage of metaplasia, while distinct radiopacity will reflect the completed formation of hard tissue (Patel et al, 2016). Areas of hard tissue formation, which appear to be mottled on conventional radiographs, can be more readily identified with CBCT. Two basic presentations of hard tissue inclusion within ECR are generally seen on CBCT:

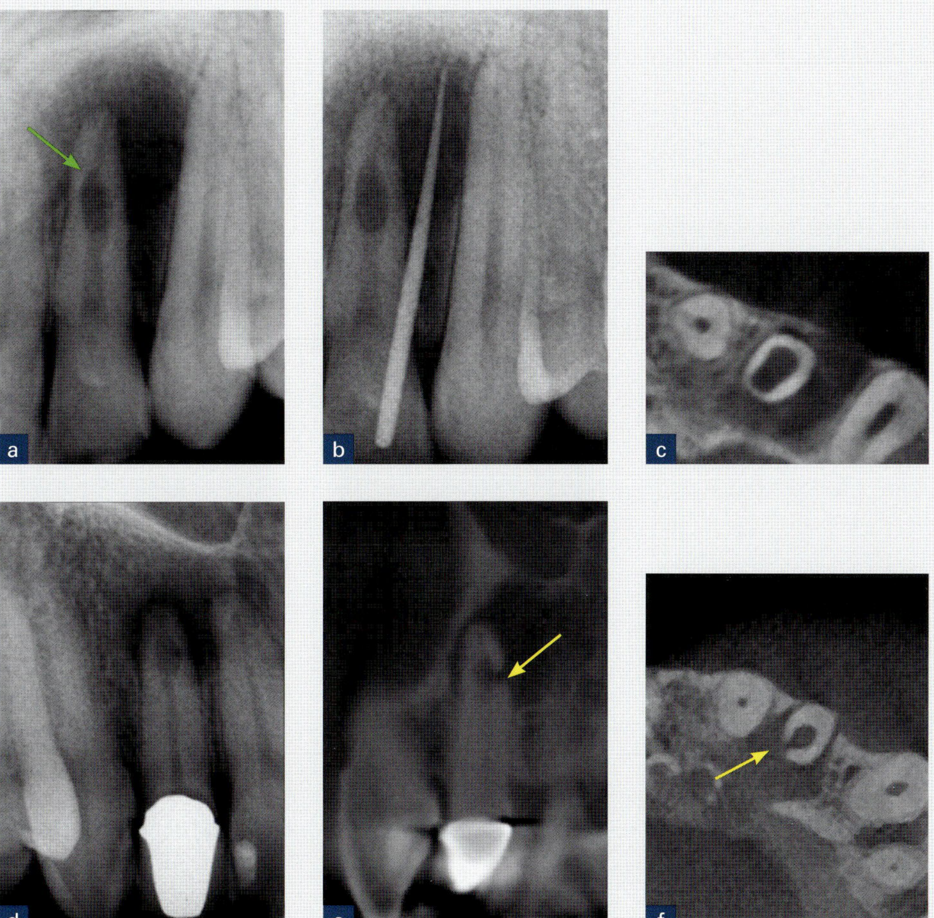

Fig 10-12 Internal root resorption. (a) A periapical radiograph of a maxillary left lateral incisor with radiographic signs of IRR (green arrow); note the ballooning out of the root canal—the defect is symmetrical, well-defined and uniformly radiolucent. (b) The radiolucency stays centred on the second (parallax) radiograph, helping to confirm the diagnosis of IRR. (c) An axial CBCT slice reveals intact canal walls. (d) A periapical radiograph of a maxillary right lateral incisor with radiographic signs of IRR. (e) Sagittal and (f) axial CBCT slices reveal that the resorptive defect has perforated (yellow arrow) the root canal wall (courtesy of Patel S, Ricucci D, Durak C, Tay F. Internal root resorption: a review. J Endod 2010;36:1107-1121).

- Radiopaque islands of hard tissue formation, which comprise a varying quantity of the lesion depending on the extent of the completed metaplastic change, interspersed by radiolucent (granulomatous) tissue.
- Radiopaque bands or streaks of hard tissue formation comprising the majority of the lesion, which are interspersed by minimal amounts of radiolucent (granulomatous) tissue.

The area of the major tissue destruction may represent the site of onset of the resorptive process, and the lesion may be confined to this area. However, narrow branches of resorption, represented on CBCT images as thin, projecting radiolucencies, often (but not always) radiate from the main site of tissue destruction in varying directions and planes within the root. These branches may be confined to the root, may penetrate the crown of the tooth, or in advanced cases may communicate with the external root surface and/or root canal space. These branches sometimes partially or completely circumscribe the root canal. If the site of the bulk tissue destruction is at a location distant from the anticipated level of epithelial attachment (which can be estimated from the CBCT scan), a radiating branch can normally be identified, extending from the lesion proper to communicate with the root's external surface at a more cervical level. It is at this point that the resorptive process is likely to have commenced, despite the comparatively minimal tissue destruction. This detailed information is essential for the predictable management of ECR (Patel and Dawood, 2007; Gunst et al, 2013).

It is often easier to define the margins of the lesion when viewed using CBCT; borders may be smooth, irregular, or a combination of both.

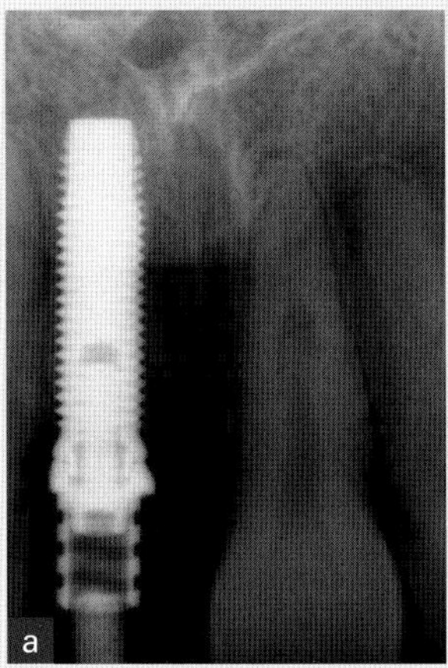

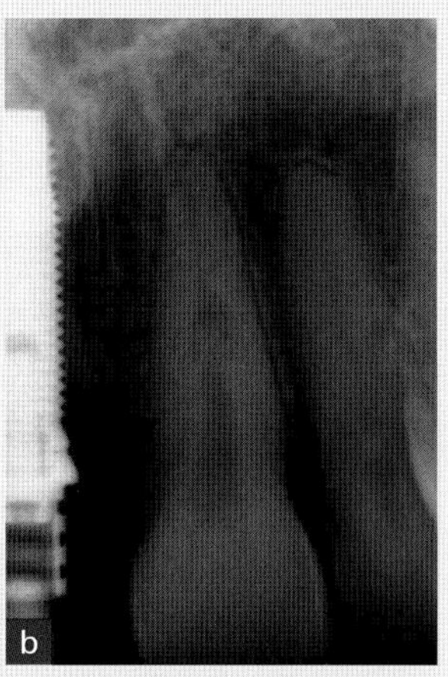

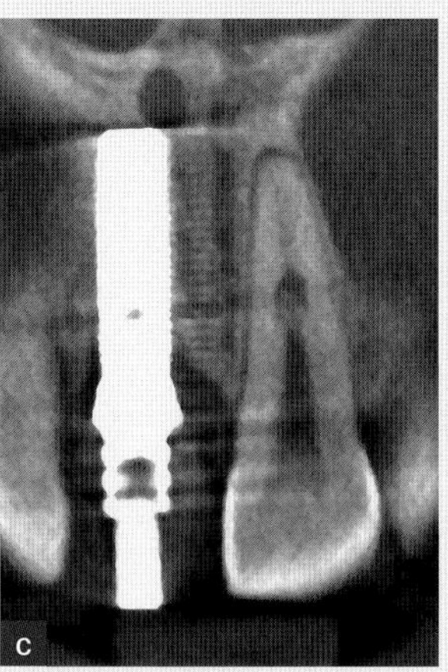

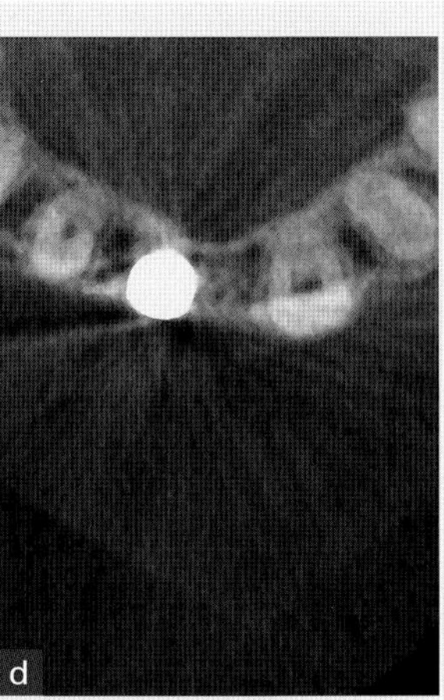

Fig 10-13 Internal root resorption. (a and b) Parallax periapical radiographs of the maxillary left central incisor reveal a well-centred radiolucency, which appears to balloon out, suggesting an internal resorptive defect. There are signs of mottling in the coronal half of the resorptive cavity, indicating internal replacement resorption. (c) A coronal CBCT slice reveals the mottling in more detail, while (d) the axial CBCT slice reveals that the mottling is on the palatal aspect of the cavity. Streaking artefacts from the adjacent relatively low-density titanium implant impair the quality of the image. This type of CBCT scan would not be advisable if the neighbouring teeth were restored with highly dense metallic materials (e.g. gold or stainless steel) (courtesy of Patel S, Ricucci D, Durak C, Tay F. Internal root resorption: a review. J Endod 2010;36:1107-1121).

Internal root resorption

Conventional radiography

The conventional radiographic appearance of internal root resorption (IRR) is variable and in reality deviates in many instances from historical descriptions of its 'typical' appearance. Gartner et al (1976) described guidelines for the radiographic diagnosis of IRR, suggesting that such lesions are 'radiolucent with uniform radiodensities', 'have smooth and clearly defined margins', and are generally 'symmetrically distributed over the root', with the walls of the root canal appearing to 'balloon out'. Ne et al (1999) described IRR lesions as oval, circumscribed radiolucencies in continuity with the root canal wall. Some cases of IRR may exhibit some or all of these features (Çalişkan and Türkün, 1997; Heithersay, 2007); however, many more cases will not (Fig 10-12).

In reality, IRR can occur at any location within the root canal system, including the pulp chamber, and may manifest radiographically as radiolucencies with variable shape, outline, border definition, radiodensity, and symmetry in relation to the root canal. Internal inflammatory resorption defects are more likely to be uniformly radiolucent, while in cases of internal metaplastic resorption the defect will appear mottled, reflecting hard tissue deposition (Fig 10-13). Either type of IRR may appear cloudy radiographically; a feature caused either by anatomical noise over the area of interest, and/or a transitional stage of metaplastic hard tissue formation within the lesion in the case of replacement resorption (Patel et al, 2016).

The margins of IRR have no typical appearance. Depending on the age of the lesion and the degree of associated tissue destruction and deposition, the lesion outline may be smooth, irregular, poorly defined, or well defined. However, anecdotal evidence would suggest a propensity for better-defined margins, which are more asymmetrically distributed over the root canal.

It is not uncommon for IRR to be misdiagnosed as ECR (Gulabivala and Searson, 1995; Schwartz et al, 2010); the defining difference is the site of resorption.

An IRR lesion will be continuous with the normal root canal walls, as it is essentially an extension of them. As such, in teeth with single canals affected by IRR, the canal walls should not be traceable through the defect (Gartner et al, 1976). This is in contrast to cases of ECR, where the lesion lies buccal or palatal/lingual to the defect and is consequently superimposed on the canal system when viewed on conventional radiographs. In cases of ECR, therefore, the canal walls should main-

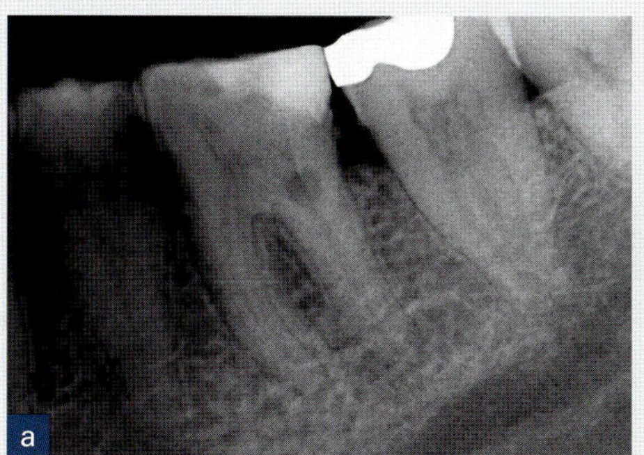

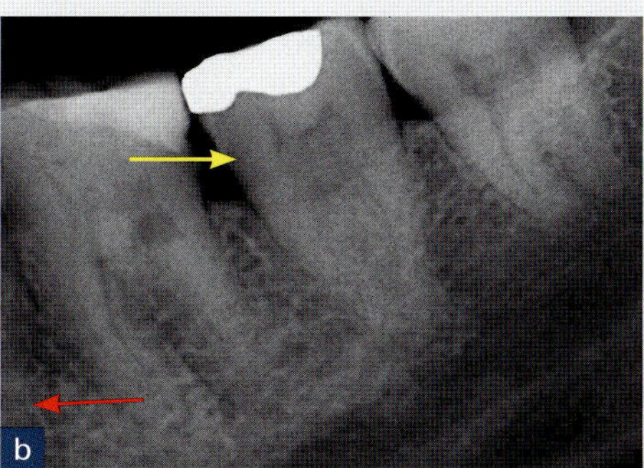

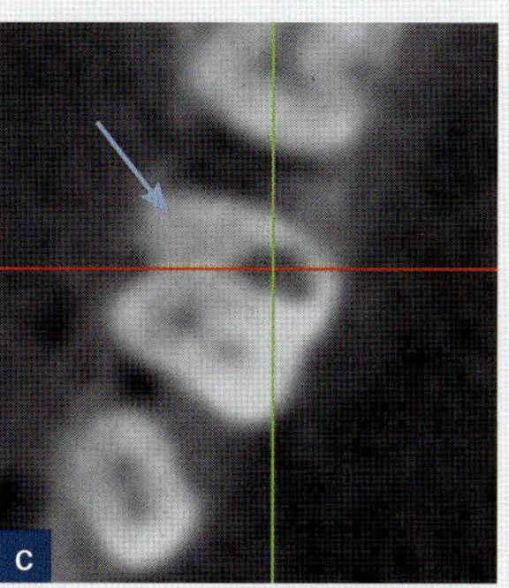

Fig 10-14 Internal root resorption. (a and b) Parallax periapical radiographs of the mandibular left first molar; note the well-defined radiolucency over the distal root. The root canal can be traced through the radiolucency, and the radiolucency moved in the opposite direction (yellow arrow) to the X-ray beam shift (red arrow); these are all 'classic' signs of ECR. (c) An axial CBCT slice reveals the true nature of the radiolucency within the distal root, and therefore a definite a diagnosis of IRR. The distolingual root canal (blue arrow) was superimposed onto the distobuccal root, hence the potential for the misdiagnosis as ECR (Patel S, Kanagasingam S, Pitt Ford T. External cervical resorption: a review. J Endod 2009b;35:616-625).

tain their normal course as they pass through the resorption defect, allowing them to be traced through it.

A parallax radiograph, with a change in the horizontal angulation of the X-ray tube head, will provide additional information regarding the nature of the lesion. In cases of IRR, when viewed on a parallax radiograph, the lesion should maintain its position relative to the root canal on both images. In cases of ECR, however, a palatally positioned lesion will move in the same direction relative to the root canal as the tube shifts (Fig 10-12). A buccal lesion will move in the opposite direction. However, these diagnostic criteria have several shortcomings (outlined below), which may impair diagnosis.

- In cases where extensive hard tissue deposition has occurred within the resorptive defect, the root canal walls may be obscured radiographically.
- An ECR lesion may perforate the root canal wall such that the lesion and the root canal are in communication.
- In teeth with multiple canals, a canal that has been unaffected by internal resorption may be superimposed onto the resorption defect on conventional radiographs (Fig 10-14).

CBCT

By overcoming the limitations of conventional radiographic imaging, CBCT allows the exact location and, therefore, the type of resorption to be confirmed (Figs 10-14 and 10-15). The dimensions of the internal resorptive defect in all planes, and the presence and position of any root wall perforations, can also be established (Fig 10-12). The walls of the defect are contiguous with those of the root canal. By eliminating anatomical noise, the true radiodensity of the IRR can be elucidated such that the presence of metaplastic hard tissue inclusions or a transitional metaplastic state (cloudy appearance on CBCT) can be ascertained (Patel et al, 2010). In cases of IRR, types of hard tissue formation (similar to those seen in ECR), can normally be identified. In cases of IRR, however, hard tissue banding/streaking is a less common occurrence, and the majority of cases of internal metaplastic resorption are characterised by islands of hard tissue formation. These are generally less diffusely spread throughout the lesion than in cases of ECR. Unlike ECR, IRR is less invasive, so the presence of projections extending from the main site of the defect is not a feature of IRR. The lesion tends to invade the root canal walls locally. The walls are generally well defined on CBCT.

Recent clinical studies have highlighted the improved accuracy of CBCT for the diagnosis of ECR and IRR (Patel et al, 2009a). In this study, a series of postgraduate endodontics students and experienced endodontists were asked to assess a series of radiographs and CBCT scans and diagnose the type of resorption (if present). CBCT was shown to be more effective and reliable than radiographs. Other studies have come to similar conclusions when assessing external surface resorption (Alqerban et al, 2009).

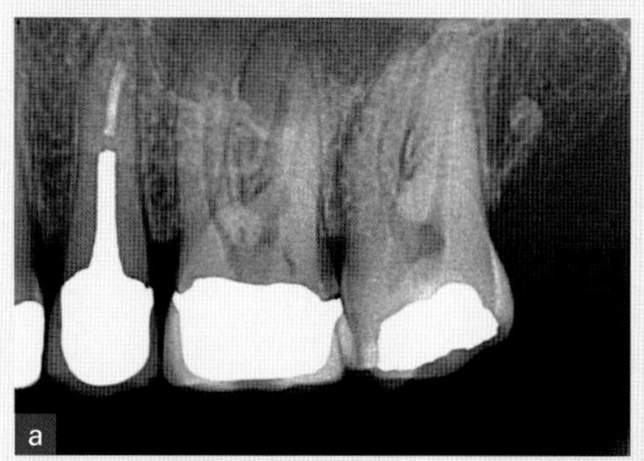
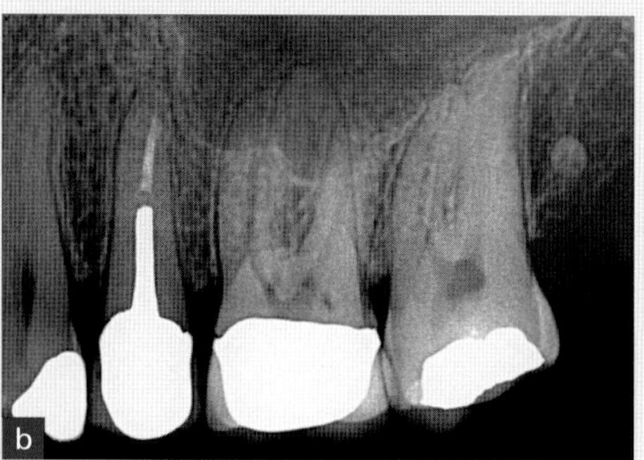
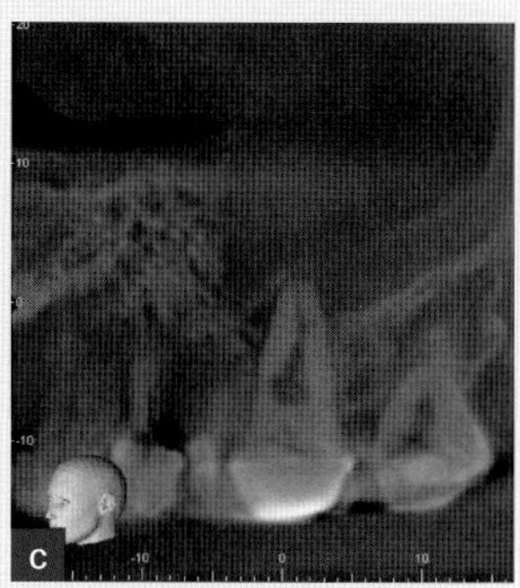
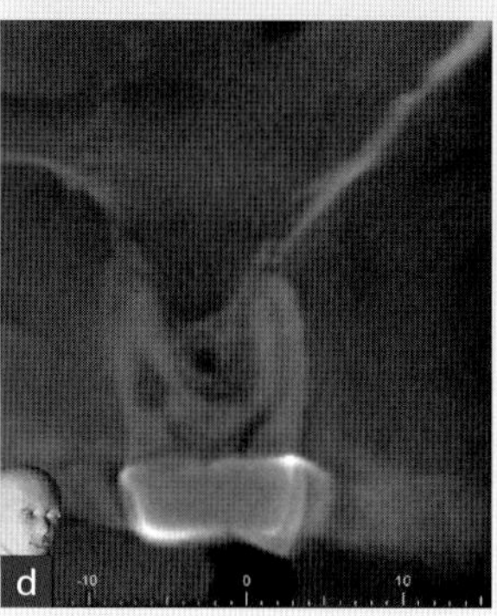
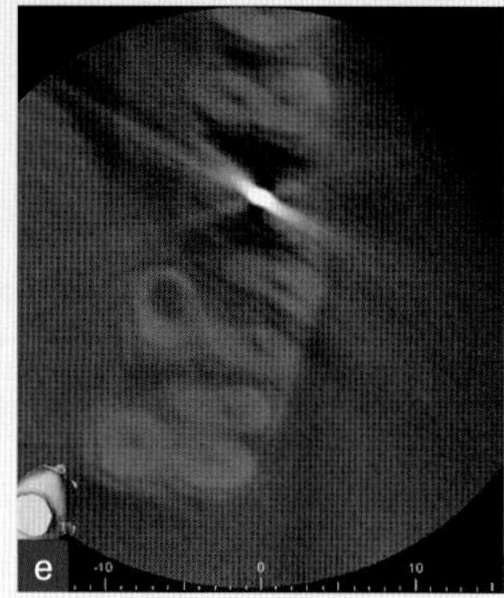

Fig 10-15 Internal root resorption. (a and b) Parallax periapical radiographs of the maxillary left molar teeth do not reveal anything untoward. (c) Sagittal, (d) coronal, and (e) axial CBCT slices reveal IRR within the palatal canal; the resorption defect is confined to the root but has not perforated it.

Conclusion

There is a considerable body of evidence to suggest that CBCT scans are more diagnostically accurate than conventional radiographs for diagnosing different types of root resorption. This should improve the likelihood of the correct treatment plan being chosen (Patel et al, 2009b; Ee et al, 2014).

However, the diagnostic yield of any given scan is CBCT-scanner specific, and this must be borne in mind before considering a CBCT scan (Patel et al, 2015); the results of one study using a specific CBCT scanner (and exposure parameters) is not necessarily transferable to other CBCT scanners (Neves et al, 2012; Da Silveira et al, 2014).

A CBCT scan should only be considered if there is insufficient information from parallax radiographs to confidently diagnose and/or manage a resorptive lesion (European Society of Endodontology CBCT position statement, 2014).

References

Alqerban A, Jacobs R, Souza PC, Willems G. In-vitro comparison of 2 cone-beam computed tomography systems and panoramic imaging for detecting simulated canine impaction-induced external root resorption in maxillary lateral incisors. Am J Orthod Dentofacial Orthop 2009;136:764–765.

Andreasen JO, Hjørting-Hansen E. Replantation of teeth. I. Radiographic and clinical study of 110 human teeth replanted after accidental loss. Acta Odontol Scand 1966a;24:263–286.

Andreasen JO, Hjørting-Hansen E. Replantation of teeth. II. Histological study of 22 replanted anterior teeth in humans. Acta Odontol Scand 1966b;24:287–306.

Andreasen FM, Pedersen BV. Prognosis of luxated permanent teeth—the development of pulp necrosis. Endod Dent Traumatol 1985;1:207–220.

Andreasen FM, Sewerin I, Mandel U, Andreasen JO. Radiographic assessment of simulated root resorption cavities. Endod Dent Traumatol 1987;3:21–27.

Andreasen JO. Review of the root resorption systems and models. Etiology of root resorption and the homeostatic mechanisms of the periodontal ligament. In: The Biological Mechanisms of Tooth Eruption and Root Resorption. Davidotch D (ed). Birmingham, UK: EBSCO Media 1988:9–21.

Bernardes RA, de Paulo RS, Pereira LO, Duarte MA, Ordinola-Zapata R, de Azevedo JR. Comparative study of cone beam computed tomography and intraoral periapical radiographs in diagnosis of lingual-simulated external root resorptions. Dent Traumatol 2012;28:268–272.

Çalişkan MK, Türkün M. Prognosis of permanent teeth with internal resorption: a clinical review. Endod Dent Traumatol 1997;13:75–81.

Chapnick L. External root resorption: an experimental radiographic evaluation. Oral Surg Oral Med Oral Pathol 1989;67:578–582.

D'Addazio PS, Campos CN, Özcan M, Teixeira HGC, Passoni RM, Carvalho ACP. A comparative study between cone-beam computed tomography and periapical radiographs in the diagnosis of simulated edodontic complications. Int Endod J 2011;44:218–224.

Da Silveira PF, Fontana MP, Oliveira HW, et al. CBCT-based volume of simulated root resorption -influence of FOV and voxel size. Int Endod J 2014: doi: 10.1111/iej.12390 [Epub ahead of print].

De Souza DV, et al. External cervical resorption: comparison of the diagnostic efficacy using two different cone beam tomography units versus periapical radiography - an in vitro investigation. Master of Clinician Dentistry dissertation, Kings College London (in progress).

Durack C, Patel S, Davies J, Wilson R, Mannocci F. Diagnostic accuracy of small volume cone beam computed tomography and intraoral periapical radiography for the detection of simulated external inflammatory root resorption. Int Endod J 2011;44:136–147.

Ee J, Fayad MI, Johnson BR. Comparison of endodontic diagnosis and treatment planning decisions using cone-beam volumetric tomography versus periapical radiography. J Endod 2014;40:910–916.

Estrela C, Bueno MR, De Alencar AH, et al. Method to evaluate inflammatory root resorption by using cone beam computed tomography. J Endod 2009;35:1491–1497.

European Society of Endodontology, Patel S, Durack C, et al. European Society of Endodontology position statement: the use of CBCT in Endodontics. Int Endod J 2014;47:502–504.

Gartner AH, Mark T, Somerlott RG, Walsh LC. Differential diagnosis of internal and external cervical resorption. J Endod 1976;2:329–334.

Goldberg F, De Silvio A, Dreyer C. Radiographic assessment of simulated external root resorption cavities in maxillary incisors. Endod Dent Traumatol 1998;14:133–136.

Gulabivala K, Searson LJ. Clinical diagnosis of internal resorption: an exception to the rule. Int Endod J 1995;28:255–260.

Gunst V, Huybrechts B, De Almeida Neves A, Bergmans L, Van Meerbeek B, Lambrechts P. Playing wind instruments as a potential aetiologic cofactor in external cervical resorption: two case reports. Int Endod J 2011;44:268–282.

Gunst V, Mavridou A, Huybrechts B, Van Gorp G, Bergmans L, Lambrechts P. External cervical resorption: an analysis using cone beam, and microfocus computed tomography and scanning electron microscopy. Int Endod J 2013;46:877–887.

Hammarström L, Lindskog S. General morphological aspects of resorption of teeth and alveolar bone. Int Endod J 1985;18: 93–108.

Heithersay GS. Invasive cervical resorption: an analysis of potential predisposing factors. Quintessence Int 1999;30:83–95.

Heithersay GS. Invasive cervical resorption. Endod Topics 2004;7:73–92.

Heithersay GS. Management of tooth resorption. Aust Dent J 2007;52(1 Suppl):S105–121.

Iqbal MK. Clinical and scanning electron microscopic features of invasive cervical resorption in a maxillary molar. Oral Surg Oral Med Oral Pathol Oral Radiol Endod 2007;103:49–54.

Kamburoğlu K, Kurşun S, Yüksel S, Oztaş B. Observer ability to detect ex vivo simulated internal or external cervical root resorption. J Endod 2011;37:168–175.

Laux M, Abbott PV, Pajarola G, Nair PNR. Apical inflammatory root resorption: a correlative radiographic and histological assessment. Int Endod J 2000;33:483–493.

Ne RF, Witherspoon DE, Gutmann JL. Tooth resorption. Quintessence Int 1999;30:9–25.

Neves FS, Vasconcelos TV, Vaz SL, Freitas DQ, Haiter-Neto F. Evaluation of reconstructed images with different voxel sizes of acquisition in the diagnosis of simulated external root resorption using cone beam computed tomography. Int Endod J 2012;45:234–239.

Patel S, Ford TP. Is the resorption external or internal? Dent Update 2007;34:218–229.

Patel S, Dawood A. The use of cone beam computed tomography in the management of external cervical resorption lesions. Int Endod J 2007;40:730–737.

Patel S, Dawood A, Wilson R, Horner K, Mannocci F. The detection and management of root resorption lesions using intraoral radiography and cone beam computed tomography—an in vivo investigation. Int Endod J 2009a;42:831–838.

Patel S, Kanagasingam S, Pitt Ford T. External cervical resorption: a review. J Endod 2009b;35:616–625.

Patel S, Ricucci D, Durak C, Tay F. Internal root resorption: a review. J Endod 2010;36:1107–1121.

Patel S, Durack C, Abella F, Shemesh H, Rog M, Lemberg K. Cone beam computed tomography in endodontics—a review. Int Endod J 2015;48:3–15.

Patel S, Durack C, Ricucci D. Root resorption. In: Cohen's Pathways of the Pulp, ed 11. Hargreaves K (ed). Oxford UK: Elsevier, 2016:660–682.

Ponder SN, Benavides E, Kapila S, Hatch NE. Quantification of external root resorption by low- vs high-resolution cone-beam computed tomography and periapical radiography: A volumetric and linear analysis. Am J Orthod Dentofacial Orthop 2013;143:77–91.

Ren H, Chen J, Deng F, Zheng L, Liu X, Dong Y. Comparison of cone-beam computed tomography and periapical radiography for detecting simulated apical root resorption. Angle Orthod 2013;83:189–195.

Schwartz RS, Robbins JW, Rindler E. Management of invasive cervical resorption: observations from three private practices and a report of three cases. J Endod 2010;36:1721–1730.

Chapter 11

Vertical Root Fractures

Shanon Patel, Simon C Harvey

Introduction

Vertical root fracture (VRF) is a term used to describe longitudinally orientated cracks or fractures originating within the tooth root. The fracture may involve proximal and/or aproximal surfaces (Pitts and Natkin, 1983; Colleagues for Excellence; American Association of Endodontists, 2008). Although VRFs are more commonly associated with endodontically treated teeth (Llena-Puy et al, 2001), they can also occur in non-endodontically treated teeth (Zadik et al, 2008; Chen et al, 2008).

An incomplete VRF may be defined as a longitudinal fracture line where there has been no separation of the root fragments; generally, these VRFs have not extended to form a communication between the root canal and the periodontal ligament. Whereas with complete VRFs the root fragments are separable (Rivera and Walton, 2007; Brady et al, 2014). By its very nature, an incomplete VRF will have a narrower width compared to a complete VRF. The prognosis of a tooth with a complete VRF is generally very poor (Zadik et al, 2008).

The prevalence of VRF is more commonly reported in endodontically treated teeth than in vital teeth (Chan et al, 1999; Cohen et al, 2003). Between 20% and 32% of endodontically treated teeth are extracted due to VRFs (Caplan and Weintraub, 1997; Chen et al, 2008).

In some instances, a diagnosis of VRF may be confirmed clinically with the aid of a dental operating microscope; for example, a complete VRF running along the pulp chamber floor, or externally on the buccal/lingual root surface. However, it is not uncommon for the diagnosis to be more challenging, especially with incomplete VRFs (Cohen et al, 2003; Chavda et al, 2014). Incorrect diagnosis may lead to inappropriate management. A recent systematic review concluded that there was a lack of evidence-based data regarding the diagnostic accuracy of commonly used clinical and conventional radiographic examinations for detecting VRFs (Tsesis et al, 2010).

Early diagnosis of VRF is essential to allow the appropriate management of the affected tooth, and ideally improve its prognosis.

Conventional radiography

Currently, periapical radiography is the imaging system of choice for assessing teeth with suspected VRFs (Junqueira et al, 2013; Bechara et al, 2013). However, due to the limitations of conventional radiographic imaging, periapical radiography will only detect a VRF if the root fragments are displaced (complete VRF) (Meister et al, 1980), and the X-ray beam passes through the fracture line (Rud and Omnell, 1970; Kambungton et al, 2012). With an extensive VRF, there may be complete separation of the fractured root fragments (Pitts and Natkin, 1983; Moule and Kahler, 1999), which may be detected radiographically (Fig 11-1).

The radiographic appearance of a VRF is dependent on the position of the fracture within the root and the degree of displacement of the fracture. The narrower the fracture line, the less likely it is to be detected (Meister et al, 1980; Brady et al, 2014). Even with the aid of parallax radiographs, complete and incomplete VRFs with minimal displacement are not readily identifiable in either endodontically treated (Patel et al, 2013) or non-endodontically treated teeth (Brady et al, 2014). The overall accuracy of both digital (solid-state and phosphor plate) and conventional radiographs in detecting VRFs is similar. There is a higher accuracy in unfilled root canals but the presence of radiodense gutta-percha and/or metal posts reduces the diag-

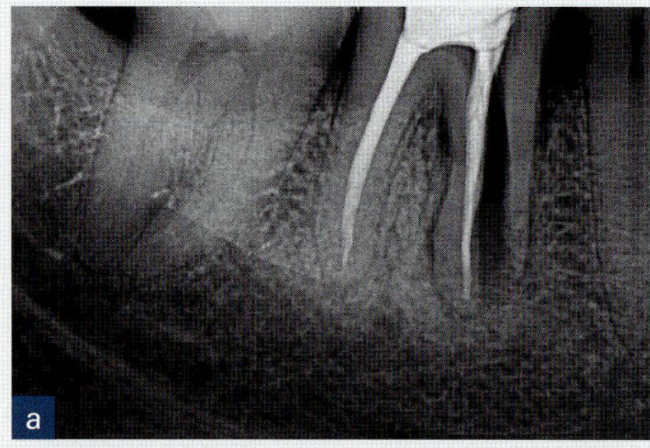

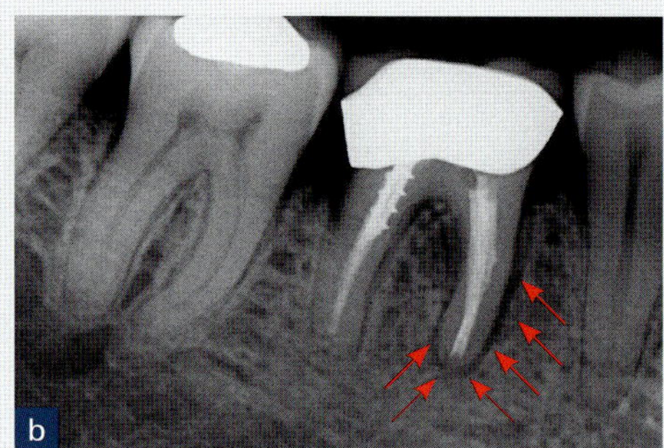

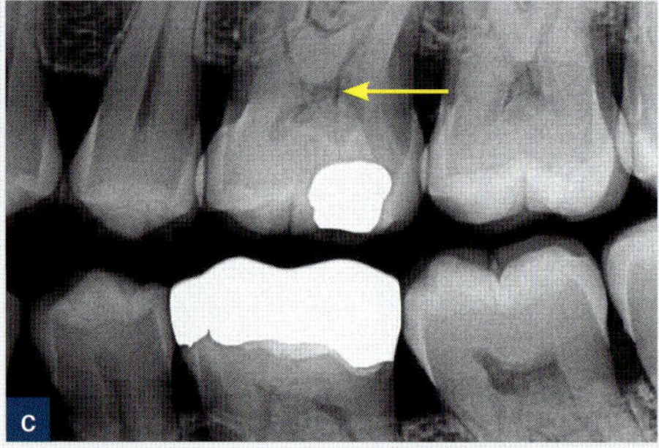

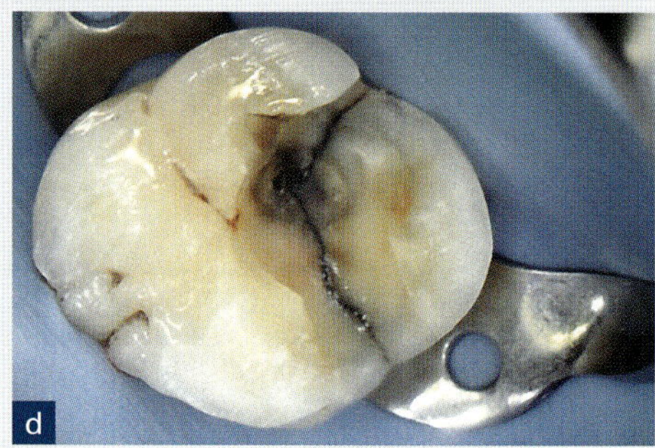

Fig 11-1 (a) Periapical radiograph of a root filled mandibular first molar. A complete separation of the mesial root indicates a complete VRF. (b) Periapical radiograph of a symptomatic root filled mandibular molar with a 'J'-shaped radiolucency (red arrows). (c) A bitewing radiograph reveals signs of a fracture (yellow arrow), which is confirmed clinically (d).

Table 11-1 Radiographic features suggestive of vertical root fractures.

- Visible separation of root
- Isolated angular bone loss at crestal level
- Widening of periodontal ligament space on one or more aspects of root
- 'J'-shaped periradicular radiolucency
- Periradicular radiolucency in furcation region
- Floating retrograde root end root filling
- Sinus tract pointing to root apex

nostic accuracy of periapical radiographs (Nascimento et al, 2015a).

Conventional radiographic systems have high specificity but low sensitivity in the detection of VRFs *ex vivo* (Tsesis et al, 2008; Patel et al, 2013). The specific type of image receptor used (plain film versus digital receptors) appears to have no significant effect on the diagnostic accuracy of periapical radiography in the detection of artificially created VRFs in single-rooted teeth (Tsesis et al, 2008; Tofangchiha et al, 2011). In contrast, one study suggested that, in multirooted teeth, digital sensors produce more diagnostically accurate images in the detection of VRFs compared to plain film radiographs (Kondylidou-Sidira et al, 2013).

Basic digital manipulation of the radiographic images (e.g. zooming in, colourising, and inverting) has been shown to improve the detection of simulated VRFs in non-root filled teeth when compared to the raw image (Nascimento et al, 2015b). However, similar image manipulation has no significant effect on diagnostic yield in root filled teeth (Kositbowornchai et al, 2001; Kamburoğlu et al, 2010; Tofangchiha et al, 2011).

It has been reported that 'floating' retrograde root end fillings that are no longer seated within the root end may be a sign of a VRF (Pitts and Natkin, 1983). However, this is more likely to occur with amalgam retrograde root end fillings than with more contemporary materials, such as mineral trioxide aggregate (MTA) and biodentine.

Although the identification of a VRF within the root is challenging, certain features in the adjacent periradicular bone may indicate a VRF (Table 11-1). These include: localised angular bone loss at the crestal level (Testori

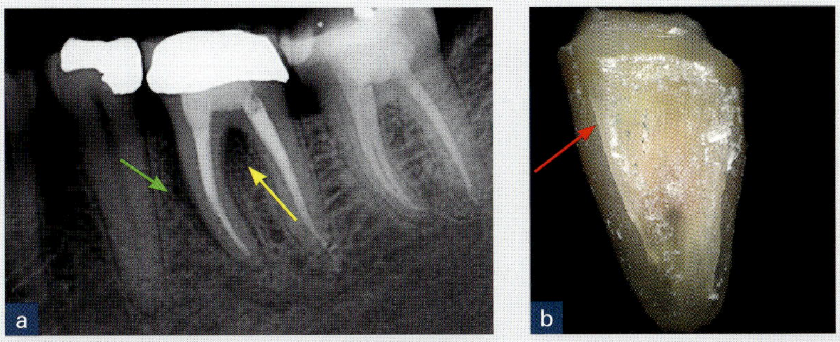

Fig 11-2 (a) Periapical radiograph of a root filled mandibular molar with a subtle radiolucency running along the mesial aspect of the mesial root (green arrow), and a radiolucency in the furcation region (yellow arrow); note a VRF cannot be seen within the root. (b) The extracted root with an incomplete VRF (red arrow).

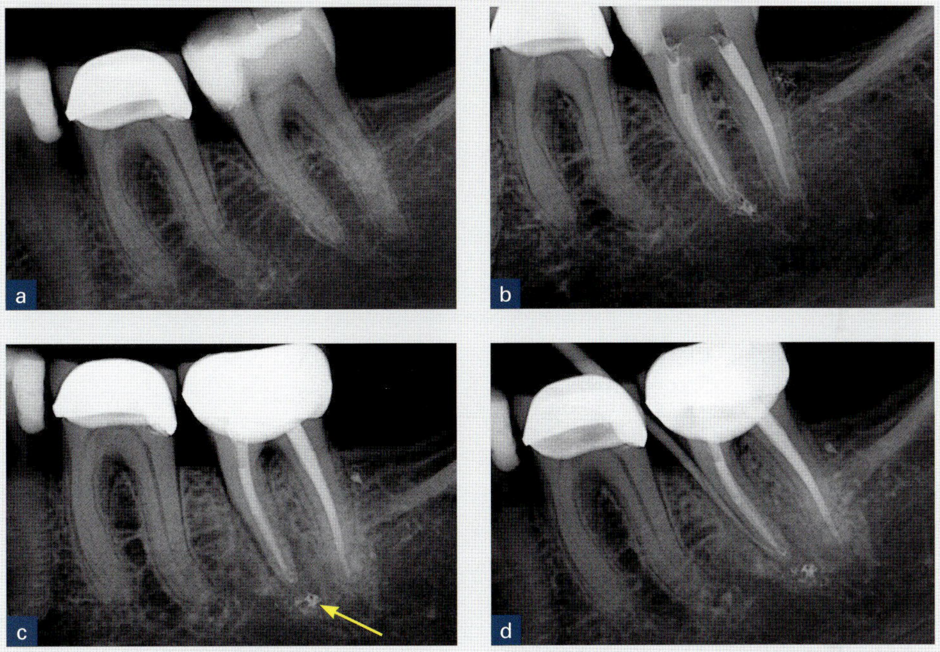

Fig 11-3 (a) Diagnostic radiograph and (b) post-obturation radiograph of a root-treated mandibular second molar; note that the periapical tissues appear to be healthy. (c) At 3 years post-treatment, the patient presents with low-grade pain localised to this tooth; the periapical radiograph reveals widening along the mesial aspect of the mesial root and an associated periapical radiolucency (yellow arrow). (d) An isolated probing depth on the mesial aspect of the tooth is tracked with a gutta-percha point.

et al, 1993; Nicopoulou-Karayianni et al, 1997; Tamse et al, 1999; Lustig et al, 2000); an extensive periradicular radiolucency, also known as a 'halo'- or 'J'-shaped periradicular radiolucency (Tsesis et al, 2010) (Figs 11-2 and 11-3); an isolated radiolucency in the furcation region of molar teeth; thickening of the periodontal ligament space on one aspect of the root or a sinus tract (Figs 11-3 and 11-4), which can be traced radiographically to the VRF (Tamse et al, 2006).

Cone beam computed tomography

There are conflicting results on the overall diagnostic accuracy of cone beam computed tomography (CBCT) when used to detect VRF (Hassan et al, 2010; Fayad et al, 2012; Neves et al, 2014).

Ex vivo studies

Ex vivo studies have demonstrated that CBCT is more accurate than periapical radiography in the detection of VRF in extracted human teeth (Hassan et al, 2009, 2010; Özer 2010; Özer et al 2011; Kamboroğlu et al, 2010). However, the diagnostic accuracy of CBCT may have been higher in these studies due to the size of the artificially created fractures (complete fractures), which were wider and more easily identifiable than clinically occurring, incomplete fractures. In a clinical situation, it has been suggested that these simulated complete VRFs would be detected clinically, and therefore a CBCT scan would not be required to confirm the diagnosis (Patel et al, 2013).

A recent series of *ex vivo* studies compared the diagnostic accuracy of CBCT and conventional radiographs for detecting incomplete and complete VRFs

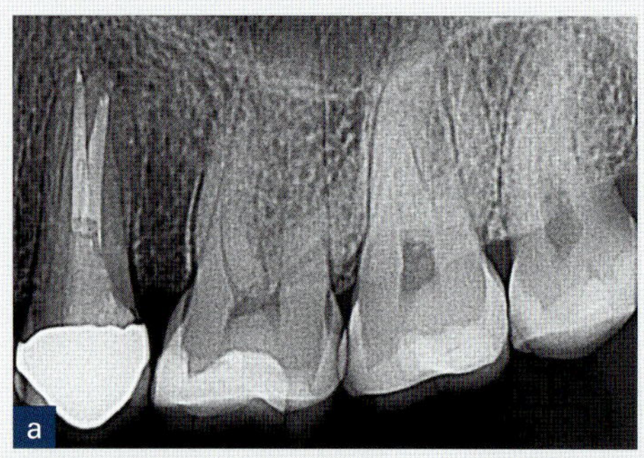

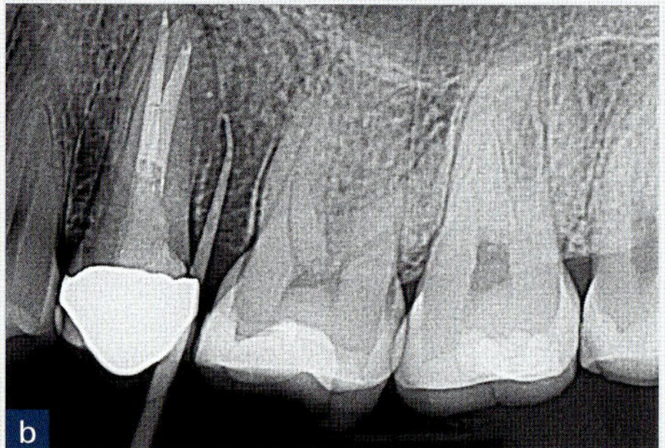

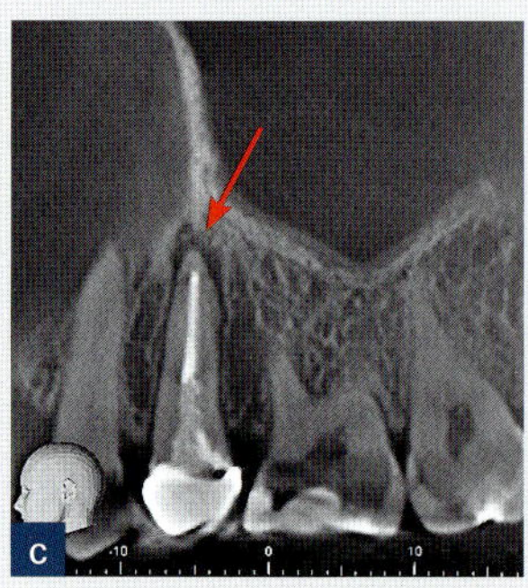

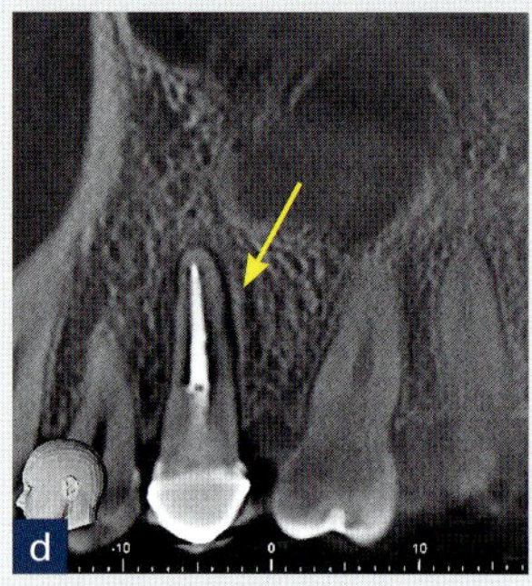

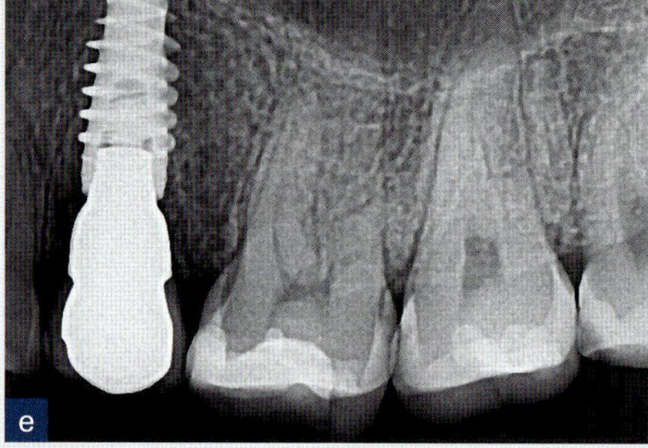

Fig 11-4 (a) Periapical radiograph of a symptomatic root filled mandibular second premolar; (b) with a gutta-percha point tracking the buccal sinus. There are no abnormal signs on either radiograph. (c and d) Reconstructed CBCT sagittal images reveal a well-defined periapical radiolucency (red arrow), and distinct widening of the periodontal ligament (yellow arrow) on the distal aspect of the root. (e) This tooth was subsequently extracted and replaced with an implant-retained crown. (Implant placement by Dr Fiona Mackillop.)

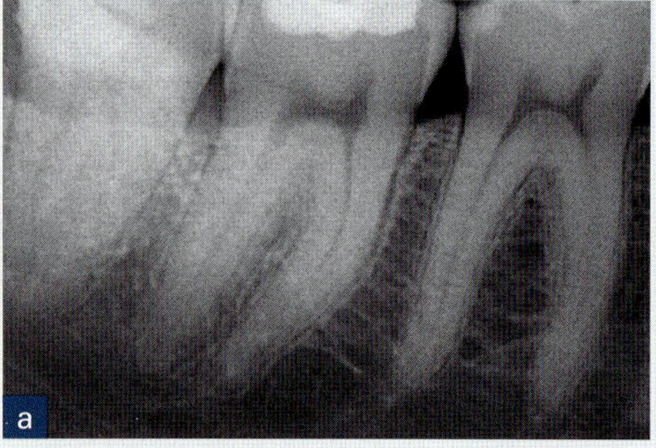

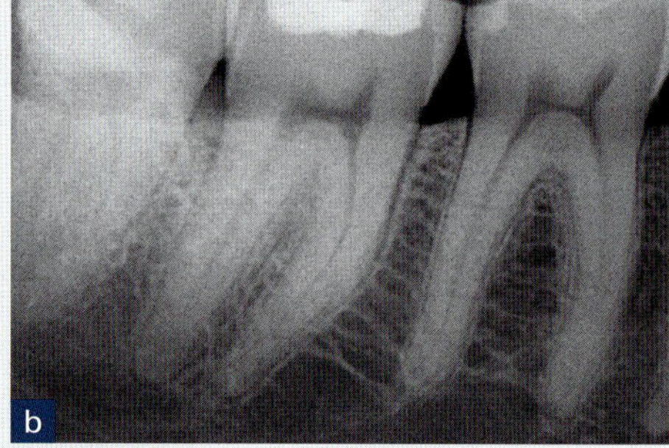

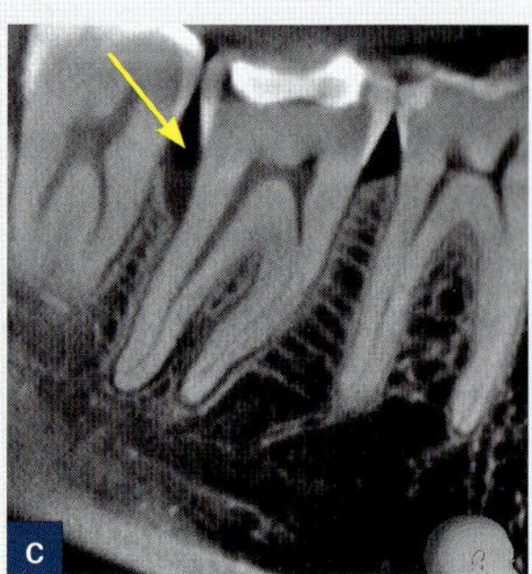

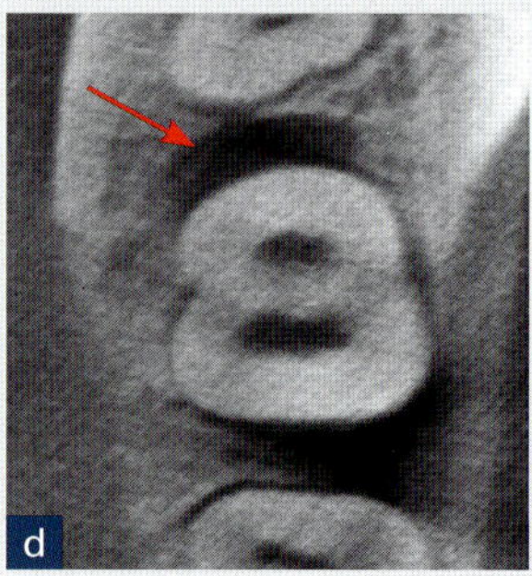

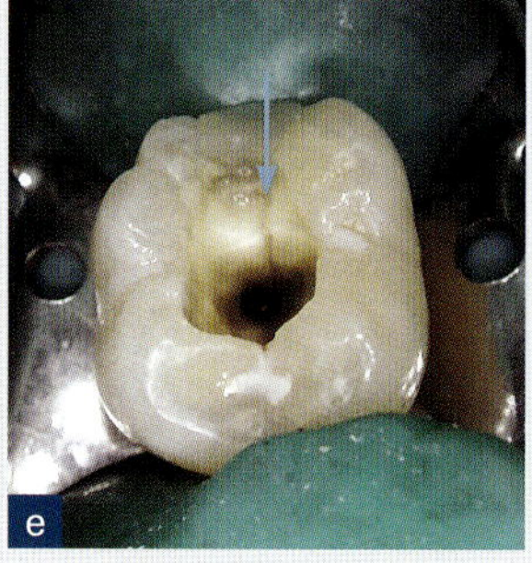

Fig 11-5 (a and b) Parallax periapical radiographs of a symptomatic mandibular second molar do not reveal anything unusual; (c) the reconstructed sagittal (yellow arrow) and (d) axial (red arrow) images reveal localised angular crestal bone loss on the distal aspect of the tooth. (e) Accessing the tooth revealed an incomplete VRF running into the root canal (blue arrow), which due to its narrow width was not evident on the CBCT scan.

with a predetermined range of widths (Patel et al, 2013; Brady et al, 2014). The fractures created in these two studies were up to four times narrower than in the study conducted by Özer (2011). The overall sensitivity of periapical radiography and CBCT in the detection of VRFs (regardless of the fracture dimensions) in teeth without root fillings was 0.63 and 0.87, respectively, while in root filled teeth it was 0.45 and 0.53, respectively. The presence of a root-filling material resulted in a reduction of specificity in both imaging techniques (Patel et al, 2013). Furthermore, Brady et al (2014) found that CBCT was more accurate than parallax periapical radiography for detecting incomplete VRFs in non-endodontically treated teeth.

As would be expected, CBCT was more accurate at detecting complete VRFs. Incomplete VRFs, wider

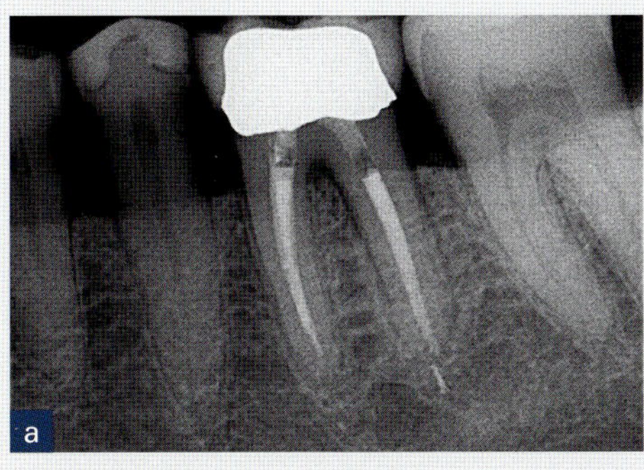
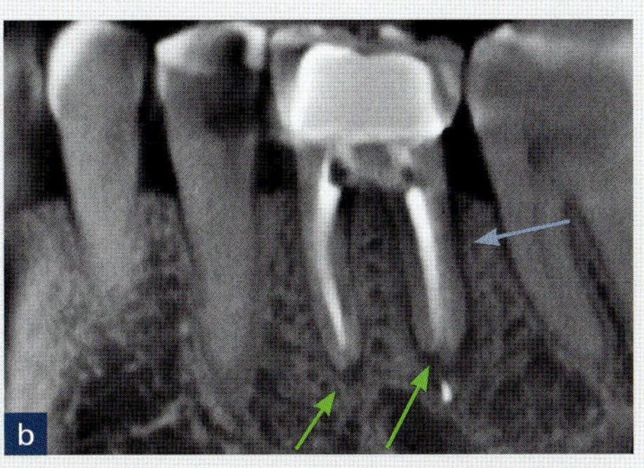
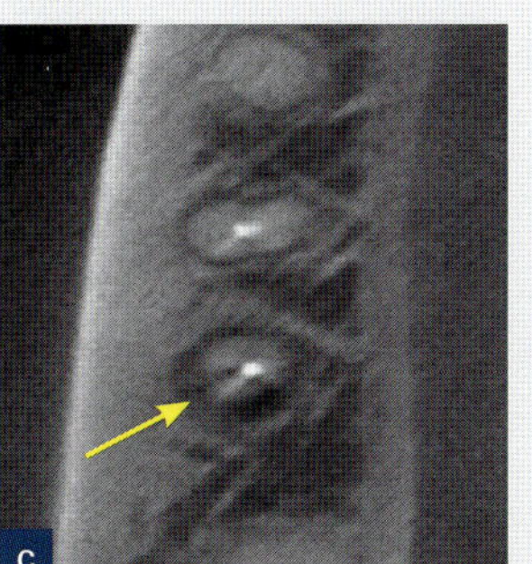
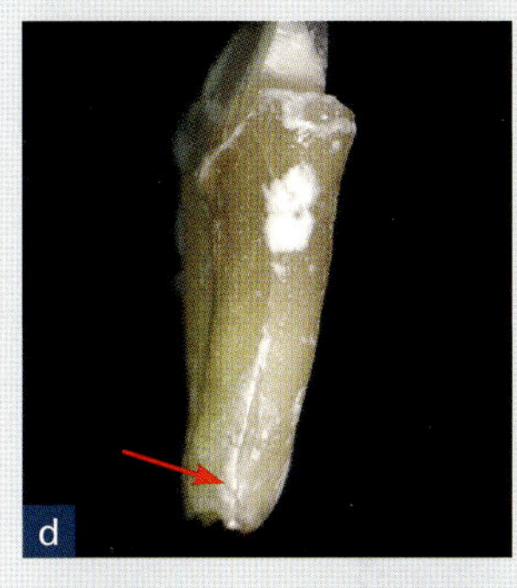

Fig 11-6 (a) Periapical radiograph of a symptomatic mandibular first molar, which had been root-treated 10 years previously; the root fillings are well compacted and to length, and there is a small amount of sealer extrusion from the distal root. (b) A reconstructed CBCT sagittal image reveals periapical radiolucencies associated with the mesial and distal roots (green arrows), and widening of the periodontal ligament (blue arrow) on the distal aspect of the distal root. (c) A reconstructed CBCT axial image reveals a fracture line (yellow arrow), while (d) the extracted distal root has a complete VRF (red arrow).

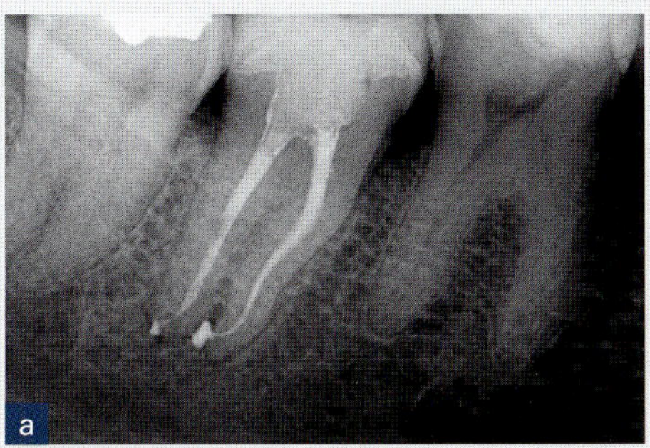
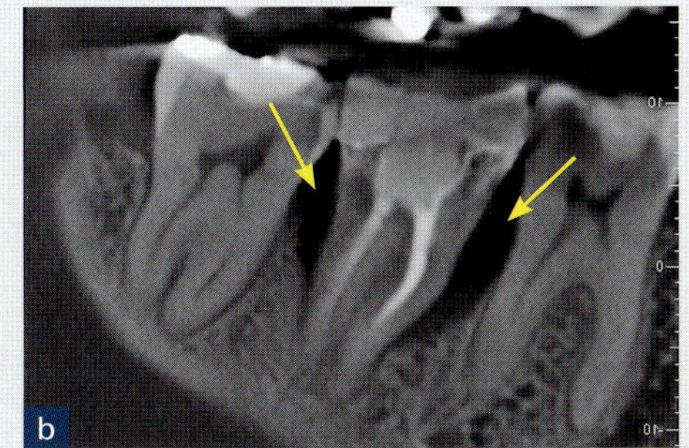
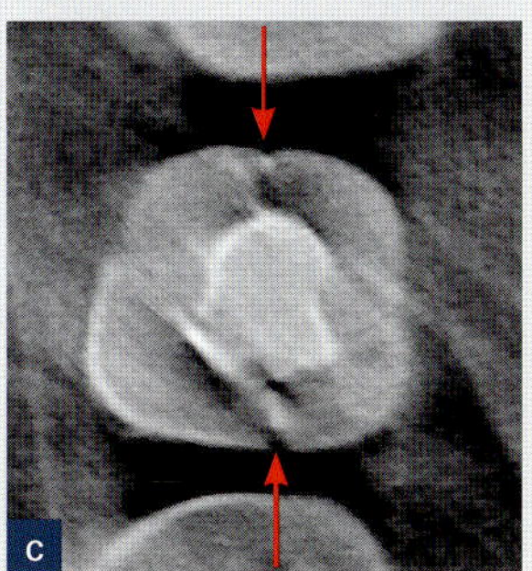
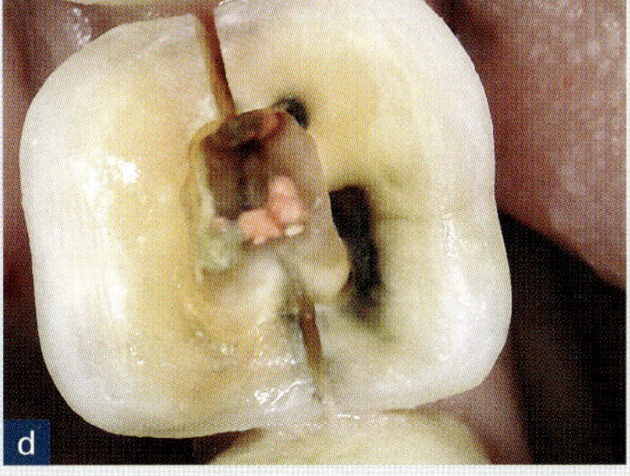

Fig 11-7 (a) Periapical radiograph of a symptomatic root-treated mandibular second molar. (b) The reconstructed sagittal CBCT slice reveals significant bone loss localised to the tooth under investigation (yellow arrows), which is only visible in a CBCT slice without the overlying cortical plate. (c) A reconstructed axial slice (coronal third of root) reveals the extent of the complete and much separated VRF (red arrows). (d) The crown was removed from the tooth, revealing the true extent of the VRF.

than 50 μm were more likely to be detected with CBCT compared to those with a width of less than 50 μm (Patel et al, 2013; Brady et al, 2014). These results are consistent with a previous study, which concluded that narrow VRFs (<0.2 mm) were not detected as easily as wider fractures (0.2 mm and 0.4 mm) on CBCT (Özer, 2010).

In vivo studies

In a clinical study, Chavda et al (2014) assessed the ability of radiographs and CBCT to assess VRFs in endodontically treated and non-endodontically treated teeth. After a conventional radiographic and CBCT assessment, these teeth were provisionally diagnosed as having a VRF and were subsequently atraumatically

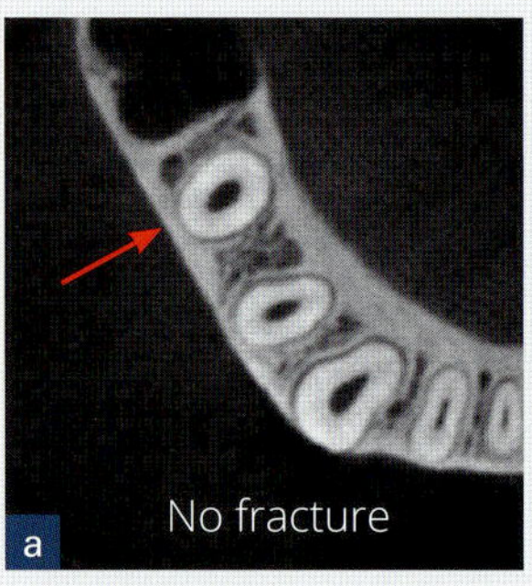

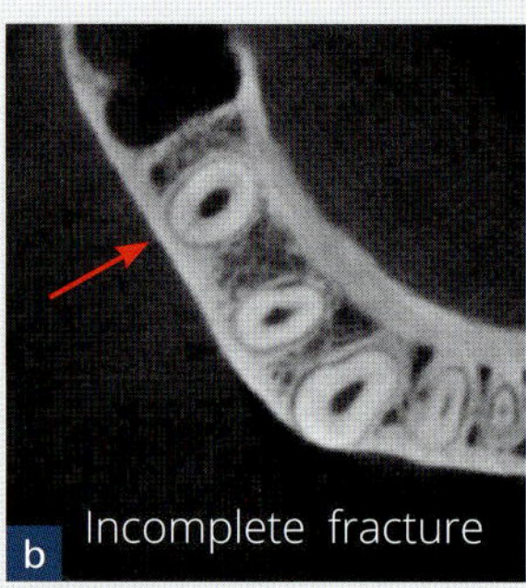

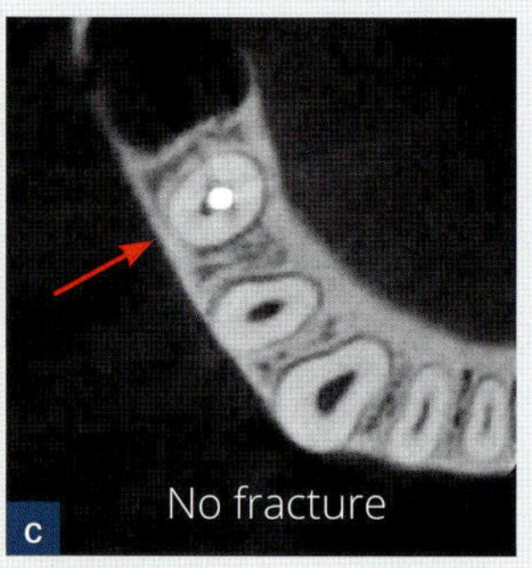

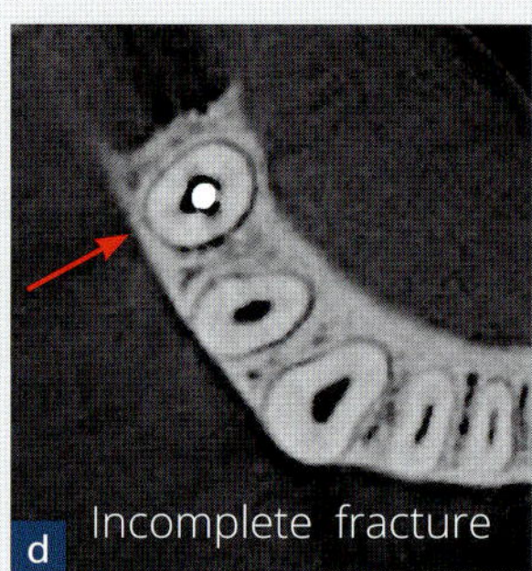

Fig 11-8 (a to d) A series of reconstructed axial CBCT slices of a dry mandible with simulated soft tissue, highlighting how image quality is compromised when radiopaque gutta-percha is placed in the root canal space; note the banding and streaking artefacts (red arrows) in (c) and (d), compared to the same tooth without a root filling.

extracted (Figs 11-5 to 11-7). The presence or absence of a VRF was confirmed by inspecting the entire cleaned root surface with the aid of a microscope following extraction. The microscopic examination of these extracted teeth was used as the reference standard. Periapical radiographs and CBCT had a high specificity of 0.92 and 0.83, respectively, but a similarly poor sensitivity of 0.16 and 0.27, respectively. Therefore, it was concluded that neither imaging system was accurate at diagnosing VRFs.

In contrast, other *in vivo* studies have concluded that CBCT is more accurate than periapical radiography for diagnosing VRFs (Edlund et al, 2011; Wang et al, 2011; Metska et al, 2012). However, in these studies, not all teeth were extracted and examined in a controlled environment. In some cases, surgical exploration and/or orthograde re-treatment was used to confirm the presence of VRFs; however, the entire root surface of the affected teeth were not assessed. Therefore, the incidence of VRFs may have been under-reported.

The inability of CBCT to detect incomplete VRFs is because the CBCT voxel dimensions are greater than the VRF width being assessed (see Chapter 4), resulting in the phenomenon of partial volume averaging (Scarfe and Farman, 2008).

The presence of a radiopaque root-filling material also impairs the diagnostic accuracy of CBCT in the detection of VRFs (Hassan et al, 2010; Khedmat et al, 2012; Neves at al, 2014). Cast posts have a similar effect (Costa et al, 2014; Junqueira et al, 2013). The reduced accuracy is due to beam hardening (Schulze et al, 2011), in which banding and streaking artefacts impair the detection within the area of interest (Fig 11-8). This makes diagnosis more challenging (Bechara et al, 2013) and may result in misdiagnosis and incorrect management (Kajan and Taromsari, 2012). It has been reported that lower radiodensity fibre posts result in fewer artefacts and therefore more diagnostically useful images (Neves et al, 2014).

The ability of CBCT to accurately diagnose VRFs will also vary according to the unique specifications and characteristics of the CBCT scanner being used (Hassan et al, 2010). Each CBCT scanner has specific hardware, software, and exposure parameters, which may also have an impact on diagnostic accuracy (Kamburoğlu et al, 2010; Melo et al, 2010). Therefore, the image quality and diagnostic accuracy of one CBCT scanner does not automatically translate to other CBCT scanners. 'Artefact reduction' algorithms in CBCT software have been shown to reduce the diagnostic accuracy of VRFs *ex vivo* in root-treated teeth (Bechara et al, 2013).

Although CBCT may not always directly reveal a VRF within the root, subtle changes within adjacent periradicular bone may be detected earlier with CBCT due to the ability of this imaging modality to overcome the limitations (i.e. anatomical noise) of conventional radiography (Figs 11-4 to 11-7).

Conclusion

Current evidence indicates that incomplete and complete VRFs cannot be readily detected with CBCT. Furthermore, imaging artefacts caused by radiodense root canal filling and/or post materials may impair the diagnostic accuracy of CBCT in the detection of VRFs. Therefore, CBCT cannot be recommended to directly detect VRFs within roots (Patel et al, 2015).

However, in cases where clinical and conventional radiographic examination are inconclusive, CBCT may be useful in detecting subtle changes in periradicular bone adjacent to the site of a suspected VRF (European Society of Endodontology CBCT position statement, 2014).

References

Bechara B, Alex McMahan C, Moore WS, Noujeim M, Teixeira FB, Geha H. Cone beam CT scans with and without artefact reduction in root fracture detection of endodontically treated teeth. Dentomaxillofac Radiol 2013;42:20120245.

Brady E, Mannocci F, Brown J, Wilson R, Patel S. A comparison of cone beam computed tomography and periapical radiography for the detection of vertical root fractures in non-endodontically treated teeth. Int Endod J 2014;47:735–746.

Caplan DJ, Weintraub JA. Factors related to loss of root canal filled teeth. J Public Health Dent 1997;57:31–39.

Chan CP, Lin CP, Tseng SC, Jeng JH. Vertical root fracture in endodontically versus nonendodontically treated teeth. Oral Surg Oral Med Oral Pathol Oral Radiol Endod 1999;87:504–507.

Chavda R, Mannocci F, Andiappan M, Patel S. Comparing the in vivo diagnostic accuracy of digital periapical radiography with cone-beam computed tomography for the detection of vertical root fracture. J Endod 2014;40:1524–1529.

Chen SC, Cheuh LH, Hsaio CK, Wu HP, Chiang CP. First untoward events and reasons for tooth extraction after nonsurgical endodontic treatment in Taiwan. J Endod 2008;34:671–674.

Cohen S, Blanco L, Berman L. Vertical root fractures. J Am Dent Assoc 2003;134:434–441.

Colleagues for Excellence. Cracking the cracked tooth code: detection and treatment of various longitudinal tooth fractures. American Association of Endodontics, 2008.

Costa FF, Pinheiro LR, Umetsubo OS, dos Santos O Jr, Gaia BF, Cavalcanti MG. Influence of cone-beam computed tomographic scan mode for detection of horizontal root fracture. J Endod 2014;40:1472–1476.

Edlund M, Nair MK, Nair UP. Detection of vertical root fractures by using cone-beam computed tomography: a clinical study. J Endod 2011;37:768–772.

European Society of Endodontology, Patel S, Durack C, et al. European Society of Endodontology position statement: the use of CBCT in Endodontics. Int Endod J 2014;47:502–504.

Fayad MI, Ashkenaz PJ, Johnson BR. Different representations of vertical root fractures detected by cone-beam volumetric tomography: a case series report. J Endod 2012;38:1435–1442.

Hassan B, Metska ME, Ozok AR, van der Stelt P, Wesselink PR. Detection of vertical root fractures in endodontically treated teeth by a cone beam computed tomography scan. J Endod 2009;35:719–722.

Hassan B, Metska ME, Ozok AR, van der Stelt P, Wesselink PR. Comparison of five cone beam computed tomography systems for the detection of vertical root fractures. J Endod 2010;36:126–129.

Junqueira RB, Verner FS, Campos CN, Devito KL, Carmo AMR. Detection of vertical root fractures in the presence of intracanal metallic post: a comparison between periapical radiography and cone-beam computed tomography. J Endod 2013;39:1620–1624.

Kajan ZD, Taromsari. Value of cone beam CT in detection of dental root fractures. Dentomaxillofac Radiol 2012;41:3–10.

Khedmat S, Rouhi N, Drage N, Shokouhinejad N, Nekoofar MH. Evaluation of three imaging techniques for the detection of vertical root fractures in the absence and presence of gutta-percha root fillings. Int Endod J 2010;45:1004–1009.

Kambungton J, Janhom A, Prapayasatok S, Pongsiriwet S. Assessment of vertical root fractures using three imaging modalities: cone beam CT, intraoral digital radiography and film. Dentomaxillofac Radiol 2012;41:91–95.

Kamburoğlu K, Murrat S, Yükel SP, Cebeci AR, Horasan S. Detection of vertical root fracture using cone-beam computerized tomography: an in vitro assessment. Oral Surg Oral Med Oral Pathol Oral Radiol Endod 2010;109:74–81.

Kondylidou-Sidira A, Fardi A, Giannopoulou M, Parisis N. Detection of experimentally induced root fractures on digital and conventional radiographs: an in vitro study. Odontology 2013;101:89–95.

Kositbowornchai S, Nuansakul R, Sikram S, Sinhawattana S, Saengmontri S. Root fracture detection: a comparison of direct digital radiography with conventional radiography. Dentomaxillofac Radiol 2001;30:106–109.

Llena-Puy MC, Forner-Navarro L, Barbero-Navarro I. Vertical root fracture in endodontically treated teeth: a review of 25 cases. Oral Surg Oral Med Oral Pathol Oral Radiol Endod 2001;92:553–555.

Lustig JP, Tamse A, Fuss Z. Pattern of bone resorption in vertically fractured endodontically treated teeth. Oral Surg Oral Med Oral Pathol Oral Radiol Endodontol 2000;90:224–227.

Meister F, Lommel TJ, Gerstein H. Diagnosis and possible causes of vertical root fracture. Oral Surg Oral Med Oral Pathol 1980;49:243–253.

Melo SL, Bortoluzzi EA, Abreu M Jr, Correa LR, Correa M (2010) Diagnostic ability of a cone-beam computed tomography scan to assess longitudinal fractures in prosthetically treated teeth. J Endod 2010;36:1879–1882.

Metska ME, Aartman IHA, Wesselink PR, Ozok AR. Detection of vertical root fractures in vivo in endodontically treated teeth by cone-beam computed tomography scans. J Endod 2012;38:1344–1347.

Moule AJ, Kahler B. Diagnosis and management of teeth with vertical root fractures. Aust Dent J 1999;44:75–87.

Nascimento HAR, Ramos ACA, Neves FS, de-Azevedo-Vaz SL, Freitas DQ. The 'Sharpen' filter improves the radiographic detection of vertical root fractures. Int Endod J 2015a;48:428–434.

Nascimento HA, Neves FS, de-Azevedo-Vaz SL, Duque TM, Ambrosano GM, Freitas DQ. Impact of root fillings and posts on the diagnostic ability of three intra-oral digital radiographic systems in detecting vertical root fractures, Int Endod J 2015b;48:864–871.

Neves FS, Sampaio F, Freitas FQ, Campos PSF, Ekestubbe A, Lofthag-Hansen S. Evaluation of cone-beam computed tomography in the diagnosis of vertical root fractures: the influence of imaging modes and root canal materials. J Endod 2014;40:1530–1536.

Nicopoulou-Karayianni K, Bragger U, Lang NP. Patterns of periodontal destruction associated with incomplete root fractures. Dentomaxillofac Radiol 1997;26:321–326.

Özer SY. Detection of vertical root fractures of different thicknesses in endodontically enlarged teeth by cone beam computed tomography versus digital radiography. J Endod 2011;36:1245–1249.

Özer SY, Ünlü G, Değer Y. Diagnosis and treatment of endodontically treated teeth with vertical root fracture: three case reports with two-year follow-up. J Endod 2011;37:97–102.

Patel S, Brady E, Brown J, Wilson R, Mannocci F. The detection of vertical root fractures in root filled teeth with periapical radiographs and CBCT scans. Int Endod J 2013;46:1140–1152.

Patel S, Durack C, Abella F, Shemesh H, Roig M, Lemberg K. Cone beam computed tomography in Endodontics—a review. Int Endod J 2015;48:3–15.

Pitts DL, Natkin E. Diagnosis and treatment of vertical root fractures. J Endod 1983;9:338–346.

Rivera EM, Walton EM. Longitudinal tooth fractures: findings that contribute to complex endodontic diagnoses. Endod Topics 2007;16:82–111.

Rud J, Omnell KA. Root fractures due to corrosion. Diagnostic aspects. Scand J Dent Res 1970;78:397–403.

Scarfe WC, Farman AG. What is cone-beam CT and how does it work? Dent Clin N Am 2008;52:707–730.

Schulze R, Heil U, Grob D, Breullmann DD, Dranischnikow E, Schwanecke U, Schoemer E. Artefacts in CBCT: a review. Dentomaxillofac Radiol 2011;40:265–273.

Tamse A, Fuss Z, Lustig J, Kaplavi J. An evaluation of endodontically treated vertically fractured teeth. J Endod 1999;25:506–508.

Tamse A, Kaffe I, Lustig J, Ganor Y, Fuss Z. Radiographic features of vertically fractured endodontically treated mesial roots of mandibular molars. Oral Surg Oral Med Oral Pathol Oral Radiol Endod 2006;101:797–802.

Testori T, Badino M, Castagnola M. Vertical root fractures in endodontically treated teeth: a clinical survey. J Endod 1993;19:87–91.

Tofangchiha M, Bakshi M, Fakhar MB, Panjnoush M. Conventional and digital radiography in vertical root fracture diagnosis: a comparison study. Dent Traumatol 2011;27:143–146.

Tsesis I, Kamburoğlu K, Katz A, Tamse A, Kaffe I, Kfir A. Comparison of digital with conventional radiography in detection of vertical root fractures in endodontically treated maxillary premolars: an ex vivo study. Oral Surg Oral Med Oral Pathol Oral Radiol Endod 2008;106:124–128.

Tsesis I, Rosen E, Tanse A, Taschieri S, Kfir A. diagnosis of vertical root fractures in endodontically treated teeth based on clinical and radiographic indicies: a systemic review. J Endod 2010;36:1455–1458.

Wang P, Yan XB, Lui DG, Zhang WL, Zhang Y, Ma XC. Detection of dental root fractures by using cone-beam computed tomography. Dentomaxillofac Radiol 2011;40:290–298.

Zadik Y, Sandler V, Bechor R, Salehrabi R. Analysis of factors related to extraction of endodontically treated teeth. Oral Surg Oral Med Oral Pathol Oral Radiol Endod 2008;106:31–35.

Index